Peter Van Bogaert
Sean Clarke

Editors

# The Organizational Context of Nursing Practice

Concepts, Evidence, and Interventions
for Improvement

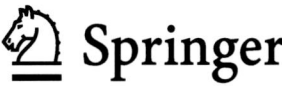 Springer

*Editors*
Peter Van Bogaert
Nursing and Midwifery Sciences
Centre for Research and Innovation in Care
Faculty of Medicine and Health Sciences
University of Antwerp
Antwerp
Belgium

Sean Clarke
William F. Connell School of Nursing
Boston College
Chestnut Hill, Massachusetts, USA

ISBN 978-3-319-71041-9      ISBN 978-3-319-71042-6   (eBook)
https://doi.org/10.1007/978-3-319-71042-6

Library of Congress Control Number: 2018930349

Printed on acid-free paper

This Springer imprint is published by Springer Nature
The registered company is Springer International Publishing AG
The registered company address is: Gewerbestrasse 11, 6330 Cham, Switzerland

# Foreword

The global health agenda for the next decade focuses on Universal Health Coverage (UHC), i.e., providing high-quality, cost-effective care and access to basic care for all. Some other leading global concerns are the attainment of the Sustainable Development Goals (SDG2030) and People Centered Care and the addressing of non-communicable diseases (NCDs). At the national level, countries are continuously focusing on how to manage the growing demand for healthcare services and their associated costs. Whether the national healthcare system is publicly or privately financed, or involves a blend of the two, costs are at the heart of funding and programmatic decisions. While there is a significant discussion about evidence-based practice and evidence-informed policy, there isn't sufficient appreciation and understanding among funders and decision makers that quality care is synonymous with cost-effective care or that investing in healthcare workers is a form of investment in cost-effective care. The 2016 UN report entitled Working for Health and Economic Growth which was tabled by the High Level Commission on Health Employment and Economic Growth makes a clear case that allocating resources to healthcare workers is an important means of promoting the economic success of nations. The report also indicates that by 2030, we will need an additional 40 million healthcare workers, of which 22 million will be in the Organization for Economic Co-operation and Development (OECD) countries (which include many of the world's most developed nations). Therefore, preparing the right number of healthcare professionals, investing in them, and retaining them should be a major concern for health system funders and decision makers.

There is a plethora of peer-reviewed publications in top journals in nursing and the health sciences more broadly that have demonstrated the impacts of well-prepared and well-managed nurse workforces can have on the patient and system outcomes. While we are well informed of the global agenda, many healthcare professionals, leaders, and experts are ill informed about the rich body of evidence that has accumulated over the last three to four decades, relating to how nursing can contribute to the global health agenda of reducing morbidity and mortality while providing important economic and social returns on all investments. Additionally, surprisingly few appear aware that extensive research and scholarly work have documented the organizational conditions that best draw forth nurses' contributions.

Thus the arrival of this book is well timed. Because nurses constitute the largest segment of the professional arm of healthcare work, it is essential to understand the existing evidence about nurses' work and nursing services as we continue to transform our healthcare systems toward greater productivity, effectiveness, and efficiency.

Ensuring that nurses are able to provide the care required by various populations should be of significant interest to governments, quasi-governmental organizations, and executives and managers at all levels of the healthcare system, whether their involvement is global, national, or local. This book deals primarily with the experiences of nurses in hospital settings, albeit across societies and across a wide range of specialties. However, the ideas reviewed across its chapters apply to virtually any setting where nurses or other allied health workers or professionals work. Whether in a hospital, community center, or primary care facility or at the level of a district level, getting the nursing workforce "right" will lead to high-quality and cost-effective care that strengthen the well-being of citizens who will in turn contribute to the economic and social well-being of their communities and countries.

This book is unique in bringing together under one cover the science (evidence) and the art (implementation) of building robust, successful, and effective systems that serve patients, communities, staff, and systems alike. It lays out the decades of research that studied the elements that constitute a positive work environment and factors that contribute to nurses' desire to stay in an organization and provide quality care. The synthesis of the research to date in this book illuminates the essential building blocks for a positive work environment. In addition to having a "one-stop" opportunity to learn about the key ingredients from conceptual and research perspectives, the book also contains numerous chapters that demonstrate how these elements have been integrated in building quality of care and a satisfied workforce.

In addressing major global and national health concerns, it is essential to have the right number and the right quality of nurses and other healthcare workers functioning effectively. Retaining the workforce and having a satisfied workforce will help to overcome the looming risks of severe nurse shortages that could jeopardize our societies' abilities to meet our populations' healthcare needs. This book should be a "go-to" reference for decision makers, policy makers, funders, and system administrators interested in the evidence base regarding work environments that will build optimal systems for staff and patients alike.

President of International Council of Nurses (ICN)
2013–2017, Geneva, Switzerland                                    Judith Shamian

# Acknowledgments

Eleven co-authors have collaborated closely on this book, sharing their expertise and describing research projects that draw upon the ideas and assumptions described in the chapters. I thank each of the contributors and all our colleagues who have been involved (directly and indirectly) in the various projects described in the book. I also thank my colleagues in the Department of Nursing and Midwifery Sciences, the Centre of Research and Innovation in Care (CRIC), and the Faculty of Medicine and Health Sciences at the University of Antwerp—the environment where we were able to build this program of work.

In 2004, Paul Van Aken gave me a book—*Keeping Patients Safe: Transforming the Work Environment of Nurses*, a report of the Institute of Medicine. I was a director of nursing at Antwerp University Hospital, and Paul, a former colleague, was at that time my chief nursing officer (CNO). Reading the book thoroughly was a revelation for me and inspired a 10-year series of studies that I first started as a doctoral student with little funding and that later emerged as a full-fledged research program supported by healthcare organizations in the two regions of Belgium, Flanders and Wallonia, as well as the Brussels-Capital Region. I am grateful to Paul and all CNOs of the hospitals and long-term care facilities who allowed me to study their facilities, as well as all the clinical nurses and nurse managers who participated in or otherwise supported our studies.

In 2008, I met Dr. Sean Clarke somewhat by fluke when he and Dr. Linda Aiken came to deliver a presentation at the Catholic University of Leuven at the invitation of Dr. Walter Sermeus. Over the past years, Sean became one of my closest personal friends and a trusted colleague who has supported and guided me in my research journey. I was an experienced practitioner but a real neophyte in research and academic life. He treated me as a peer and helped me gain confidence and trust in my abilities to set up research projects. He also provided guidance as I built my academic career. Therefore, I was very pleased to involve Sean as a co-editor in this work as a continuation of our mutual collaboration. Sean is a sharp, independent thinker and researcher who always goes to the heart of problems and issues by asking the right questions; he is always looking for the right answers based on evidence and solid study designs.

The Antwerp University Hospital received their initial Magnet Recognition® as the first hospital in Belgium and the continent of Europe, in October 2017 after an 8-year organic journey to nursing excellence and improved patient outcomes. In our journey many colleagues were inspiring and paramount for our persistent mission starting with the CEO Johnny Van der Straeten and the hospital management committee, hospital administrators, nursing leaders, nursing managers, and above all clinical nurses supported by their interprofessional colleagues such as physicians and other healthcare workers as well as ancillary staff. Especially, our gratitude goes to Nancy Van Genechten who was the driving force of two nursing councils "mentoring" and "patient safety and infection control" and a member of the hospital ethics committee. Unfortunately, we lost Nancy; she passed away the last year of our journey to the initial Magnet Recognition®. We will keep strong remembrance of her passion, expertise, and energy supporting our clinical nurses, nurse managers, and physicians in their aims to provide excellence in care. Moreover, our deepest respect goes to all colleagues of the American Nurses Credentialing Center, as they called us, along with Paul Van Aken and Danny Van heusden our Magnet Program Director, the three Van's from Belgium; they treated us most encouraging and gave us strong confidence in our aims, especially, Jan Moran former director and Rebecca Graystone current director of Magnet Recognition Program® and their staff of program analysts, Cheryl Schmitz our senior Magnet program analyst, and Dr. Donna Havens chair of the Commission on Magnet Recognition®.

My wife and I lost three of our four parents last year over a 6-month period. All were in their 80s (82, 86, and 89) and all three died having had extensive involvement with the healthcare system: my father-in-law at home very much supported around the clock by my 83-year-old mother-in-law and my mother and father receiving treatment in a residential aged care facility. As a family, we experienced both the best and the worse the healthcare could offer them. As a healthcare provider and administrator, I could make rationalizations for the deficits in care we witnessed, but as a son, I was deeply disappointed. We were so grateful for the opportunity to learn from our parents' resilience in coping with their frailty and from their unwillingness to ever give up. The latter seems to be a trait emblematic of the generation that came of age during World War II; I saw it in the early days of my clinical career. I dedicate this book to the memory of our parents and to the importance of doing better for all our patients.

Peter Van Bogaert

As he says, Dr. Peter Van Bogaert and I met a decade ago—somewhat by chance—and I have had the privilege of collaborating with him ever since. It has been an enormous honor to watch his growth as a researcher and research leader over the years and to witness the rapid development of the University of Antwerp's Department of Midwifery and Nursing and Antwerp University Hospital's movement toward evidence-informed and data-driven nursing management. I thank him for his friendship and for the opportunity to collaborate on great projects with his network of hardworking, insightful, and exceptionally kind and welcoming colleagues and trainees.

As we hurtle through incredible change in healthcare systems around the world, the study of nurses' work lives and work environments is more important than ever. I thank the many collaborators I have worked with over the years in education, practice, and research, in the United States, Canada, Europe, Asia, and Australia, for their inspiration of their tireless work to make healthcare better. Like Peter and the authors of the chapters in this volume, they do critical work that impacts the lives of patients and healthcare workers every day. I especially thank Dr. Linda Aiken who opened the door to this field for me and who, as one of the most innovative thinkers and leaders in nursing health services research, has had an incalculable impact on the field and the careers of countless researchers.

Peter and Sean would both like to thank the Springer team for the support, trust, and opportunity to publish this work, especially Nathalie Lhorset-Poulain, Senior Publishing Editor, for her dedication to this project and commitment to advancing nursing and nursing research.

Sean Clarke

# Contents

# Contributors

**Sean Clarke** William F. Connell School of Nursing, Boston College, Chestnut Hill, MA, USA

**Sarah De Schepper** Centre of Expertise Psychological Wellbeing in Patient Care, Karel De Grote University College, Antwerp, Belgium

**Erik Franck** Nursing and Midwifery Sciences, Centre for Research and Innovation in Care (CRIC), Faculty of Medicine and Health Sciences, University of Antwerp, Antwerp, Belgium

Karel De Grote University College, Antwerp, Belgium

**Nina Geuens** Centre of Expertise Psychological Wellbeing in Patient Care, Karel De Grote University College, Antwerp, Belgium

Nursing and Midwifery Sciences and Centre, Research and Innovation in Care (CRIC), Faculty of Medicine and Health Sciences, University of Antwerp, Antwerp, Belgium

**Filip Haegdorens** Emergency Department, Antwerp University Hospital, Antwerp, Belgium

Nursing and Midwifery Sciences, Centre for Research and Innovation in Care (CRIC), Faculty of Medicine and Health Sciences, University of Antwerp, Antwerp, Belgium

**Juliet MacArthur** Research and Development, NHS Lothian, Edinburgh, UK

University of Edinburgh, Edinburgh, UK

**Koenraad Monsieurs** Faculty of Medicine and Health Sciences, University of Antwerp, Antwerp, Belgium

Emergency Department, Antwerp University Hospital, Antwerp, Belgium

**Leen Roes** Centre of Expertise Psychological Wellbeing in Patient Care, Karel De Grote University College, Antwerp, Belgium

**Stijn Slootmans** Chief Medical Officer Department, Antwerp University Hospital, Antwerp, Belgium

Nursing and Midwifery Sciences, Centre for Research and Innovation in Care (CRIC), Faculty of Medicine and Health Sciences, University of Antwerp, Antwerp, Belgium

**Olaf Timmermans** Nursing and Midwifery Sciences, Centre for Research and Innovation in Care (CRIC), Faculty of Medicine and Health Sciences, University of Antwerp, Antwerp, Belgium

HZ University College of Applied Sciences, Vlissingen, Netherlands

**Paul Van Aken** Nursing Department, Antwerp University Hospital, Antwerp, Belgium

**Peter Van Bogaert** Department of Nursing and Midwifery Sciences, Centre for Research and Innovation in Care (CRIC), Faculty of Medicine and Health Sciences, University of Antwerp, Antwerp, Belgium

**Danny Van heusden** Nursing Department, Antwerp University Hospital, Antwerp, Belgium

Nursing and Midwifery Sciences, Centre for Research and Innovation in Care (CRIC), Faculty of Medicine and Health Sciences, University of Antwerp, Antwerp, Belgium

**Bart Van Rompaey** Nursing and Midwifery Science, Centre for Research and Innovation in Care (CRIC), Faculty of Medicine and Health Sciences, University of Antwerp, Antwerp, Belgium

**Martijn Verspuy** Nursing Department, Antwerp University Hospital, Antwerp, Belgium

Medical Sciences, University of Antwerp, Antwerp, Belgium

Nursing and Midwifery Sciences, Centre for Research and Innovation in Care (CRIC), Faculty of Medicine and Health Sciences, University of Antwerp, Antwerp, Belgium

**Mark White** Nursing and Midwifery Planning and Development Unit, HSE, Kilkenny, Ireland

School of Health Sciences, Waterford Institute of Technology, Waterford, Ireland

Faculty of Nursing, Royal College of Surgeons, Dublin, Ireland

# Part I

# Concepts and Evidence

# Introduction

Peter Van Bogaert and Sean Clarke

Nearly two decades ago, the current era in research and practice in patient safety and quality began. A crisis in nurse workforces in health-care systems around the world had been declared, and the idea of "work environment" was about to be taken up by leaders and researchers throughout the nursing profession. Today, no one questions the need to deal with specific safety hazards and human factors concerns in health care. However, it is now recognized that communication and teamwork greatly influence patient safety. Moreover, work environments are now recognized as a key predictor of both nurses' experience at work and of the quality of care they are able to deliver. Therefore, work environment interventions hold great promise for addressing broad ranges of clinical care delivery challenges in an efficient way.

Not surprisingly, recurring themes have emerged in a literature that overlaps but is in many ways distinct from research in related fields in the social and administrative sciences and in other professions. Research consistently points to fundamental psychological and social elements of nurses' work and to their experiences of providing nursing care in complex organizational environments. However, despite a better understanding of causes and effects of poor experiences at work than ever before and a track record of success in implementing a number of initiatives based on best management practices (such as the Magnet movement), nurse leaders in many organizations still struggle to identify and implement practical strategies for addressing work environment strategies.

This book begins with a review of the conceptual base for research in this area, analyzing key concepts that are the major independent and dependent variables—or

P. Van Bogaert (✉)
Nursing and Midwifery Sciences, Centre for Research and Innovation in Care (CRIC),
Faculty of Medicine and Health Sciences, University of Antwerp, Antwerp, Belgium
e-mail: peter.vanbogaert@uantwerpen.be

S. Clarke
William F. Connell School of Nursing, Boston College, Chestnut Hill, MA, USA
e-mail: clarkese@bc.edu

© Springer International Publishing AG 2018
P. Van Bogaert, S. Clarke (eds.), *The Organizational Context of Nursing Practice*,
https://doi.org/10.1007/978-3-319-71042-6_1

the modifiable factors and the outcomes—of studies in the field. Next, evidence is reviewed concerning on work environments in international context, and a framework is offered for understanding this literature and its findings. Most of the remainder of the book is an exploration of practical strategies for improving nurses' work environments supported by research and illustrated with firsthand experiences of the authors, the majority of whom are members of a team of university-affiliated academics and clinical nursing leaders from a community in Flanders, Belgium.

Our intent was to provide an international audience with a new integrated perspective tying together theory, research findings, specific applications, and practical guidelines for implementing organizational interventions. We hope it is useful to students, clinicians, and nurse managers and leaders seeking an overview of this field of scholarship, which can be intimidatingly vast but offers incredible promise for charting the future of nursing care delivery settings.

# Concepts: Organization of Nursing Work and the Psychosocial Experience of Nurses

Peter Van Bogaert and Sean Clarke

**Abstract**

In this chapter, the intuitive link between balanced, healthy, and supportive psychosocial work environments and a variety of vitally important patient, nurse, and organizational outcomes is discussed with reference to a number of clearly defined and well-researched concepts. Among the essential concepts that ground the rest of the book is the notion of a bundle of factors that provide a context for nurses' work and are known collectively as the *practice environment*. Landmark studies that focused specifically on nurses' experiences of their work environments in exemplary hospitals examined so-called Magnet hospitals, leading to a framework that describes the practice environment and its linkage with professional well-being, occupational stress, and quality of practice and productivity. Many ideas and models have obvious connections to the notion of practice environment such as Job Demand–Control–Support model, worklife dimensions and burnout, concepts related to burnout such as compassion fatigue, and work engagement as a mirror image concept of burnout, as well as notions of empowerment and authentic leadership. These concepts have been chosen for discussion here based on critical masses of evidence pointing to their usefulness in healthcare management and specifically in the management of nursing services. Together all of these concepts and supporting research and scholarship speak to a common point: intentional leadership approaches, grounded in a comprehensive understanding of nurses' psychosocial experiences of their work, are essential to nurses' abilities to respond to complex patients' needs in rapidly changing healthcare contexts and socioeconomic conditions.

P. Van Bogaert (✉)
Nursing and Midwifery Sciences, Centre for Research and Innovation in Care (CRIC),
Faculty of Medicine and Health Sciences, University of Antwerp, Antwerp, Belgium
e-mail: peter.vanbogaert@uantwerpen.be

S. Clarke
William F. Connell School of Nursing, Boston College, MA, USA
e-mail: clarkese@bc.edu

© Springer International Publishing AG 2018
P. Van Bogaert, S. Clarke (eds.), *The Organizational Context of Nursing Practice*,
https://doi.org/10.1007/978-3-319-71042-6_2

**Keywords**

Nurse shortage • Practice environment • Magnet hospitals • Magnet recogniton program • Mortality and comorbidity • Burnout • Work engagement • Compasion fatigue and compassion satisfaction • Empowerment • Authentic leadership

## 2.1 Introduction

In this chapter, the intuitive link between balanced, healthy, and supportive psychosocial work environments and a variety of vitally important patient, nurse, and organizational outcomes is discussed with reference to a number of clearly defined and well-researched concepts. Among the essential concepts that ground the rest of the book is the notion of a bundle of factors that provide a context for nurses' work and are known collectively as the *practice environment*. Landmark studies that focused specifically on nurses' experiences of their work environments in exemplary hospitals are described. This work on so-called Magnet hospitals was the basis of the American Nurses Credentialing Center Magnet Recognition Program® in the United States and internationally. Magnet hospitals are believed to attract and retain professional nurses and achieve favorable patient outcomes through excellence in the management of nursing services and notably through the promotion of positive practice environments.

The Magnet Hospital framework describes the practice environment and its linkage with professional well-being, occupational stress and quality of practice and productivity. Many ideas and models have obvious connections to the notion of practice environment such as Karasek and Theorell's Job Demand–Control–Support model, Maslach and her colleagues' work on worklife dimensions and burnout, concepts related to burnout such as compassion fatigue (Kelly and colleagues), and work engagement (Schaufeli and Bakker) as a mirror image concept of burnout, as well as Kanter's notions of empowerment and authentic leadership (Laschinger and colleagues). These concepts have been chosen for discussion here based on critical masses of evidence pointing to their usefulness in healthcare management and specifically in the management of nursing services. Indeed, most of these ideas have been discussed in the nursing literature for some time. Together all of these concepts and supporting research and scholarship speak to a common point: intentional leadership approaches, grounded in a comprehensive understanding of nurses' psychosocial experiences of their work, are essential to nurses' abilities to respond to complex patients' needs in rapidly changing healthcare contexts and socioeconomic conditions.

## 2.2 Practice Environment: An Empirically Supported Concept

### 2.2.1 Early Research Initiatives to Understand and Anticipate Cycles of Nurse Shortages

Recurring nurse shortages in the United States and other Western countries have plagued hospitals and other healthcare organizations for over a century. In the early

1980s, the American Academy of Nursing (AAN) appointed a task force of leading administrators and researchers to contribute fresh ideas on this problem, which affects nurses, hospitals, and ultimately patients. *Magnet hospitals: Attraction and Retention of Professional N*urses, (the orginal study), first published in 1983 (McClure et al. 2002), was the first publication from that work and spurred many research initiatives in the United States, Canada, and beyond. At the core of the original Magnet research was the observation that despite nurse shortages, some hospitals were consistently more successful in attracting and retaining staff nurses than neighboring hospitals; there were some hospitals that in fact appeared to be immune to cyclical nurse shortages (Aiken 2002). The first study sought to identify (1) important variables in hospitals and nursing services that attracted and retained professional nurses and (2) the particular combination of variables that produced model(s) of hospital nursing practice where nurses experienced high professional and personal satisfaction that promoted recruitment and retention of qualified staff (McClure and Hinshaw 2002). Further, as the authors stated: "This work was expected to yield a variety of successful approaches that could be reviewed, adopted, and/or modified by other institutions eager to resolve their nurse shortages" (McClure et al. 2002). The promise of translating the learnings from the research project on a wider scale was ultimately fulfilled in the early 1990s with the development of the American Nurses Credentialing Center (ANCC) Magnet Nursing Services Recognition Program® (Urden and Monarch 2002). In tandem with the growth of the program later called Magnet Recognition Program® and somewhat independently of it, researchers began to study the organizational context of nursing practice and the impact on outcomes such as job satisfaction, nurse attraction and retention and nurse-assessed quality of care, and nurse burnout and on patient outcomes such as mortality and surgical complications (Aiken et al. 2008; Estabrooks et al. 2005; Friese et al. 2008, Tourangeau et al. 2007).

The original Magnet hospital study identified relevant factors for future study, such as management style and leadership, organizational structure, staffing, personnel policies, quality of patient care, teaching, image of nursing, professional development, orientation, and career development. Forty-one hospitals were identified as the *original (reputational) Magnet hospitals* after 165 hospitals in 8 designated regions of the United States were initial nominated by Fellows of the American Academy of Nursing and were ultimately selected after interviews with staff nurses and directors of nursing.

The interviews in the original Magnet hospital study revealed that the directors of nursing in Magnet hospitals were clear about their *philosophy and the value systems* in terms of *high-quality care* for patients in their hospitals (McClure et al. 2002). They were aware of the institution's *mission* and the need to get the message across the nursing staff as well as the importance of programs and practices to meet needs for *adequate and competent staff*, *career development*, and consideration of *personal lives*. From the staff nurses' point of view, the directors were on target in terms of their high level of concern for actual nursing practice. Staff nurses identified specific factors that reflected the operationalization of a philosophy and value system such as *adequate numbers of competent colleagues*, *flexibility in scheduling*, educational programs for *professional growth*, and *recognition as individuals*. Moreover, staff nurses credited *supportive administrators and middle managers* for the positive climate in their hospital, leaders' work to support personal and professional goals alongside organizational ones as well as *collegial and collaborative relationships*. Directors of nursing in these hospitals expected to participate fully in management decisions at the executive level in all matters pertaining to patient care and the role of nurses in the institution. The roles of nursing in these facilities were conceived as increasingly autonomous and multifaceted including *teaching* and *coordination of care*. Staff nurses expected workers in auxiliary services to provide support for the work instead of substitute for them. Staff nurses were keen to be treated as career-oriented *professionals* and were convinced that nursing as a profession was important for the benefit of patients as well as hospitals. Certainly, these hospitals were not stress-free, but staff nurses experienced support from administrators in issues such as medical dominance that might have been anticipated in the face of expanding competencies among staff nurses. Ultimately, both staff nurses and nursing leaders, with the director of nursing at the summit, were advocates for high-quality patient care. In these hospitals, some ongoing shifting of power in favor of nurses was noted. The combination of elements put in place by administrators, leaders, and staff nurses as just described created a positive and supportive practice environment for nurses.

These findings, published in 1983 or almost 35 years ago, were visionary at the time and are still fresh and inspiring. Much research speaks to their continuing relevance for the profession and for leaders and clinicians in nursing. As mentioned earlier, in 1993 a formal program, the ANCC Magnet Recognition program®, was established as a voluntary form of external professional nurse peer review available to hospitals and nursing homes based on established standards of nursing care and nursing service administration (Aiken 2002). Recognition was available first in the United States and later internationally. Meanwhile research began to study the hospitals designated under the new criteria and explore whether and how they had organizational traits and outcomes comparable to those identified in the original Magnet study (Aiken et al. 2000).

Directly from this report, a 65-item questionnaire, the Nursing Work Index (NWI), was developed based on Korman (1971) work and Locke (1973) need fulfillment theory proposing that job satisfaction and productivity are the products of the presence of various attributes and the relative importance of those attributes to individuals' work-related and personal needs (Kramer and Schmalenberg 2004). The NWI contained items describing various workplace characteristics described in the original Magnet study (Kramer and Hafner 1989). The NWI was tested on a random sample of Magnet hospitals and nurses. Magnet hospitals were compared with excellent companies; data were used to test a causal model for outcomes of job satisfaction and nurse effectiveness, to describe attributes of nurses working in hospitals with different external systems, and to ascertain impact of congruence in values on nurse job satisfaction and effectiveness (Kramer and Schmalenberg 2002). Nurses were asked to rate their agreement–disagreement that various elements/characteristics were (1) present in their current job situation, (2) important to their job satisfaction, and (3) important in quality of care on 4-point scales. The Nursing Work Index was further adjusted to the 37 most chosen items by 4000 staff nurses over a 17-year study period, and in an additional study, staff nurses of 14 Magnet hospitals were asked to list the 10 characteristics/items that were most important to provide quality patient care (productivity). A causal model study showed that both recruitment and retention are highly correlated with job satisfaction and that more than 80% of nurse job satisfaction is attributable to being able to give quality patient care. They therefore eliminated the nurse job satisfaction component and focused only on quality care productivity (Kramer and Hafner 1989). Eight items were selected by two-thirds of the 279 staff nurse respondents and identified as the Essentials of Magnetism (Kramer and Schmalenberg 2002, 2004) (Box 2.1).

---

**Box 2.1 Eight Essentials of Magnet Hospital**
1. Working with other nurses who are clinically competent.
2. Good nurse—physician relationships and communication.
3. Nurse autonomy and accountability.
4. Supportive manager and supervisor.
5. Control over nursing practice and practice environment.
6. Support for education.
7. Adequate nurse staffing.
8. Concern for the patient is paramount in this organization.

---

The authors developed further a multi-item 8 Essentials of Magnetism (EOM) tool generated from participant observations and interviews, and psychometric properties were established with staff nurses of 16 Magnet and 10 non-Magnet hospitals that evaluate what is essential for productivity of quality of care and work environments that attract and retain nurses or a *healthy work environment* (Kramer and Schmalenberg 2004). Follow-up studies with 10,514 staff nurses in 34 hospitals (18 Magnet hospitals and 16 comparison hospitals) showed an adapted valid and reliable measure (EOMII) of the quality of work environment from a staff nurse perspective. Differences in ratings of the Magnet essentials and outcome variables such as job satisfaction and nurse-assessed quality of care have been noted, where Magnet hospital staff nurses report the most productive work environments (Schmalenberg and Kramer 2008). Kramer and Schmalenberg have argued that the 65-item Nursing Work Index is outdated, originated as a tool designed for use with individuals rather than aggregated unit level data, lacked a theoretical basis, and measured the presence of attributes without regard to the steps or components of the processes or the respondent's definition of the underlying concepts (Schmalenberg and Kramer 2007). They argue that the EOM tool measures both the components of the work environment and the composite work environment because 90% of the items are written from a clinical unit perspective and the remaining 10% are organizational and unit based. Overall, the EOM is a process measurement instrument that assesses the health of the unit work environment. A healthy, productive unit work environment is one that enables nurses to engage in the eight processes/professional practices identified by nurses in Magnet hospitals as most essential to delivery of quality patient care (de Brouwer et al. 2014).

## 2.2.2    Studying Nurse Practice Environments with Adapted Versions of the Nursing Work Index

Further initiatives have been taken to generate evidence regarding why the original Magnet hospitals, and later the ANCC designated Magnet hospitals, offer a very promising model for the development of nurse professional environments in the United States and internationally. As the ANA research initiative started to understand and prevent cyclical hospital nurse shortages over time, the research on nurse workforce shortages has been integrated with research on hospital organization and its impact on nurse and patient outcome by the Center for Health Outcomes and Policy Research at the University of Pennsylvania (Aiken 2002) and later other US and international research initiatives. The center was eager to identify strategies to study how modifiable organizational traits of hospitals affect patient and nurse outcomes. As Aiken and colleagues noticed in a rapidly changing healthcare system, there are ample opportunities to make use of targets of possibilities or natural experiments in which a number of hospitals have various organizational elements that can be studied in comparison with conventionally organized hospitals (Aiken et al. 1997). The original Magnet hospitals and later the ANCC Magnet hospitals were a logical platform for studying differences in hospital organizational traits as well as the organizational context of nursing practice associated with better outcomes for patients and nurses (Aiken et al. 2000). In addition, two natural experiments in hospital organizational reform—the unfolding AIDS epidemic as well as the rapid spread of hospital reengineering in the 1990s—provided important opportunities to study to what extent and how hospital organizational characteristics affect nursing practices and in turn nurse and patient outcomes. Interestingly, through the AIDS epidemic, nurses had in a number of US urban hospitals the discretion and opportunity to redesign general medical units into dedicated AIDS units driven by the basic principles of professional nursing practice as well as organizational traits common to Magnet hospitals. Meanwhile in the 1990s, a wave of reengineering initiatives in US hospitals emerged based on fundamental rethinking and radical redesign of business processes. It was originally hoped that these initiatives would achieve dramatic improvements in critical, contemporary measures of performance such as cost, quality, service, and speed (Walston et al. 2000). These changes in the organizational context of hospitals were often associated with rigorous cost-cutting, rightsizing, and downsizing and were a special target of the Institute of Medicine's (IOM) report *To Err is Human: Building a Safer Health System* (Kohn et al. 2000). The report described many structural flaws in health systems resulting from poor management practices, including underestimating the importance of professional nursing practice (Page 2004). The document ultimately became the founding documents for a powerful international patient safety agenda that continues to this day. Besides heightening awareness of potential flaws of healthcare professionals that are inevitable consequences of the human condition, the report called attention to the disconnect between frontline workers at the sharp end of patient safety and management levels identified as the blunt end and the risks created by this divide in terms of healthcare that produces bad patient outcomes.

The University of Pennsylvania's Center for Health Outcomes and Policy Research led an unprecedentedly large research project examining the attributes and outcomes of a large representative group of hospitals in five countries with different organized and financed healthcare systems: the United States, Canada, England, Scotland, and Germany (Aiken et al. 2001). US and international research on hospital organizational context of nursing practice received an important boost from the development of the *Nursing Work Index Revised (NWI-R)* and later the *Practice Environment Scale of the Nursing Work Index (PES-NWI)*. Aiken and colleagues used the original NWI to study professional nurse practice environment in hospitals (Aiken 2002). However, instead of examining job satisfaction by comparing nurses' ratings of the importance of various elements with the same nurses' ratings of the presence of those elements in their current jobs, in the NWI-R, nurses only rate their agreement or disagreement regarding *the presence of various organizational features* on a 57-item modified version of the scale (Aiken and Patrician 2000). Conceptually and empirically derived subscales were developed to measure various core organizational attributes identified in literature as characterizing an environment supportive of professional nurse practice (Baggs et al. 1992; Grindel et al. 1996; Hoffart and Woods 1996; Knaus et al. 1986): (1) *autonomy*, (2) *control over the work environment*, (3) *relationship with physicians, and* (4) *organizational structures*. Because of the modification of the NWI to a revised instrument, the NWI-R, that evaluates the hospital organizational context instead of job satisfaction and quality patient care, additional nurse-reported constructs such as job satisfaction and quality of care were added. Moreover, inspired by concern about difficulties to attract and retain qualified staff in dedicated AIDS units because of the stresses inherent in caring for young adults with a fatal and potentially communicable disease, additional measures such as nurse burnout (Maslach Burnout Human Service Survey or MBI-HSS) and turnover intentions were also added in research designs (Aiken 2002). Furthermore, former experiences with administrative discharge data analyses on mortality and comorbidity (Needleman et al. 2002) inspired the development of the *failure to rescue concept* or death that occurs after a patient develops a complication in the hospital that was not present on admission (Silber et al. 2000). Clarke and Aiken (2003) applied practice environment ideas to the failure to rescue concept, hypothesizing that surveillance of patients' conditions by nurses would be affected by staffing adequacy,

---

**Box 2.2 Nursing Work Index Revised or NWI-R and Practice Environment Scale of the Nursing Work Index or PES-NWI**
- NWI-R: 57 items and 4 subscales—(1) nurse autonomy, (2) nurse control over the work environment, (3) nurse relations with physicians, and (4) organizational structures.
- PES-NWI: 31 items and 5 subscales—(1) nurse participation in hospital affairs; (2) nursing foundations for quality of care; (3) nurse manager ability, leadership, and support of nurses; (4) staffing and resource adequacy; (5) collegial nurse–physician relations.

- One approach to scoring draws upon the item ratings of 1 for general disagreement to 4 for general agreement. When the mean item scores across all of the nurses in an institution and all of the items in a subscale are higher than the scale midpoint (2.50), that subscale is considered to be positively rated. The work environments of organizations or organizational subunits are considered unfavorable if scores are ≥2.50 on only one or no subscales, mixed if scores ≥2.50 on two or three subscales, and favorable if ≥2.50 on four or five subscales.
- Nurses in Magnet hospitals rate practice elements more highly than nurses working in non-Magnet facilities, suggesting that organizational characteristics that support nursing practice are present to a greater extent in Magnet hospitals. These higher subscales mean scores are related to empowering characteristics in the work environment, trust in management, and ultimately professional well-being through job satisfaction, lower turnover intentions, and lower feelings of burnout measured and analyzed with study populations in the United States and Canada.
- Study results show that nurses reported more positive job experiences and fewer concerns with care quality, and patients had significantly lower risk of death and failure to rescue in hospitals with better care environments measured with PES-NWI.

administrative support, and nurse–physician relations and that practice environment features should be important explanatory factors for differences between hospitals in patient rescue rates (Box 2.2).

Lake (2002) presented a parsimonious set of 31 items from the NWI grouped into 5 subscales derived from factor analyses that she called the Practice Environment Scale (PES): (1) *nurse participation in hospital affairs*; (2) *nursing foundations for quality of care*; (3) *nurse manager ability, leadership, and support of nurses*; (4) *staffing and resource adequacy*; and (5) *collegial nurse–physician relations*. Reference values for original Magnet hospitals are available for both the NWI-R and PES-NWI sets of subscales. Lake defines the nursing practice environment as the organizational characteristics of a work setting that facilitate or constrain professional nursing practice such as the nature of relationships with managers and physicians and the status of nurses within the hospital hierarchy. Given the complex, unpredictable nature of nurses' work, Lake argues that a professional model, also known as the goal-centered model, emphasizes individual qualifications and collegial control systems and is preferable to a bureaucratic model, also known as the task-centered model which emphasizes control exercised through hierarchical authority and formal rule enforcement. The author preferred to develop, based on an existing real-work set, the NWI, instead of new set with theoretically relevant organizational characteristics. A composite measure, in addition to subscales representing distinct domains of the nursing practice environment, was presented based on factor analyses. The PES-NWI is an organizational measure, but a target level of organization, either the hospital or the nursing unit, has not been explicit. The author noticed that empirical evidence may reveal at what level nurses interpret some items or subscales. The construct validity showed significant higher mean scores of nurses in Magnet hospitals compared with those of the non-Magnet hospitals. However, as the author mentioned, differences in hospital size and ownership between the Magnet and non-Magnet hospital samples may account for some of the observed difference in practice environment scores. Lake and Friese (2006) later described a three-level classification, *favorable, mixed, and unfavorable*, that sorts hospitals according to how many subscales have scores suggesting agreement of the nurses that characteristics related to an underlying construct are present in the facility. A fairly generous standard was used to identify favorable ratings: values above 2.50—the theoretical midpoint—were considered favorable because they were on the side of agreement that the features were present in the current job situation. Hospitals where nurse ratings were above 2.50 on only one or no subscales were classified as having unfavorable practice environments, on two or three subscales as mixed practice environments, and on four or five subscales as favorable. The following study of 156 Pennsylvania Hospitals (Lake and Friese 2006) shows that the nurse practice environments of the small samples of Magnet hospitals were superior to those of the Pennsylvania sample. About 17% of the hospitals had favorable practice environments, and hospitals with better practice environments had higher RN-to-bed ratios. However, hospitals within the favorable category of practice environments had a wide variation in staffing that supports the thesis that staffing and practice environment are distinct concepts. Practice environment differences were not associated with hospital characteristics; however, at the time the data analyzed were gathered, Magnet hospitals tended to be large institutions with intensive medical education missions that were located in urban areas.

### 2.2.3 Research Insights Regarding Hospital Nurse Practice Environments

Various studies use the NWI-R or PES-NWI to evaluate nurse work environments comparing Magnet hospitals, the original and ANCC designated, and non-Magnet hospitals and the extent that Magnet hospital characteristics are presents in the United States and Canada. Aiken et al. (2000) compared 7 ANCC Magnet hospitals with 13 original Magnet hospitals. Study findings confirmed that ANCC Magnet hospital designation identified hospitals that provided practice environments that were as good as or better than those at the original Magnet hospitals in terms of professional nursing practice (autonomy 3.01 vs 2.86, $p < 0.001$; control over the practice setting 2.95 vs 2.65, $p < 0.001$; and nurse relations with physicians 3.03 vs 2.98, $p = 0.10$) and nurses' assessment of the quality of care delivered to their patients (rated as excellent 43 vs 21%, $p < 0.001$). Nurses in ANCC Magnet hospitals were more satisfied with their jobs (rated as very satisfied 33 vs 22% and dissatisfied 16 vs 28%, $p < 0.0001$) and less likely to suffer from job-related burnout (rated burned out from their job 20.4 vs 29.9%, $p < 0.001$, and emotionally drained from their work 42.2 vs 52.9%, $p < 0.001$). In addition, nurses in ANCC Magnet hospitals had significant higher educational preparation as well as nurse-to-patient ratios than in original Magnet hospitals. The authors mentioned that the original Magnet hospitals are not immune to changes in the health system. Some have been adversely affected, but many have, despite vast organizational change, continued fostering elements of professional practice that distinguish them from non-Magnet hospitals. Havens compared in her study 19 ANCC Magnet hospitals with 24 non-Magnet hospitals based on chief nurse executives' (CNEs) reports (Havens 2001). Both hospital groups were comparable with the general hospital characteristics in the United States dealing with the same health system and socioeconomic context. CNEs were invited to serve as organizational informants, and results of their reports suggested that the two hospital groups were characterized by different nursing infrastructure organization, leadership features, and support for the hospital structures. The ANCC Magnet hospitals had far more likely a discrete nursing department as part of the organizational structure, which may indicate certain value and respect for nursing as a vital and distinct clinical discipline. The ANCC group of CNEs reported that nursing was visible as a distinct professional clinical discipline in their hospital and that nurses had control over nursing practice and the nursing practice environment more than a comparison group of CNEs. The two groups of CNEs reported differences in the nature and extent of the implementation of restructuring and reengineering strategies within the previous 5 years. Interestingly, the ANCC hospitals implemented more changes to expand the CNE role than the comparison hospitals. The authors concluded that organizational structure provides the framework in which nurses' practice appears to contribute to the total ambiance of the hospital. Thus, if the role of the CNE is to develop and maintain the context in which care is delivered, then it is not surprising that the variance in the role, power, and position of the role of the CNE and the nursing department in the organization is associated with variance in reports of quality of the practice environment and patient and staff outcomes. In a mixed design including a quantitative survey study and a qualitative study based on interviews with nursing leaders (Upenieks 2002), comparing two Magnet hospitals with two non-Magnet hospitals, clinical nurses of the first had more autonomy (3.10 vs 2.64, $p < 0.001$) and control over their practice (2.79 vs 2.34, $p < 0.001$), characterizing their work environment as one support from administration and their organizational structures (2.93 vs 2.40, $p < 0.001$) with favorable physician relations (3.13 vs 2.78, $p < 0.01$) more often than nurses of the latter settings. Factors that influenced nurse leader effectiveness included a strong commitment to nursing, recognition of professional nursing practice, leadership visibility, and support of an autonomous climate.

Kanter's structural theory of organizational behavior (Kanter 1993) asserts that certain work empowerment structures have the potential to explain differences in individual responses to situations in the work environment: structural access to sufficient information; support of subordinates, peers, as well as supervisors; and opportunities to learn and develop. This would suggest that nurses in an empowering work environment have the ability to mobilize all necessary resources, both human and material, to support the best care for their patients. Furthermore, they have access to the information they need and that they have opportunities for learning, which stimulates their personal development and fosters supportive relationships with supervisors, peers, and subordinates. Moreover, informal and formal networks of alliances within the organization provide such nurses with opportunities to achieve their goals and ensure professional discretion and visibility. The revised Conditions for Work Effectiveness Scale assesses empowerment, power, and opportunity components of Kanter theory. Upenieks (2003a) used the CWEQ-II scale (mean scale scores ranging from 1 or low to 5 or high) in another study using the same design. She found that clinical nurses in Magnet hospitals experienced higher levels of empowerment due to greater access to work empowerment structures in their work environment such as opportunity, information, and resources compared with clinical nurses of non-Magnet hospitals. Differences in leadership effectiveness between Magnet hospitals and non-Magnet hospitals accounted for the differences in empowerment scores (3.55 vs 2.63, $p < 0.001$). Moreover, Magnet hospitals encompass nurse leaders who are people-oriented, visible, and empowering and that this type of leadership style is conducive to creating an environment that is supportive, autonomous, and collaborative among other leadership traits (Upenieks 2003b).

Laschinger et al. (2001a) performed a study with a stratified random sample of nurses who worked on medical and surgical hospital wards in Ontario, Canada. The study tested a model positing that if nurses perceived their work environments, afforded a high degree of autonomy, control over the practice environment, and strong collaborative nurse–physician relationships (measured with the NWI-R), they would have high levels of trust in management (assessed with the 12-item Interpersonal Trust at Work Scale) and low levels of burnout (measured using MBI-HSS) and ultimately would report high levels of job satisfaction and positive evaluations of the care delivered in their work setting. Study results confirmed that both trust in management and emotional exhaustion were important mediators of job satisfaction and assessed quality of care. The authors concluded that high levels of organizational trust are inevitable when employees feel that their managers have created work conditions that make them confident in their ability to act based on their expert judgment. Moreover, in a secondary analyses of data from three studies—two with staff nurses ($n = 496$) and one with nurse practitioners ($n = 55$)—in Ontario hospitals, Laschinger et al. (2003) showed that access to empowering work conditions (measured with the CWEQ-II scale) and Magnet hospital characteristics (measured with the NWI-R) together were predictive of nurses' satisfaction with their job.

In 2003, 13,000 Ontario nurses were surveyed to explore how they evaluated their hospital work environments using the NWI-R and experienced their positions (Tourangeau et al. 2005). Medical and surgical nurses evaluated their professional practice environments as poor. Nurses rated foundations for quality of care and nurse–physician relationships most favorably, although there was significant room for improvements for both these areas. The lowest-rated aspects of the nursing practice environment were adequacy of staffing and other resources required to provide patient care and managers' ability and support. Authors suggested that administrators could actively consult with nursing staff to obtain frontline perspectives of the amounts and kind of staffing and other resources considered adequate to meet patient care needs. Overall, nurses reported that their managers were not effectively leading and managing within their hospitals and that they did not provide adequate support, leadership, praise, or recognition. The authors suggested that nurse managers may not have adequate management and leadership knowledge and skills. Moreover, certain hospital organizational structures, such as large span of control, impede a manager's ability to provide adequate leadership and support to nursing staff. Further analyses of these data revealed that nurse intention to remain employed was predicted by job satisfaction, personal characteristics of nurses, work group cohesion and collaboration, and organizational commitment of nurses (indicated by the NWI-R scale of nurses' participation in hospital affairs). The authors suggested that nurse burnout and nurse managers' ability and support have a direct effect on job satisfaction and through the latter an indirect effect on intention to remain employed.

### 2.2.4 Hospital Nurse Practice Environments and Comorbidity, Failure to Rescue, and Mortality

In the same study, Tourangeau et al. (2007) investigated also hospital administrative discharge data to answer the research question: what are the nursing-related determinants of risk-adjusted 30-day mortality for acute medical patients of 19 hospitals in the Ontario province of Canada. A 30-day mortality is identified as the occurrence of death within 30 days of admission and preferable to inpatient mortality as there can be a lag time between hospital admission and deleterious effects of care (Chassin et al. 1989). Lower 30-day mortality rates were associated with higher % of registered nurses (RNs) and higher % of baccalaureate-prepared nurses in the staff mix, lower nursing staff dose (total inpatient clinical nursing worked hours—all categories) per weighted patient case, higher nurse-reported adequacy of staffing and resources, higher uses of care maps or protocols to guide patient care, and higher nurse-reported quality of care. Results suggest that certain structures or *having the right things* and processes or *doing the right things* of hospital care are relevant, explaining variances in patient outcome such as mortality. Interestingly, lower nurse-reported adequacy of manager ability and support and higher nurse burnout (emotional exhaustion) were also predictors of lower 30-day mortality. Overall, nurses across study hospitals rated their support from the nurse managers as low, and authors suggest that managers in low-mortality hospitals may have focused their energies on enabling other hospital structures and processes, such as securing resources or promoting patient care initiatives that supported lower mortality than providing direct support to nursing staff. Likewise, higher levels of nurses' emotional exhaustion could act as motivator enabling nurses to detect and intervene promptly with serious patient complications that could have led to unnecessary patient death if left unattended or detected too late. These factors explained 45% of variance in risk- and case-mix-adjusted 30-day mortality.

Estabrooks et al. (2005, 2011) investigated variations in 30-day mortality in 49 hospitals in the Canadian province of Alberta. Adjusted for individual patient characteristics and comorbidities and other institutional characteristics, higher proportion of baccalaureate-prepared nurses, a richer skill mix of nursing staff (RN to non-RN ratio), better nurse–physician relationships, and lower casual and temporary employment were associated with lower patient mortality. The institutional and hospital nursing characteristics explained 36.9% of variation in hospital mortality. Both studies performed in Canadian hospitals suggested (albeit in inconsistent forms) that organizational context of nursing practice is not only potentially relevant for nurses' professional well-being but also for quality of patient care and patient outcomes. Various study limitations explain these inconsistencies, and later studies provided broader insights.

Friese et al. (2008) investigated the effect of nursing practice environment on outcomes of hospitalized cancer patients undergoing surgery of 164 hospitals in the US state of Pennsylvania. Nurse staffing (nurse-to-patient ratio), educational preparation (the proportion of baccalaureate-prepared nurses), and the PES-NWI were calculated from a survey of nurses, aggregated to the hospital level, and analyzed as predictors for 30-day mortality, complications, and failure to rescue. PES-NWI subscales were categorized as described by Lake and Friese (2006) as *unfavorable* (mean subscale score $\geq$2.50 on 0 or 1 subscale), *mixed* (mean subscale scores $\geq$2.50 on 2 or 3 subscales), and *favorable* (mean subscale scores $\geq$2.50 on 4 or 5 subscales). Failure to rescue defined as death within 30 days of hospital admission for patients who have experienced a postoperative complication is more highly associated with hospital characteristics than 30-day mortality and complication rates (Needleman et al. 2002). Complications were identified using a set of 21 secondary diagnosis codes and procedure codes and conditions not identified in prior admission (Silber et al. 1995). Adjusted for patient and hospital characteristics, unfavorable nurse practice environments had significantly increased odds of death and failure to rescue. The study confirms significant variation in nurse practice environments and patient outcomes across acute care hospitals. The relationship between nurse practice environments and outcomes persists after adjusting for differences in patients and hospitals. Authors found it quite striking that distinct but related concepts such as staffing, education, and practice environment remained significant predictors of 30-day mortality when estimated simultaneously. Moreover, one in five hospitals had favorable working conditions according to nurse assessments, meaning that four out of every five hospitals studied appeared to show room for improvements within the control of hospital administration. In over 7% of studied hospitals, nurses reported caring for eight or more patients on their last shift, and fewer than 25% of hospitals had a majority of baccalaureate-prepared nurses. Authors noticed that these organizational characteristics are modifiable and strongly associated with better outcomes.

Aiken et al. (2008) investigated 168 Pennsylvania hospitals in the United States to analyze the net effects of nurse practice environments on nurse and patient outcomes after accounting for nurse staffing and education. Outcomes included nurse job satisfaction, burnout, intent to leave, and reports of quality of care, as well as mortality and failure to rescue in patients. Nurse staffing was measured as the mean number of patients assigned to staff nurses who reported caring for at least 1 but less than 20 patients on their last shift. The educational profile of staff nurses in each hospital was calculated as the percentage of baccalaureate-prepared staff nurses. Three of the five PES-NWI subscales that did not overlap empirically with the selected nurse staffing and education measures were chosen for the analysis: nursing foundation for quality of care; nurse manager ability, leadership, and support; and collegial nurse–physician relations. Hospitals above the median on all three subscales, on one or two subscales, and on none of the subscales were classified as having *better, mixed,* and *poor* care environments. Six nurse survey measures that were analyzed as outcomes included job satisfaction, burnout (MBI-HSS emotional exhaustion scale), and intent to leave their job within the next year and three questions related to nurses' perceptions on quality of care. Patient deaths within 30 days of hospital admission and failure to rescue among patients with complications were included as patient outcomes. Study results show that nurses reported more positive job experiences and fewer concerns with care quality, and patients had significantly lower risk of death and failure to rescue in hospitals with better care environments. Authors conclude that care environment elements must be optimized alongside staffing and education to achieve high quality of care and that nurse leaders have at least three major options for improving nurse retention and patient outcomes: improving RN staffing, moving to a more educated nurse workforce, and improving the care environment. All of this work points to higher levels of characteristics associated with Magnet hospitals associated with better patient outcomes.

### 2.2.5 Scientific Framework of ANCC Magnet Recognition Program®

A national *Magnet Recognition Program*® in the United States was initiated in 1993 by the American Nurses Association (ANA) guided by the groundbreaking 1983 study on Magnet hospitals and organized by the American Nurses Credentialing Center (ANCC). Since the incorporation in 1991, ANCC has provided formal systematic mechanism whereby individuals and organizations may voluntarily seek credentials that recognize quality in professional practice and continuing education (Urden and Monarch 2002). The Magnet Recognition Program® is an integral division of the ANCC. The ANCC has both an *accreditation* division that validates whether an organization meets established continuing educational standards and a *certification* division that validates if an individual RN possesses the requisite knowledge, skills, and abilities to practice in a defined specialty. *Recognition* is a third credentialing process to evaluate an organization's adherence to excellence-focused standards. The forces of magnetism gleaned from the original study (McClure et al. 2002) were those elements that contributed to an organizational culture that permitted patients to receive excellent care from nurses practicing in an excellent healthcare environment (Urden and Monarch 2002). The *Nursing Administration: Scope and Standards of Practice* (ANA 1996) was a foundational document from the outset of the program, along with the subsequent versions of the Magnet Manual that guide organizations to their eligibility for recognition, evaluation methods for all criteria as well as acceptable sources of evidence for each force. The recognition process starts with an application, followed by written documentation within a year, a site visit, and finally a decision of the Commission on Magnet (COM) that recognizes each hospital that meets all criteria for Magnet recognition for a period of 4 years. (Redesignation is possible after 4 years.) In 1998 and 2000, the program was expanded to include long-term care facilities and accommodated applications from international healthcare organizations, respectively. After 25 years, the term *Magnet hospitals* has been equated with *excellence*. At that time almost 300 hospitals were designated facilities, and applications had grown 32% per year on average for the previous 5 years (Triolo et al. 2006; Wolf et al. 2008).

In 2004 the COM launched a comprehensive evaluation of the Magnet Recognition Program®. Guided by recommendations for changes, a new model was developed to bring greater clarity to how the forces worked systematically, to reinforce and synergize excellence in nursing practice, and to reduce redundancy to provide greater focus and simplify the application process for organizations. A multivariate structural analysis was performed on 164 sources of evidence rated by 2–4 appraisers of 147 Magnet facilities. Factor and cluster analyses reveal seven domains or clusters of evidence: (1) leadership, (2) resource utilization and development, (3) nursing model, (4) safe and ethical practice, (5) autonomous practice, (6) research, and (7) quality processes (Wolf et al. 2008). Although the forces had served the program well, evidence showed that 7 domains could capture the 14 forces, a breakthrough finding. The COM proposed an additional domain dedicated to outcomes because Magnet designation was until then primarily focused on structure and processes, with the assumption that outcomes will follow. The designation process lacked specific, minimal criteria for evaluating outcomes. Thirty experts reviewed the new Magnet domains and examined sources of evidence that supported these domains. Ultimately, the COM adopted a model that comprises five components:

(1) *Transformational leadership* or leading people to where they need to be to meet the demands of the future, by listening, challenging, influencing and affirming as the organization makes its way into the future, giving birth to new ideas and innovations in practice environments that need to be stable though transforming.

(2) Structural empowerment or operationalizing the mission, vision, and values and achieving the necessary outcomes; staff needs to be developed, directed, and empowered to accomplish the organizational goals and achieve desired outcomes; once the structure has been established and hardwired into place, good outcomes should result.

(3) Exemplary professional nursing practice or understanding the independent and dependent role of nursing, the application of that role with patients, families, communities, and the interdisciplinary team and the application of new knowledge and evidence; the goal is more than the establishment of a strong professional practice, it is what that professional practice can subsequently achieve.

(4) *New knowledge, innovations, and improvements* or systems that are constantly evolving and therefore must be redesigned and redefined to be successful in the future; organizations in designation cycle should reinforce structure and process focusing on outcomes that are tracked, trended, and improved over time as well as benchmarked against high-performing organizations.

---

**Box 2.3 From the Forces of Magnetism to the Magnet Model** (Wolf et al. 2008)
- 14 Forces of Magnetism:

  (1) Quality of leadership, (2) organizational structures, (3) management style, (4) personnel policies and programs, (5) professional models of care, (6) quality of care, (7) quality improvement, (8) consultation and resources, (9) autonomy, (10) community and the hospital, (11) nurses as teachers, (12) image of nursing, (13) interdisciplinary relationships, and (14) professional development

- Magnet Hospital Model:

  (1) Transformational leadership

  Domain of evidence: (1) leadership
  Forces of magnetism: (1) nursing leadership and (3) management style

  (2) Structural empowerment

  Domain of evidence: (2) resource utilization and development
  Forces of magnetism: (14) professional development, (12) image of nursing, (2) organizational structure, (4) policies and programs, and (10) community

  (3) Exemplary professional nursing practice

  Domains of evidence: (3) professional practice model, (4) safe and ethical practice, and (5) quality processes
  Forces of magnetism: (5) models of care, autonomy, (13) interdisciplinary relations, (8) resources and consultations, and (11) nurses as teachers

  (4) New knowledge, innovation, and improvement

  Domain of evidence: (7) research
  Force of magnetism: (7) quality improvement

  (5) Empirical quality outcomes

  Domain of evidence: (8) outcomes
  Force of magnetism: (6) quality of care

(5) *Empirical quality outcomes* categorized into clinical outcomes, patient and family outcomes, and organizational outcomes, collected routinely and quantitatively benchmarked; the report card of a Magnet organization will demonstrate graphically to what extent the organization is on track (Wolf et al. 2008) (Box 2.3).

Wolf and Greenhouse (2006) published a study that indicates the primary and secondary priority forces of Magnet needed to achieve high-performing nursing teams. The authors argue that nursing staff perceives their practice environment differently, depending on the developmental level described by Nelson and Burns (1984). These authors define organizational traits in terms of teams being *reactive, responsive, proactive, and high performing*. Their High-Performance Programming Model provides the hallmarks of each level supporting managers and team members to identify their own work environments. Reactive teams are described as having a crisis mentality, minimal teamwork, small cliques, and a focus on survival, paranoia, distrust, and pessimism. In a responsive team, staff exhibits an ability to handle most situations effectively, supported by staff cohesiveness and, where team members follow rules, is focused on achieving near-term goals with a feeling of health. A proactive team can anticipate and handle difficult situations, where team members see the future as a choice to be made, within a strong shared vision and values and begin to use innovative and creative approaches. Finally, a high-performance team has a high level of synergy among team members with high energy and spirit, high creativity, and innovation, where staff is capable of going beyond expectations. Through surveys (the American Nurses Association Magnet survey) completed by nurses at six hospitals in Pittsburgh (US) as well as categorizing hospital units by hospital executives of patient care, three forces of Magnet were significantly different between reactive teams and responsive teams: organizational structure, management style, and interdisciplinary relations. Between responsive and proactive teams, six Magnet forces were significantly different: policies and programs; professional models of care; quality of care, consultation, and resources; autonomy; and interdisciplinary relations. Achieving an organizational context that supports excellent nursing practice and outcomes is complex and will take years of dedication and perseverance grounded on strong fundamentals primarily to begin with and to evaluate the

---

**Box 2.4 Road Map for Creating a Magnet Work Environment** (Wolf and Greenhouse 2006)
- Primary Priority Forces of Magnet in High-Performing Teams
  - Organizational structures are flat; unit-based decision-making prevails; there is strong nursing representation in the organizational committee structure.
  - Hospitals and nursing leaders use a participative management style, incorporating feedback from staff at all levels of the organization; feedback is encouraged and valued; nursing leaders are visible, accessible, and committed to communicating effectively with staff.
- Interdisciplinary relationships or characterized as positive; mutual respect is exhibited among all disciplines.

- Secondary Priority Forces Magnet in High-Performing Teams
  - Personnel policies and program or salaries and benefits are competitive or creative, and flexible staffing models are used; staff is involved in personnel policies; significant clinical promotional opportunities exist.
  - Professional models of care or transformational model gives nurses the authority and responsibility for patient care; nurses are accountable for their own practice; nurses are the coordinators of care.
  - Quality of care or nurses perceive they are providing high-quality care; providing quality care is seen as an organizational priority.
  - Consultation and resources; experts, especially advanced practice nurses, are available and used; peer support is given within and outside the nursing division.
  - Autonomy or nurses are permitted and expected to practice autonomously, consistent with standards; independent judgment is expected within multidisciplinary approach to care.

organizational structure, the existing management style, and current the interdisciplinary relationships, and secondarily other forces such as proposed in this study will be the next priority (Box 2.4).

### 2.2.6 Practice Environment: A Core Concept in the Organizational Context of Nursing Practice Internationally

Originally developed in the United States to better understand nurse turnover and why certain hospitals appeared immune to shortage, practice environment has become a core concept. More than 30 years of research shows that nurse practice environments have a very important role, distinct from but related to the concepts of nurse staffing and nurse education mix and other variables in the broader category of the organizational context of nursing practice. Nursing practice is potentially complex and unpredictable and vulnerable to resource structures and fluctuations, especially to human resources and how these resources are organized. International researchers were also interested in the concept and eager to investigate in what extent the ideas and instruments could be adopted in other socioeconomic context and health systems. The NWI-R and PES-NWI were replicated first in the United States (Choi et al. 2004; Erickson et al. 2004; Li et al. 2007) and Canada (Estabrooks et al. 2002), and soon translated versions of the instrument have been tested and used, among others, in Canada, Iceland, Switzerland, and Belgium (McCusker et al. 2004; Gunnarsdóttir et al. 2009; Schubert et al. 2007; Van Bogaert et al. 2009a, b). Most of these studies find consistent but not identical clustering of items under common themes. These themes or subscales showed that in comparison with the US

Magnet hospitals, nurses' agreements of statements were rather moderate or poor and predicted various outcomes such as job satisfaction, intention to leave the current employer and the nursing profession, work-related injuries, nurse burnout, nurse-reported quality of care, nurse reports of wrong medication, nosocomial infections, complaints of patients and families, and verbal abuse. These studies make it clear that across countries with different cultures and histories, nursing and healthcare leaders face similar issues with respect to workforce supply, quality of care, and financial constraints (Clarke and Aiken 2008). Using common research protocols to investigate structures, processes, and outcomes of variables in hospital nursing across countries, studying the aspects of practice environments most important to patients and nurses in large numbers of hospitals will be a window of opportunity to provide more insights and knowledge. Soon international studies were set up such as RN4CAST in Europe.

RN4CAST was one of the largest nurse workforce studies conducted in Europe that will add accuracy of forecasting models and generate new approaches to more effective management of nursing resources in Europe (Sermeus et al. 2011). A multi-country, multilevel, cross-sectional design studied forecasting models including how features of hospital work environments impact nurse recruitment, retention, and patient outcomes using 4 data sources such as nurse, patient, and organizational surveys as well as routinely collected hospital administrative discharge data in 12 European countries. The main results suggested that deficits in hospital care quality were common to all countries (Aiken et al. 2012). Nursing staffing and the quality of the hospital work environment measured with the PES-NWI were significantly associated with patient satisfaction, quality and safety care, and workforce outcomes. Whether patients rated their hospital as excellent or would recommend their hospital was significantly associated with nurses' ratings of their hospital work environment and reports of nursing staffing. Consequently, the authors suggested that managers' skepticism regarding nurses' complaints around objective clinical observations of care quality might need to be tempered since nurses' assessments concur with those made independently by patients. Moreover, nurses in every country indicated lack of confidence that hospital management would solve identified problems in patient care. Aiken et al. (2012) mentioned that the United States has recently implemented several high-profile initiatives to achieve safe nurse staffing and improve work environments. At that time more than 20 US states had enacted or were considering legislation to regulate nurse staffing. They also cited Magnet Hospital Recognition®, which promotes improved work environment to almost 400 or 7% of US hospitals. Magnet status is internationally recognized in Australia, New Zealand, and Singapore, among others. However, Europe does not have a single Magnet hospital or an equivalent recognition of nursing excellence. The authors of the RN4CAST study concluded that improvement of hospital work environments is necessary for improving safety and quality of hospital care and to increase patient satisfaction. Moreover, further results showed associations between nursing staffing and bachelor-prepared nurses with inpatient dying within 30 days of admission (Aiken et al. 2014). Patient mortality data were obtained focusing on postoperative patients discharged from study hospitals in the year most proximate to the nurse survey for which data were available. Nurse staffing was calculated from survey data by dividing the number of patients by the number of nurses that each nurse reported were present on their ward on their last shift. Low ratios suggested more favorable staffing. Nurse education was calculated by the % of all nurses in each hospital that reported that the highest academic qualification they had earned was a bachelor's degree or higher. These results show that variation in hospital mortality is associated with differences in nursing staffing levels and educational qualifications.

Another paper from the RN4CAST study analyzed data from 11 countries, 352 hospitals, and more than 2000 nursing units, and almost 23,500 nurses showed associations between unfavorable nurse perceptions of their work environments (in terms of managerial support for nursing care, good physician–nurse relations, nurse participation in decision-making, and organizational priorities on care quality) and nurse burnout at both the nursing unit and the hospital levels (Li et al. 2013). The authors concluded that nurse work environment dynamics are related to nurses' burnout experiences at both the *nursing unit and the hospital level*. The correlation structure among the three burnout outcomes varies across countries but is stable between hospitals within countries and between nursing units within hospitals. These findings provide a motivation for nurses and physicians within nursing units to partner up and for nurse leaders from bedside to boardroom to further develop their managerial skills. Moreover, there is a clear need toward an integrated vision on promotion of care quality in tune with the workforce according to these RN4CAST researchers.

Just about the same period when the research on nurse shortages and the organizational context of nursing practice was set up, research on burnout was developed and provides until now numerous studies and rich insights and knowledge on determinants associated to employers' professional well-being and productivity relevant for nursing practice and healthcare.

## 2.3 Burnout, Compassion Fatigue, and Work Engagement: Cycles of Loss and Gain

### 2.3.1 Development of the Burnout Concept and Empirical Findings

The Nurses' Early Exit or NEXT-Study, conducted in the first decade of this millennium, investigated the reasons, circumstances, and consequences surrounding premature departure from the nursing profession. It was carried out across Europe in Belgium, Finland, France, Germany, Great Britain, Italy, the Netherlands, Poland, Sweden, and Slovakia. Of particular interest in this study were the consequences of the decision to leave as a nurse, their healthcare institution, and the healthcare system (www.next.uni-wuppertal.de). Burnout was found to be one of the most important risk factors for leaving nursing along with poor quality of teamwork. Intention to leave the nursing profession in the coming year increased twofold to threefold in nurses with high burnout scores. The authors identified in addition that patients receiving care within units having adequate staff, good administrative support for nursing care, and good relations between physicians and nurses, perceived by the nursing staff, were more than twice as likely, compared with other patients, to report high satisfaction with their care and their nurses reported significant lower burnout (Estryn-Béhar et al. 2007). The six-item scale Copenhagen Burnout Inventory (CBI) was chosen to measure *personal burnout*. Item examples are: Do you feel tired?, do you think "I can't take it anymore?," and do you feel weak and susceptible to illness? The CBI originally consists of three parts, namely, personal burnout, work burnout, and client burnout. According to Borritz and Kristensen (2001), personal burnout is a state of prolonged physical and psychological exhaustion.

A recently published systematic review concluded that the majority of the articles included revealed high levels of work-related stress, burnout, job dissatisfaction, and poor health are common within the nursing profession supported by studies suggesting that nurses experience longer working hours as well as frequent direct, personal, and emotional contact with a large number of patients in comparison with other health professionals (Khamisa et al. 2013). After Aiken (2002), hearing concerns about difficulties recruiting and retaining qualified staff for dedicated AIDS units where young adults were treated for a fatal and potentially communicable disease, added burnout along with turnover intentions to their study design, nurse burnout became an important study variable in research related to the organizational context of nursing practice. Leiter and Maslach (2009) studied the mediating role of burnout between areas of worklife and nurse turnover intentions. Mediation refers to situations where variables have an intermediate position between predictors and outcome variables. Study results confirm the relationship among the three burnout dimensions: emotional exhaustion predicts depersonalization or cynicism, which predicts reduced personal accomplishment or efficacy. Areas of worklife such as the extent nurses experience limited value congruence predict all three burnout dimensions, while perceived workload and lack of fairness just emotional exhaustion and depersonalization, respectively. The extent nurses experience lack of control predicts other areas of worklife such as lack of fairness and the latter limited value congruence. Burnout predicts turnover intentions directly by depersonalization or cynicism and indirectly by the remaining burnout dimensions. The study reveals burnout as a critical mediator for nurses' intentions to leave their job.

The most frequently used instrument to measure burnout was developed by Maslach et al. (1996), the Maslach Burnout Inventory Human Service Survey or MBI-HSS, and defined *burnout as a syndrome of emotional exhaustion, depersonalization, and reduced personal accomplishment*. These authors consider *increased emotional exhaustion as key aspect of burnout where emotional resources are depleted; workers feel they are no longer able to give of themselves at a psychological level. A second aspect of the burnout syndrome is depersonalization as negative, cynical attitudes and feelings about one's client. A third aspect of the burnout syndrome, reduced personal accomplishment, refers to the tendency to evaluate oneself negatively, particularly with one's work with clients. The consequences of burnout are potentially very serious for workers, their clients, and the larger institution in which they interact.* Authors' initial research on the burnout syndrome involved interviews, surveys, and field observations of employees in a wide variety of human service professions including healthcare, social services, mental health, criminal justice, and education between 1977 and 1985. The MBI-HSS is designed to assess the three aspects of the burnout syndrome as separate subscales or dimensions. The emotional exhaustion subscale assesses feelings of being emotionally overextended and exhausted by one's work. The depersonalization subscale measures an unfeeling and impersonal response toward recipients of one's services, treatment, or instruction. The personal accomplishment subscale assesses feelings of competence and successful achievement in one's work with people. The frequency, which with the respondents experience feelings related to each subscale, is assessed using a 7-point Likert scale ranging from *never* to *everyday*. Burnout is conceptualized as a continuous variable ranging from low to moderate to high (Maslach et al. 1996, pp. 4 and 5), and research contributed to the establishment of demographic norms as well as occupational specific norms although norms vary across cultures, work settings, and occupational groups (Maslach et al. 1996, p. 35). Initial research began in the United States and Canada and later internationally with many translations of the MBI-HSS showing similar psychometric properties across cultures but differences in average levels of burnout. For example, Europeans show lower average scores in comparison with average scores of North Americans (Schaufeli and Enzmann 1998).

The authors developed a second version of the Maslach Burnout Inventory General Survey or MBI-GS to measure burnout in occupational groups without direct personal contact with service recipients or with casual contact with people. The MBI-GS measures respondents' relationship with their work, not necessarily as a crisis in one's relationship with people at work. It has three subscales: exhaustion or references to fatigue, cynicism reflects indifference or distant attitude to work, and professional efficacy encompasses social and nonsocial aspects of accomplishments. The MBI-GS measures respondents' relationship with their work on a continuum from engagement to burnout. Engagement is an energetic state in which one is dedicated to excellent performance of work and confident of one's effectiveness. In contrast, burnout is a state of exhaustion in which one is cynical about the value of one's occupation and doubtful of one's capacity to perform (Maslach et al. 1996, pp. 20 and 21).

Maslach and her coauthors developed a structural model of burnout that incorporates various predictors of burnout such as demands and workload, interpersonal conflict among colleagues, ineffective coping styles, low social support from coworkers and supervisors, and limited autonomy and decision involvement. These predictors are all associated with feelings of exhaustion, cynicism, and diminished efficacy and in turn reduced organizational commitment, increased turnover and absenteeism, and physical illnesses (Maslach et al. 1996, pp. 36 and 38). In addition, drawing on the long-standing notion that stress results from a misfit between the individual and the job, Maslach and colleagues proposed the greater the mismatch within six areas, the greater the likelihood of burnout. These areas of worklife are *workload, control, reward, community, fairness,* and *values congruence* (Maslach et al. 1996, p. 42). Experiences of workload and the extent of control, the first two areas of worklife, are key aspects of the Demand–Control model of job stress (Karasek and Theorell 1992), and reward calls upon the power of reinforcement to shape behavior (Leiter and Maslach 2009). Community refers to social support and interpersonal relationships as resources, while fairness refers to equity and social justice in organizations, and finally value congruence refers to the cognitive–emotional power of agreement between personal and organizational goals and expectations (Leiter and Maslach 2009).

Research shows that jobs can be categorized in terms of job demands and job control (Karasek and Theorell 1992; Van der Doef and Maes 1998, 1999). Four groups of jobs can be identified: low demand/low control, low demand/high control, high demand/high control, and high demand/low control. The latter job subgroup has a potential risk for high job strain, psychological distress, and illness. The first two subgroups have a potential risk for decreased motivation and low strain, respectively. High-demand and high-control jobs are potentially challenging an increase in motivation and learning. Study shows that job control acts as a buffer for the negative consequences of high job demands (Ibrahim and Ohtsuka 2014; Adriaenssens et al. 2017).

Research over 25 years has revealed the complexity of the construct and places the individual prolonged stress experience within a larger organizational context of people's relation to their work (Maslach et al. 2001). The focus on engagement, the positive antithesis of burnout, gave new perspectives on interventions to alleviate burnout, and the social focus of burnout and its specific ties to the work domain make a distinct and valuable contribution to people's health and well-being. Schaufeli and Buunk (2003) describe a clear difference between job stress and burnout. Job stress occurs when job demands do not match the person's adaptive resources, while in contrast burnout can be considered as a final stage in a breakdown in adaptation that results from the long-term imbalance of demands and resources, from prolonged job stress. Burnout includes the development of negative attitudes and behaviors toward recipients, the job, and the organization, whereas job stress is not necessarily accompanied by such attitudes and behaviors. Authors notice that anybody can experience stress, while those who entered their careers enthusiastically with high goals and expectations can only experience burnout. In addition, some personal characteristics such as anxiety, neuroticism, and lack of hardiness seem to be associated with burnout.

A later study of Maslach and Leiter (2008) using the MBI-GS and the Areas of Worklife Scale or AWS (Leiter and Maslach 1999) in a longitudinal design had the basic premise that if an individual is experiencing some early signs of burnout (exhaustion only or cynicism only), then that information is sufficient for consideration of actions to prevent burnout and build engagement. People's psychological relationships to their jobs have been conceptualized as a continuum between the negative experience of burnout and the positive experience of engagement with three interrelated dimensions: exhaustion—energy, cynicism—involvement, and inefficacy—efficacy. Authors argue that the practical significance of this burnout—engagement continuum is that engagement represents a desired goal for any burnout interventions. Study results show that engagement is the more normative experience in the workplace, and occupational problems are likely to be temporary and more easily resolved if the person maintains a good relationship with the job. In this study, lack of fairness (one of the areas of worklife) such as favoritism, unjustified inequities, or cheating turns out to be the critical incongruity or tipping point to develop into burnout over time. Lack of fairness is also associated with depersonalization in a nurse population studying a mediation model describing the impact of areas of worklife that predicts nurse turnover through burnout as described above (Leiter and Maslach 2009).

### 2.3.2 Development of the Concept of Work Engagement and Empirical Findings

Another group of researchers have proposed work engagement as an independent, distinct (albeit related) concept negatively correlated with burnout, rather than representing the opposite of the three burnout dimensions of emotional exhaustion, depersonalization, and personal accomplishment (Schaufeli and Bakker 2003). Engagement scholars believe that work engagement is a positive and fulfilled work-related state of mind characterized by vigor, dedication, and absorption and have developed tools to measure it such as the Utrecht Work Engagement Scale (UWES). Bakker et al. (2011a) argue that measures of work engagement should capture both positive and negative aspects of psychological state, and response anchors should be designed to accommodate both short-term and longer-term time frames. However, it has been argued that burnout and work engagement are not inverses of each other (although they can coexist to some extent), and thus the Maslach Burnout Inventory and the Oldenburg Burnout Inventory are not valid measures of work engagement (Schaufeli and Salonova 2011).

A recent systematic review of the engagement literature revealed a need for a conceptually consistent definition and measurement of work engagement to permit the study of organizational behavior, including work performance and healthcare organizational outcomes (Simpson 2009). Several conceptual papers discussed the concept of work engagement and summarizing research on its most important antecedents (Bakker et al. 2011a, b; Schaufeli and Salonova 2011). In particular, job demands and job resources have shown associations with job strain and motivational processes, respectively (Bakker and Demerouti 2007; Salanova and Schaufeli 2008; Schaufeli et al. 2009; Bakker et al. 2011b). Increases in job demands such as work overload, emotional demands, and work–home interference and decreases in job resources such as social support, autonomy, opportunities to learn, and feedback predict burnout. Unbalanced job demands and job resources were identified as part of *a strain process or loss cycle*, and increases in job resources were found to predict work engagement in *a motivational process or gain circle*. Similarly, a longitudinal study of Finnish healthcare personnel confirmed that job resources were better predictors of work engagement, especially vigor and dedication, than job demands (Mauno et al. 2007). A study performed in long-term facilities' work shows that engagement measured by vigor, dedication, and absorption has a mediating relationship between service climate and patient-centered behavior (Abdelhadi and Drach-Zahavy 2012). Of the three dimensions of work engagement, absorption plays a pivotal role in the relationships here. The latter finding is in contrast with the results of an earlier qualitative study suggesting that absorption may not affect nurses' turnover intentions (Freeney and Tiernan 2009). The authors of that paper argue that nurses leave certain specialties because of difficulties detaching themselves emotionally from their work; they proposed that absorption would be related to turnover rather than retention. A study investigating the association between nurses' individual characteristics, job features, and work engagement found that job satisfaction, quality of working life, lower social dysfunction, and lower stress associated with patient care predicted vigor and dedication. The authors suggested that organizational strategies to reduce stress associated with patient care and to improve social and communication skills might enhance nurses' vigor and dedication (Jenaro et al. 2011). Another study showed positive associations between nurses' role, stress, and feelings of burnout as well as negative associations on work engagement after controlling for personal resources (optimism, hardy personality, and emotional competence) and social and demographic variables (Garrosa et al. 2011). Both these studies are consistent with Bakker et al. (2011b) hypothesis that when employees perceive that their organizations provide a supportive, involving, and challenging climate that accommodates their psychological needs, they are more likely to be engaged. The authors argue that work environments can facilitate climates for engagement and in addition can be interpreted as collective engagement (Salanova and Schaufeli 2008). In a cross-sectional survey design using the UWES, work engagement was studied in a representative test group of hospital-based ward teams, who had recently commenced the latest phase of the national "Productive Ward" (PW) initiative in Ireland and compared them to a control group. The findings demonstrate how quality improvement activities that support nurses' capacity to provide more direct patient care eliminating waste and activities without added value for patients, as integrated by the PW program, appear to positively impact the work engagement (the vigor, absorption, and dedication) of ward-based teams. The use and suitability of the UWES as an appropriate measure of "engagement" in quality improvement interventions were confirmed. The authors argue that engagement of nurses and frontline clinical teams is a major component of creating, developing, and sustaining a culture of improvement (White et al. 2014). In a longitudinal study design with a large population of health employees, Armon et al. (2012) found that changes in the levels of job demands, job control, and social support over time predicted subsequent certain changes in levels of vigor over time. The growth of interest in work engagement is potentially a reflection of widespread recognition that is making effective use of employee skills and knowledge with proper support and resources and is imperative in rapidly changing economies and organizations (Leiter and Bakker 2010). Laschinger and colleagues' empirical studies showed that nurses perceptions of sufficient support (e.g., peers and supervisors) and sufficient resources needed to do the job, in accordance with opportunities to be involved in joint decision-making, are linked with job satisfaction, commitment, engagement, productivity, and quality of care (Laschinger et al. 2004, 2009; Laschinger and Finegan 2005).

### 2.3.3 Balancing Effort and Reward and Recognition as Predictors of Compassion Fatigue and Compassion Satisfaction

Kelly et al. (2015) study the impact of meaningful recognition on compassion fatigue and compassion satisfaction in a Magnet-designated 700-bed teaching hospital. Compassion fatigue has been defined as a state of physical or psychological distress in caregivers, which occurs as a consequence of an ongoing and snowballing process in a demanding relationship with needy individuals (Coetzee and Klopper 2010). Compassion fatigue is a concept that combines burnout described by three dimensions such as emotional exhaustion, depersonalization, and personal accomplishment and secondary trauma stress. Secondary trauma stress identified by Stamm (2010) occurs from pressure, anxiety, and various negative feelings that are linked with caring for people who have directly experienced a traumatic situation, in particular, nurses and other healthcare workers who provide direct care, have frequently prolonged, continuous, and intense contact with patients and families, and are undergoing stressful life changes with a potential risk of compassion fatigue and in turn undermining relationships with patients and their families (Coetzee and Klopper 2010). Compassion fatigue has been associated with a "helper syndrome" that results from continuous disappointing situations and leads to moral distress (Figley 1995; van Mol et al. 2015). Compassion fatigue was described for the first time in the early 1990s as the loss of compassion in result of repeated exposure to suffering during work and, later, defined as secondary traumatic stress resulting from a deep involvement with a primarily traumatized person, because of the *more friendly framing*. From this time on, compassion fatigue has interchangeably been referred to as secondary and posttraumatic stress or vicarious trauma (Figley 1995; van Mol et al. 2015).

Instead of compassion fatigue, compassion satisfaction, however, encompasses nurses' pleasure and gratitude that develops from caregiving for patients through activities that help strengthen their passion for caring for patients (Simon et al. 2005) as a gain circle. The authors studied the impact of the DAISY Award. This award formally recognizes nurses for their extraordinary contributions and is offered through the nonprofit organization the DAISY Foundation (https://www.daisyfoundation.org/daisy-award). The foundation was formed after cofounders Mark and Bonnie Barnes experienced an extended hospitalization and loss of their 33-year-old son to an autoimmune disease (Kelly et al. 2015). In hospitals that participate in the program, patients and colleagues can nominate nurses to be honored. Nurses who are nominated receive their nomination form, as well as recognition from their employer. From the nominees, a single awardee is selected and honored in front of his or her colleagues. At the study hospital, nominees receive a DAISY pin and their nomination form from their direct supervisor, and awardees are recognized on their unit in front of their colleagues. To date approximately almost hospitals participate in the DAISY recognition program in 15 countries (Kelly et al. 2015). Compassion fatigue and compassion satisfaction were measured in the study by a well-known instrument the Professional Quality of Life Scale (ProQOL) (Stamm 2010). The study results show that the younger generations of nurses are experiencing burnout and secondary trauma stress, potentially contributing to their decision of leaving the positions and possibly the profession. Fortunately, the research shows that meaning-ful recognition through the DAISY Award and increasing satisfaction have the potential to combat compassion fatigue by increasing compassion satisfaction. The authors expressed their worries that nurses who gain experience are more likely to have higher compassion fatigue and compassion satisfaction and could be a major cause for turnover and lack of retention. Meaningful recognition provided by the DAISY Award is linked with lower compassion fatigue and higher compassion sat-isfaction even when nurses are nominated. Authors refer to other beneficial mean-ingful recognition initiatives such as peer and supervisor feedback.

These study findings are in line with the findings of the European NEXT study. A prospective study with 1-year follow-up showed that high effort—reward imbal-ance at the baseline, measured with a dedicated instrument, has an elevated risk of intention to leave the profession (Li et al. 2011). The study assumption is based on the postulate that unbalanced reciprocity in transaction results in a stressful experi-ence. Therefore, a balance between what nurses give (effort) and what nurses receive (reward) is preferable and necessary to monitor. Reward implicates financial reward as well as esteem, recognition, and career opportunities including job security. Besides extrinsic efforts, intrinsic effort was measured as a component of overcom-mitment, a personal pattern of excessive coping with work demands. The discrep-ancy between high efforts spent and low reward received in turn is what matters most. Nurses experiencing high level of overcommitment are expected to exagger-ate their efforts beyond levels usually considered, in combination with increased susceptibility to reward frustration as described in a theoretical assumption (Siegrist et al. 2004). The authors conclude that a comprehensive approach combining both individual and organizational directed interventions would be a promising way to promote healthy workplace and job performance. In addition, results of studies guided by social exchange theory suggest that burnout often develops in organiza-tions where nurses are in emotionally charged and unbalanced relationships with patients in terms of costs and benefits or investments and outcomes (Schaufeli and Buunk 2003; Schaufeli et al. 2006). This studied lack of reciprocity or disturbed balance between give and take confirmed that burnout develops when nurses per-ceive an unbalanced relationship with colleagues and the organization as well. Emotional exhaustion appears to be related to lack of reciprocity at all three levels: in contact with patients and colleagues as well as toward the institution.

A systematic review on the prevalence of compassion fatigue and burnout among healthcare professionals in intensive care units selected 40 of the 1623 identified publications, which included 14,770 respondents, which met the selection criteria (van Mol et al. 2015). Two studies reported the prevalence of compassion fatigue as 7.3 and 40%; five studies described the prevalence of secondary traumatic stress ranging from 0 to 38.5%. The reported prevalence of burnout in the ICU varied from 0 to 70.1%. A wide range of intervention strategies emerged from the recent litera-ture search, such as different work schedules, educational programs on coping with emotional distress, improved communication skills, and relaxation methods. The authors conclude that policy-makers should introduce interventions to prevent the negative consequences of emotional distress suggesting to perform longitudinal experimental studies to examine the emotional distress among ICU professionals in relation to their communication skills and educational sessions on stress.

### 2.3.4  Coping and Prevention of Burnout: What Do We Learn from Intervention Studies

Le Blanc et al. (2007) conducted an intervention study on 29 oncology wards to evaluate the effect of a team-based burnout intervention program combining a staff support group with a participatory action research approach. The first intervention was to organize regular meetings during which care providers had the opportunity to share personal work-related experiences and feelings with colleagues in a supportive and nonjudgmental environment. The authors argued that social support is crucial in the care provider adaptation in working with cancer patients. Empathic concern and active care from one's coworkers can reduce greatly the effects of accompanying stress and help prevent burnout. The second intervention was focused on the participation and experience of care providers of the oncology wards (participatory action research) and aimed to take users' local contexts as a starting point for the research and share control over the research and knowledge generation process with the nursing staff. It would thus appear that a better understanding of work stress in a local context can be developed and translated into effective interventions. The ultimate goal in work stress intervention in this study was building an organization's capacity to solve self-identified problems. Study findings showed that subjects in the experimental group felt significantly less exhaustion and depersonalization than care providers in the control group immediately after the program ended as well as 6 months later. The authors argued that the intervention not only had an impact on reducing arousal addressing perceptions of job demands, preventing further energy depletion or exhaustion, but also had positive effects on perceptions of job resources—such as job control and within-team interpersonal support relationship—which have found to be related to motivational outcome measures such as depersonalization. The authors concluded that shared responsibility for the quality of work environment and mutual support are effective means of maintaining staff morale among professionals in highly demanding, specialized occupations.

Awa et al. (2010) performed a review of burnout intervention programs evaluating 25 primary intervention programs. Seventeen (68%) were person-directed interventions, among them cognitive behavioral training, adaptive coping, relaxation therapy, and psychosocial skill and communication training. Two (8%) were organization-directed and six (24%) were a combination of both intervention types such as cognitive behavioral and management skill training and social support. Eighty percent of all programs led to a reduction in burnout. Person-directed interventions reduced burnout in the short term (6 months or less), while a combination of both person- and organization-directed interventions had longer-lasting positive effects (12 months and over). In all cases, positive intervention effects diminished in the course of time. The authors of the review proposed that positive effects can be extended by refresher courses at appropriate intervals after the end of the initial program, and future studies should use better designed and evaluated randomized controlled trials, with comparable participants, appropriate baseline data, and at least two post-intervention measurement points. Nowrouzi et al. (2015) performed a literature review of workplace interventions aiming to create healthy work environments and improve nurses' quality of worklife by managing occupational stress and burnout prevention. The authors noted that the studies included in this review were all based in workplaces and focused mainly on individual strategies. Occupational stress research often lacks a comprehensive theoretical framework that includes both individual and organizational factors. In addition, these Canadian authors argue that any nurse retention strategy should be linked to organizational structures and functions to take advantage of existing partnerships and increase efficiencies. For example, health policy should be directed at upgrading health facilities and improving the work environment as part of a national health facility expansion plan. Furthermore, management style, incentives and career structures, educational opportunities, salary scales, and recruitment and retention practices were some of the organizational factors that can influence the geographic distribution of health resources. As Schaufeli and Buunk (2003) mention, almost every author on the subject acknowledges that a combination of individual and workplace approaches is likely the most effective; the vast majority of burnout interventions have been conducted on the individual level. Therefore, Awa et al. (2010) propose properly planned intervention programs that include aspects of both person-directed and organization-directed prevention measures. Nowrouzi et al. (2015) conclude that future studies should incorporate random assignment to treatment and control groups and report the results of all outcomes. In addition, the continued use of meta-analytic techniques to synthesize research findings should be pursued. As more primary studies are conducted, systematic reviews should be updated to reassess results.

The concepts of burnout, compassion fatigue, and later work engagement provide broad insights about the organizational context of nursing practice and in addition provide nurses and leaders with keys to better understand what is happening to them, their teams, and institutions as well as their patients. Leadership is therefore essential to open opportunities and capacity to create healthy and productive work environments.

## 2.4 Empowerment and Authentic Leadership: To an Adaptive Healthy Work Environment and Productivity

### 2.4.1 Development of Empowerment Concept and Empirical Findings

Organizational empowerment, a construct based on Kanter (1993) model of structural or workplace empowerment, has been empirically applied in several research projects. Structural empowerment, described as nurses' access to relevant information, support, and resources needed to do the job, and opportunities to learn and grow are linked with job satisfaction, commitment, productivity, and burnout

(Kanter 1993; Laschinger et al. 2001b, 2003; Laschinger and Finegan 2005). Kanter described workplace social structures that enable employees to mobilize human and material resources to accomplish meaningful work, and sources of empowerment will determine the extent to which employees have developed an organizational network of alliances (e.g., development of informal power), and jobs that have a large degree of discretion are visible and important to organizational goals (e.g., having formal power). Kanter's theoretical framework defines structural empowerment as the following work characteristics: formal and informal power, access to information, opportunities to learn and personal development, and supportive relationships (e.g., superiors, peers, and subordinates).

A Canadian study found that staff nurses' perception of empowerment, supervisor incivility, and cynicism most strongly predicted low job satisfaction and job commitment. Furthermore, emotional exhaustion, cynicism, and supervisor incivility most strongly predicted nurse turnover intentions (Laschinger et al. 2009). Kanter thus described empowerment structurally, whereas Spreitzer (1995) considered it a psychological response to conditions within the practice environment that lead nurses to experience a certain degree of *meaning* (I value my work), *competence* (I make a difference at work), *self-determination* (I have control over my work), *and impact* (I am confident/competent that I can do my work well), essential motivational aspects of nurses' worklife and productivity (Dahinten et al. 2014). Various studies have described the effect that conditions for nurse structural empowerment have on the experience of empowerment linking nurse structural and/or psychological empowerment with job satisfaction, commitment, engagement, and spirit at work, as well as work effectiveness, unit effectiveness, and quality of work (Laschinger et al. 2004; Wagner et al. 2013; Laschinger et al. 2014; Yang et al. 2013; Eo et al. 2014; Wang and Liu 2015).

A cross-sectional survey conducted among nurses in the Netherlands demonstrated the impact of structural and psychological empowerment on innovative behavior; informal power and the extent of impact were found to be the most relevant determinants in the latter study (Knol and Van Linge 2009). Similarly, another survey-based study of mental health staff members found that structural conditions such as opportunity and resources were important for creating support for evidence-based practice (Engström et al. 2015). Lethbridge et al. (2011) conducted an integrative literature review and described links between structural empowerment, psychological empowerment, and reflective thinking as means of assisting undergraduate nursing students to become effective professionals in both their academic and future practice careers. A Korean study of staff nurses showed that empowerment mediated the relationship between job characteristics, transformational leadership, and work effectiveness (Eo et al. 2014), while a Canadian study (Wagner et al. 2013) showed the impact of resonant leadership and individual empowerment on spirit at work (e.g., nurses' individual experiences that energized their work), job satisfaction, and organizational commitment. Wong and Laschinger (2013) confirmed the mediating role played by nurse empowerment through authentic leadership in nurse performance and job satisfaction. Authentic leadership has been described as "a pattern of transparent and ethical leader behavior that encourages openness in sharing information needed to make decisions while accepting input from those who follow" (Avolio et al. 2009).

### 2.4.2 The Pivotal Role of Authentic Leadership

Clinical teams are prone to various negative factors that can undermine their capacity to perform their daily tasks well and to meet complex patients' needs as well as organizational goals. Referring to practice experiences and learning from a number of studies, nurse practice environments are complex to understand, and it is not always clear how to support clinical teams effectively. The introduction of new graduates in clinical teams requires careful attention because their transition to professional practice can be stressful, leading to early career burnout and decreased emotional well-being (Van Bogaert 2016). Laschinger's and colleagues' study (Laschinger et al. 2015) provides insights into new graduates' feelings about burnout and mental health status. The study tested a model linking authentic supervisor leadership with areas of worklife and occupational coping efficacy, predicting burnout and mental health of new nursing graduates. Moreover, the study introduced interpersonal strain as a third component of burnout alongside emotional exhaustion and cynicism. Authentic leadership was defined and measured as the extent to which new graduates evaluated their leaders as self-aware and transparent, as well as by acting through moral–ethical perspective and through balanced processes. Areas of worklife were measured as the extent to which respondents experienced workload, control, rewards, community and fairness, and valued congruence (Leiter and Maslach 2011). Previous insights linked authentic leadership to a positive fit between nurses' job expectations and actual levels of the six basic areas of worklife and found also that person–job fit among the six areas of worklife fully mediated the influence of authentic leadership on nurses' work engagement (Bamford et al. 2013). Study results show that authentic leadership had a positive effect on areas of worklife, and the latter, in turn, had a positive effect on occupational coping self-efficacy, resulting in lower burnout, such as lower levels of emotional exhaustion and cynicism as well as less interpersonal strain, which ultimately was associated with favorable new mental health of graduates. The study adds to previous studies around authentic leadership to support nurses' psychosocial and practice environment in the capacity to achieve excellent care as well as professional well-being (Wong and Laschinger 2013).

Laschinger et al. (2015) describe authentic leaders as positive, transformational, moral leaders who are true to themselves and aim to bring out the best in themselves and others. They communicate their genuine selves to others through four key behaviors: relational transparency and presenting themselves as who they truly are, balanced processing and considering differing points of view before making decisions, moral/ethical behavior and acting in accordance with internal moral and ethical values, and self-awareness and having insight about self and influence on others (Avolio and Gardner 2005; Walumbwa et al. 2008). Importantly, authentic leaders foster the development of their followers' intrapersonal resources such as psychological capital or their sense of optimism, hope, resiliency, and self-efficacy. These positive psychological resources support followers' self-awareness and self-regulatory behaviors, contributing to positive self-development and confidence (Avolio and Gardner 2005). Authors argue that authentic leadership theory has gained empirical support in both the management and nursing literature. In nursing, nurses who perceive their leaders to engage in authentic behaviors feel empowered and supported in their jobs (Laschinger et al. 2012).

MacPhee et al. (2014) and Dahinten et al. (2014) evaluated a leadership program for novice first-line nurse leaders in Western Canada: the Nursing Leadership Institute. The leadership program consists of a 4-day residential workshop with didactic leadership content and interactive learning sessions; a year-long innovation project of relevance to the leaders' respective organizations; mentorship from senior nursing leaders; organizational supports, such as release time for project work; and an online knowledge network to facilitate connections among leaders (MacPhee and Bouthillette 2008; MacPhee et al. 2012). The program targets novice first-line nurse leaders with less than 3 years' experience because of their critical roles and responsibilities within healthcare facilities. Study results show in a first part (MacPhee et al. 2014) that the program was directly associated with leaders' perceptions of using more empowering behaviors based on sociopsychological theory (Conger and Kanungo 1988) and capture five major categories of leader-empowering behaviors such as meaningful work, participation in decision-making, facilitating goal accomplishment, autonomy, and removing bureaucratic barriers (Hui 1994). Leader-empowering behaviors were also associated with feelings of being structurally empowered, mediated through feelings of being psychologically empowered, although as the authors mentioned the source of empowerment needs further investigation. In a second part (Dahinten et al. 2014) study results show that the leaders' program participation was directly associated with greater staff organizational commitment 1 year after the program. Both program attendance and leader-empowering behaviors were found to act as independent catalysts for staff empowerment, with structural empowerment partially mediating the effects of leader-empowering behaviors on organizational commitment. But the results showed some unclear findings because of limited sample and variability in measurements. Authors identified a discrepancy between leaders' own assessment of empowering behaviors and staff nurse's assessment of leader-empowering behaviors. The authors refer to many unknown factors and processes that remain to be more fully explored, such as the antecedents to the leader empowerment process and the role(s) of psychological empowerment. Relational leadership is a social process influenced by many organizational factors. Moreover, the authors cite the work of Edmonstone and Western (2002) who argue that leaders cannot control or manipulate the culture of their organization but can only influence and shape its direction as it emerges (Dahinten et al. 2014).

In this chapter, we began with reviewing research attempting to explain nurse shortages that eventually led to the emergence of a concept, the *nurse practice environment*, measured with an instrument, the NWI-R, that evaluates the presence of certain organizational traits from the original Magnet hospital research which have been found to be predictive of various nurse and patient outcomes. We continued by presenting a concept, *burnout*, measured primarily using the MBI-HSS that describes the negative emotional and mental state of nurses providing care to their patients under chronically stressful conditions, reflecting the fit of six key areas of worklife with their needs and in turn predicting their health conditions, turnover intentions, and productivity in *a potential loss cycle*. A second concept related to burnout but almost its inverse, *engagement*, measured with the UWES, is a positive and fulfilled work-related state associated with certain resources such as social support, autonomy, and opportunities to learn and receive feedback: *a potential motivational process or gain circle*. Finally, an essential element for sustaining gain rather than loss cycles is *empowerment* or the extent nurses have control and autonomy in decision-making as well as support of peers and supervisors and the impact of another concept nurse managers' and leaders' *authentic leadership* behavior on staff empowerment. Both concepts have a crucial and promising role in the various aspects that creates an organizational context of nursing practice to a healthy and productive work environment.

## 2.5    Further Research Initiatives

Based on these conceptual and empirical insights and specifically the work of Laschinger and Leiter (2006), Leiter and Laschinger (2006) and Kowalski et al. (2010), we developed two models: a burnout model and an engagement model in three phases.

The first phase was the development of preliminary burnout model tested in an acute care hospital population of staff nurses ($n = 401$) showing that feelings of burnout influenced by nurse practice conditions (determined by *unfavorable perceived* interprofessional relations with physicians, hospital management, and organizational support as well as the conditions within the unit or nurse management at the unit level) have subsequent effects on job dissatisfaction, turnover intentions, and unfavorable reported quality of care (Van Bogaert et al. 2009a, b) (Fig. 2.1).

In the next phase, two models were tested—a burnout model and a work engagement model developed with the same variables as the preliminary model. Additionally, a nurse-assessed workload variable was tested with a psychiatric hospital population of nurses and other healthcare workers such as licensed practice nurses/unregulated caregivers ($n = 357$). Findings in the burnout model showed that feelings of burnout were influenced by nurse practice conditions (determined by *unfavorable perceived* interprofessional relations with physicians, hospital management, and organizational support and the conditions within the unit or nurse management at the unit level) as well as *unfavorable* nurse-reported *workload* and

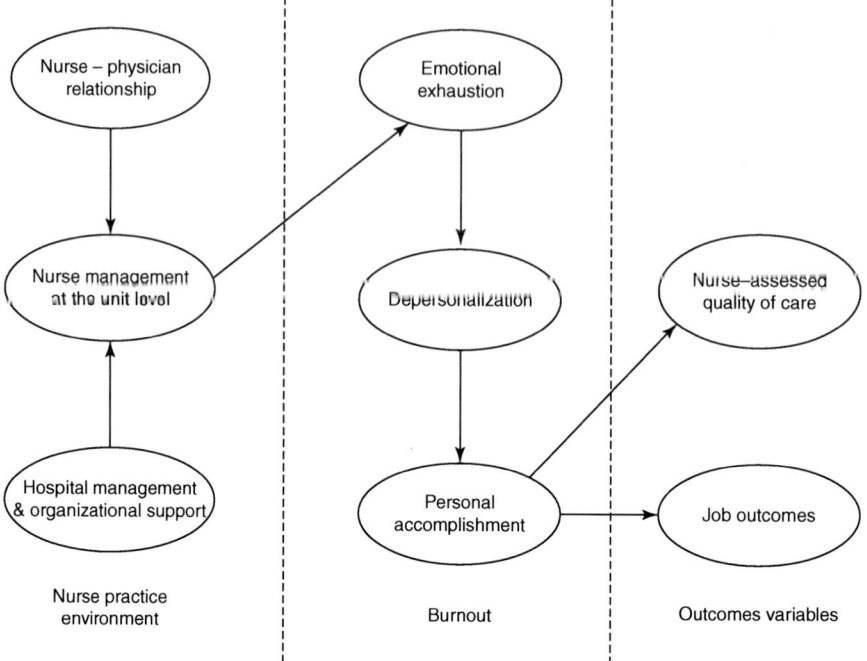

**Fig. 2.1** Model preliminary phase (hypothesis)

subsequently had unfavorable effects on reports of quality of care. Although counterintuitive, *unfavorable reported workload* had a direct positive effect on job satisfaction and low turnover intentions as well as an inverse impact between hospital management and quality of care.

Instead, in the work engagement model, feelings of engagement are influenced by nurse practice conditions—determined by *favorable perceived* interprofessional relations with physicians, hospital management, and organizational support and the conditions within the unit (nurse management at the unit level)—and *favorable* nurse-reported *workload*—consequently has a favorable effect on reported quality of care. However, an inverse impact between hospital management and organizational support and nurse-reported quality of care was identified (Van Bogaert et al. 2013a, b) (Fig. 2.2).

In a final phase (Van Bogaert et al. 2013c, 2014), both the burnout model and the work engagement model describe the organizational context of nursing practice using six variables: three independent variables and three mediating variables (see Model 1 and Model 2 as described in the next chapter). The independent variables are captured by the nurse practice environment dimensions: nurse—physician relations, nurse management at the unit level, and hospital management and organizational support. The nurse practice dimensions reflect two levels, the direct care context and frontline leadership, as well as higher management and leadership level and structural support, and in addition the interprofessional relationship with physicians. We assume that

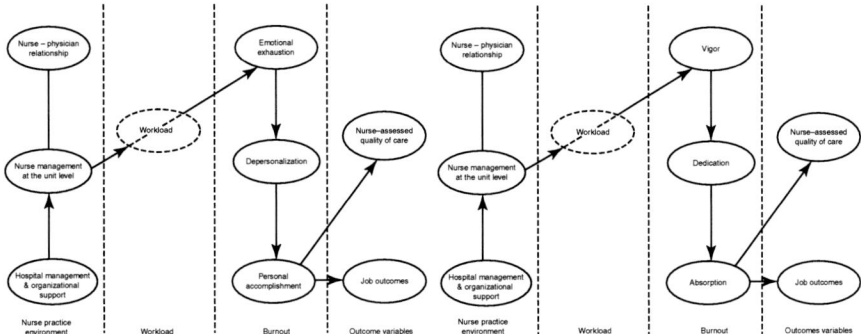

**Fig. 2.2** Next-generation models (hypothesized)

both the higher management level and the interprofessional relationship will have an impact on the direct care context and frontline leadership. In the model, nurse management at the unit level plays a mediating and pivotal role to the three mediating variables, although direct pathways of the other two dimensions. The mediating variables or nurse work characteristics are related to the empowerment concept: how nurses assess workload and their extent of autonomy (decision latitude) and whether they collaborate and share values (social capital) within their team. Six variables describe the outcome variables with three mediating variables, the three burnout dimensions or the three work engagement dimensions (e.g., burnout model—work engagement model) and finally the outcome variables with job outcomes (job satisfaction and turnover intentions) and nurse reports of quality of care (at the unit, the last shift and the hospital). Again nurse management at the unit level plays a mediating role through the nurse work characteristics between independent variables and outcome variables as well as burnout or work engagement plays a mediating role between the six independent variables and the outcome variables.

In detail it means the following two models:

In our burnout model (see left hypothesized model (Fig. 2.3) and Model 1 in next chapter), independent variables of nurse practice environment predict the mediating variables of burnout dimensions, as well as job outcomes and nurse-assessed quality of care (dependent variables). In addition, workload, decision latitude, and social capital close to the concept of empowerment have a mediating position between the nurse practice environment and burnout dimensions. Nurse–physician relations and hospital management—organizational support impact nurse management at the unit level. Nurse management at the unit level has a strong direct impact on job outcomes and nurse-assessed quality of care as well as on decision latitude and social capital. Hospital management—organizational support has a direct impact on personal accomplishment and an indirect impact on the outcome variables through workload and burnout dimensions. Nurse–physician relations show an indirect impact on the outcome variables through decision latitude. Social capital has an inverse impact on feelings of emotional exhaustion, and decision latitude supports feelings of personal accomplishments. Personal accomplishment, impacts indirectly

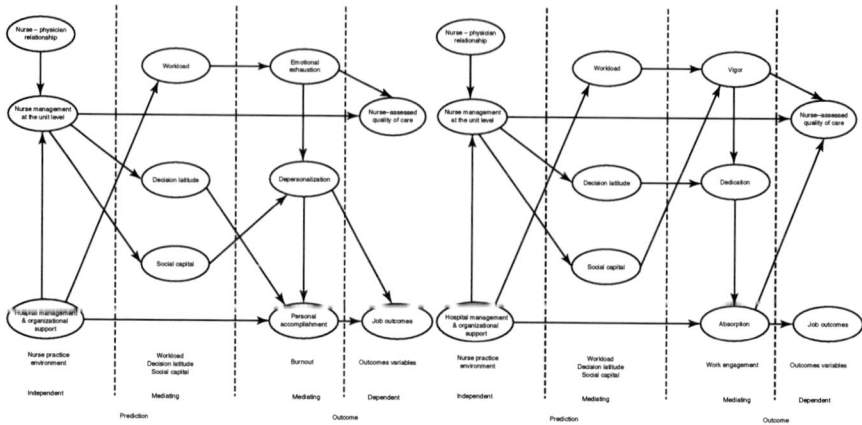

**Fig. 2.3** Final phase models (hypothesized)

by emotional exhaustion and directly by depersonalization, has a direct impact on job outcomes and nurse-assessed quality of care (Fig. 2.3).

In our engagement model (see right hypothesized model (Fig 2.3) and Model 2 in the next chapter), the independent variables of nurse practice environment predict the mediating variables of work engagement dimensions, as well as job outcomes and nurse-assessed quality of care (dependent variables). In addition, workload, decision latitude, and social capital have a mediating position between the nurse practice environment and work engagement dimensions. Nurse–physician relations and hospital management–organizational support impact nurse management at the unit level. Nurse management at the unit level has a strong direct impact on job outcomes and nurse-assessed quality of care as well as on decision latitude and social capital. Hospital management—organizational support has an indirect impact on the outcome variables through workload and work engagement dimensions. Nurse–physician relations show an indirect impact on the outcome variables through decision latitude. Social capital impacts feelings of vigor, and decision latitude supports feelings of dedication. Absorption, impacts indirectly by vigor and directly by dedication, has a direct impact on nurse-assessed quality of care.

In the next chapter, we present the retest of the burnout model and engagement model with an acute hospital dataset and two nursing home datasets and qualitative findings that buttress findings of both models as well as descriptive and multilevel analyses. In addition, we present a longitudinal study with five measurement period evaluating hospital transformation process and the implementation of the Productive Ward Program in a university acute care hospital.

## References

Abdelhadi N, Drach-Zahavy A. Promoting patient care: work engagement as a mediator between ward service climate and patient-centred care. J Adv Nurs. 2012;68(6):1276–87.
Adriaenssens J, Hamelink A, Van Bogaert P. Predictors of occupational stress and well-being in first-line nurse managers: a cross-sectional survey study. Int J Nurs Stud. 2017;73:85–92.

Aiken LH. Superior outcomes for magnet hospitals: the evidence base. In: McClure ML, Hinshaw AS, editors. Magnet hospitals revisited: attraction and retention of professional nurses. Kansas City: American Nurses Association; 2002. p. 61–81.

Aiken LH, Patrician PA. Measuring organizational traits of hospitals: the Revised Nursing Work Index. Nurs Res. 2000;49(3):146–53.

Aiken LH, Sochalski J, Lake ET. Studying outcomes of organizational change in health services. Med Care. 1997;35(11 Suppl):NS6–18.

Aiken LH, Havens DS, Sloane DM. The magnet nursing services recognition program. Am J Nurs. 2000;100(3):26–35; quiz 35.

Aiken LH, Clarke SP, Sloane DM, Sochalski JA, Busse R, Clarke H, Giovannetti P, Hunt J, Rafferty AM, Shamian J. Nurses' reports on hospital care in five countries. Health Aff. 2001;20(3):43–53.

Aiken LH, Clarke SP, Sloane DM, Lake ET, Cheney T. Effects of hospital care environment on patient mortality and nurse outcomes. J Nurs Adm. 2008;38(5):223–9.

Aiken LH, Sermeus W, Van den Heede K, Sloane DM, Busse R, McKee M, Bruyneel L, Rafferty AM, Griffiths P, Moreno-Casbas MT, Tishelman C, Scott A, Brzostek T, Kinnunen J, Schwendimann R, Heinen M, Zikos D, Sjetne IS, Smith HL, Kutney-Lee A. Patient safety, satisfaction, and quality of hospital care: cross sectional surveys of nurses and patients in 12 countries in Europe and the United States. BMJ. 2012;344:e1717.

Aiken LH, Sloane DM, Bruyneel L, Van den Heede K, Griffiths P, Busse R, Diomidous M, Kinnunen J, Kózka M, Lesaffre E, McHugh MD, Moreno-Casbas MT, Rafferty AM, Schwendimann R, Scott PA, Tishelman C, van Achterberg T, Sermeus W, RN4CAST Consortium. Nurse staffing and education and hospital mortality in nine European countries: a retrospective observational study. Lancet. 2014;383(9931):1824–30.

American Nurse Association. Scope of standards for nurse administrators. ANA task force on standards for organized nursing services, 1994–1996. Kansas City: American Nurses Publishing; 1996.

Armon G, Shmuel S, Shirom A. The relationship of the job demands-control-support model with vigor across time: testing for reciprocality. Appl Psychol Health Well Being. 2012;4(3):276–98.

Avolio BJ, Gardner WL. Authentic leadership development: getting to the root of positive forms of leadership. Leadersh Q. 2005;16(3):315–38.

Avolio BJ, Walumbwa FO, Weber TJ. Leadership: current theories, research, and future directions. Annu Rev Psychol. 2009;60:421–49.

Awa WL, Plaumann M, Walter U. Burnout prevention: a review of intervention programs. Patient Educ Couns. 2010;78(2):184–90.

Baggs JG, Ryan SA, Phelps CE, Richeson JF, Johnson JE. The association between interdisciplinary collaboration and patient outcomes in a medical intensive care unit. Heart Lung. 1992;21(1):18–24.

Bakker AB, Demerouti E. The job demands-resources model: state of the art. J Manage Psychol. 2007;22(3):309–28.

Bakker AB, Albrecht SL, Leiter MP. Key questions regarding work engagement. Eur J Work Organ Psy. 2011a;20(1):4–28.

Bakker AB, Albrecht SL, Leiter MP. Work engagement: further reflections on the state of play. Eur J Work Organ Psy. 2011b;20(1):74–88.

Bamford M, Wong C, Laschinger HK. The influence of authentic leadership and areas of worklife on work engagement of registered nurses. J Nurs Manage. 2013;21(3):529–40.

Borritz M, Kristensen TS. Copenhagen burnout inventory: normative data from a representative Danish population on personal burnout and results from the PUMA study. In: Personal burnout, work burnout, and client burnout. Copenhagen: National Institute of Occupational Health; 2001.

Chassin MR, Park RE, Lohr KN, Keesey J, Brook RH. Differences among hospitals in medicare patient mortality. Health Serv Res. 1989;24(1):1–31.

Choi J, Bakken S, Larson E, Du Y, Stone PW. Perceived nursing work environment of critical care nurses. Nurs Res. 2004;53(6):370–8.

Clarke SP, Aiken LH. Failure to rescue. Am J Nurs. 2003;103(1):42–7.

Clarke SP, Aiken LH. An international hospital outcomes research agenda focused on nursing: lessons from a decade of collaboration. J Clin Nurs. 2008;17(24):3317–23.

Coetzee SK, Klopper HC. Compassion fatigue within nursing practice: a concept analysis. Nurs Health Sci. 2010;12(2):235–43.

Conger JA, Kanungo RN. The empowerment process: integrating theory and practice. Acad Manag Rev. 1988;13(3):471–82.

Dahinten VS, Macphee M, Hejazi S, Laschinger H, Kazanjian M, McCutcheon A, Skelton-Green J, O'Brien-Pallas L. Testing the effects of an empowerment-based leadership development programme: part 2 - staff outcomes. J Nurs Manag. 2014;22(1):16–28.

de Brouwer BJ, Kaljouw MJ, Kramer M, Schmalenberg C, van Achterberg T. Measuring the nursing work environment: translation and psychometric evaluation of the essentials of magnetism. Int Nurs Rev. 2014;61(1):99–108.

Edmonstone J, Western J. Leadership development in health care: what do we know. J Manag Med. 2002;16(1):34–47.

Engström M, Westerberg Jacobson J, Mårtensson G. Staff assessment of structural empowerment and ability to work according to evidence-based practice in mental health care. J Nurs Manag. 2015;23(6):765–74.

Eo Y, Kim YH, Lee NY. Path analysis of empowerment and work effectiveness among staff nurses. Asian Nurs Res. 2014;8(1):42–8.

Erickson JI, Duffy ME, Gibbons MP, Fitzmaurice J, Ditomassi M, Jones D. Development and psychometric evaluation of the professional practice environment (PPE) scale. J Nurs Scholarsh. 2004;36(3):279–85.

Estabrooks CA, Tourangeau AE, Humphrey CK, Hesketh KL, Giovannetti P, Thomson D, Wong J, Acorn S, Clarke H, Shamian J. Measuring the hospital practice environment: a Canadian context. Res Nurs Health. 2002;25(4):256–68.

Estabrooks CA, Midodzi WK, Cummings GG, Ricker KL, Giovannetti P. The impact of hospital nursing characteristics on 30-day mortality. Nurs Res. 2005;54(2):74–84.

Estabrooks CA, Midodzi WK, Cummings GG, Ricker KL, Giovannetti P. The impact of hospital nursing characteristics on 30-day mortality. J Nurs Adm. 2011;41(7–8 Suppl):S58–68.

Estryn-Béhar M, Van der Heijden BI, Ogińska H, Camerino D, Le Nézet O, Conway PM, Fry C, Hasselhorn HM, Next SG. The impact of social work environment, teamwork characteristics, burnout, and personal factors upon intent to leave among European nurses. Med Care. 2007;45(10):939–50.

Figley CR. Compassion fatigue: coping with secondary traumatic stress disorder in those who treat the traumatized. Palo Alto: Psychology Press; 1995.

Freeney YM, Tiernan J. Exploration of the facilitators of and barriers to work engagement in nursing. Int J Nurs Stud. 2009;46(12):1557–65.

Friese CR, Lake ET, Aiken LH, Silber JH, Sochalski J. Hospital nurse practice environments and outcomes for surgical oncology patients. Health Serv Res. 2008;43(4):1145–63.

Garrosa E, Moreno-Jiménez B, Rodríguez-Muñoz A, Rodríguez-Carvajal R. Role stress and personal resources in nursing: a cross-sectional study of burnout and engagement. Int J Nurs Stud. 2011;48(4):479–89.

Grindel CG, Peterson K, Kinneman M, Turner TL. The practice environment project. A process for outcome evaluation. J Nurs Adm. 1996;26(5):43–51.

Gunnarsdóttir S, Clarke SP, Rafferty AM, Nutbeam D. Front-line management, staffing and nurse-doctor relationships as predictors of nurse and patient outcomes. a survey of Icelandic hospital nurses. Int J Nurs Stud. 2009;46(7):920–7.

Havens DS. Comparing nursing infrastructure and outcomes: ANCC magnet and nonmagnet CNEs report. Nurs Econ. 2001;19(6):258.

Hoffart N, Woods CQ. Elements of a nursing professional practice model. J Prof Nurs. 1996;12(6):354–64.

Hui C. Effects of leader empowerment behaviors and followers' personal control, voice, and self-efficacy on in-role and extra-role performance: an extension and empirical test of

Conger and Kanungo's empowerment process model. Indianapolis: Indiana University; 1994.

Ibrahim RZAR, Ohtsuka K. Review of the job demand-control and job demand-control-support models: elusive moderating predictor effects and cultural implications. Southeast Asia Psychol J. 2014;1:10–21.

Jenaro C, Flores N, Orgaz MB, Cruz M. Vigour and dedication in nursing professionals: towards a better understanding of work engagement. J Adv Nurs. 2011;67(4):865–75.

Kanter RM. Men and women of the corporation. 2nd ed. Basis Books: New York; 1993.

Karasek R, Theorell T. Healthy work: stress, productivity and the reconstruction of working life. New York: Basic Books; 1992.

Kelly L, Runge J, Spencer C. Predictors of compassion fatigue and compassion satisfaction in acute care nurses. J Nurs Scholarsh. 2015;47(6):522–8.

Khamisa N, Peltzer K, Oldenburg B. Burnout in relation to specific contributing factors and health outcomes among nurses: a systematic review. Int J Environ Res Public Health. 2013;10(6):2214–40.

Knaus WA, Draper EA, Wagner DP, Zimmerman JE. An evaluation of outcome from intensive care in major medical centers. Ann Intern Med. 1986;104(3):410–8.

Knol J, Van Linge R. Innovative behavior: the effect of structural and psychological empowerment on nurses. J Adv Nurs. 2009;65(2):359–70.

Kohn LT, Corrigan JM, Donaldson MS. To err is human: building a safer health system. Washington DC: National Academy Press; 2000.

Korman AK. Industrial and organizational psychology. Englewood Cliffs: Prentice-Hall; 1971.

Kowalski C, Ommen O, Driller E, Ernstmann N, Wirtz MA, Köhler T, Pfaff H. Burnout in nurses - the relationship between social capital in hospitals and emotional exhaustion. J Clin Nurs. 2010;19(11-12):1654–63.

Kramer M, Hafner LP. Shared values: impact on staff nurse job satisfaction and perceived productivity. Nurs Res. 1989;38(3):172–7.

Kramer M, Schmalenberg C. Staff identify essentials of magnetism. In: Margaret LM, Ada SH, editors. Magnet hospitals revisited: attraction and retention of professional nurses. Kansas City: American Nurses Association; 2002. p. 25–59.

Kramer M, Schmalenberg C. Development and evaluation of essentials of magnetism tool. J Nurs Adm. 2004;34(7–8):365–78.

Lake E. Development of practice environment scale of the nursing work index. Res Nurs Health. 2002;25:176–88.

Lake ET, Friese CR. Variations in nursing practice environments: relation to staffing and hospital characteristics. Nurs Res. 2006;55(1):1–9.

Laschinger HK, Finegan J. Empowering nurses for work engagement and health in hospital settings. J Nurs Adm. 2005;35(10):439–49.

Laschinger HK, Leiter P. The impact of nursing work environments on patient safety outcomes: the mediating role of burnout engagement. J Nurs Adm. 2006;36(5):259–67.

Laschinger HK, Finegan J, Shamian J. The impact of workplace empowerment, organizational trust on staff nurses' work satisfaction and organizational commitment. Health Care Manag Rev. 2001a;26(3):7–23.

Laschinger HK, Finegan J, Shamian J, Wilk P. Impact of structural and psychological empowerment on job strain in nursing work settings: expanding Kanter's model. J Nurs Adm. 2001b;31(5):260–72.

Laschinger HK, Almost J, Tuer-Hodes D. Workplace empowerment and magnet hospital characteristics: making the link. J Nurs Adm. 2003;33(7-8):410–22.

Laschinger HK, Finegan JE, Shamian J, Wilk P. A longitudinal analysis of the impact of workplace empowerment on work satisfaction. J Organ Behav. 2004;25(4):527–45.

Laschinger HK, Leiter M, Day A, Gilin D. Workplace empowerment, incivility, and burnout: impact on staff nurse recruitment and retention outcomes. J Nurs Manag. 2009;17(3):302–11.

Laschinger HK, Wong CA, Grau AL. The influence of authentic leadership on newly graduated nurses' experiences of workplace bullying, burnout and retention outcomes: a cross-sectional study. Int J Nurs Stud. 2012;49(10):1266–76.

Laschinger HK, Wong CA, Cummings GG, Grau AL. Resonant leadership and workplace empowerment: the value of positive organizational cultures in reducing workplace incivility. Nurs Econ. 2014;32(1):5–15, 44; quiz 16.

Laschinger HK, Borgogni L, Consiglio C, Read E. The effects of authentic leadership, six areas of worklife, and occupational coping self-efficacy on new graduate nurses' burnout and mental health: a cross-sectional study. Int J Nurs Stud. 2015;52(6):1080–9.

Le Blanc PM, Hox JJ, Schaufeli WB, Taris TW, Peeters MC. Take care! The evaluation of a team-based burnout intervention program for oncology care providers. J Appl Psychol. 2007;92(1):213–27.

Leiter MP, Bakker AB. Work engagement: introduction. In: Bakker AB, Leiter MP, editors. Work engagement: a handbook of essential theory and research. New York: Psychology Press; 2010. p 1–9.

Leiter MP, Laschinger HK. Relationships of work and practice environment to professional burnout: testing a causal model. Nurs Res. 2006;55(2):137–46.

Leiter MP, Maslach C. Six areas of worklife: a model of the organizational context of burnout. J Health Hum Serv Adm. 1999;21(4):472–89.

Leiter MP, Maslach C. Nurse turnover: the mediating role of burnout. J Nurs Manag. 2009;17(3):331–9.

Leiter MP, Maslach C. Areas of worklife survey manual. 5th ed. San Francisco: Mind Garden Inc.; 2011.

Lethbridge K, Andrusyszyn MA, Iwasiw C, Laschinger HK, Fernando R. Structural and psychological empowerment and reflective thinking: is there a link. J Nurs Educ. 2011;50(11):636–45.

Li YF, Lake ET, Sales AE, Sharp ND, Greiner GT, Lowy E, Liu CF, Mitchell PH, Sochalski JA. Measuring nurses' practice environments with the revised nursing work index: evidence from registered nurses in the Veterans Health Administration. Res Nurs Health. 2007;30(1):31–44.

Li J, Galatsch M, Siegrist J, Müller BH, Hasselhorn HM, European NEXTSG. Reward frustration at work and intention to leave the nursing profession–prospective results from the European longitudinal NEXT study. Int J Nurs Stud. 2011;48(5):628–35.

Li B, Bruyneel L, Sermeus W, Van den Heede K, Matawie K, Aiken L, Lesaffre E. Group-level impact of work environment dimensions on burnout experiences among nurses: a multivariate multilevel probit model. Int J Nurs Stud. 2013;50(2):281–91.

Locke EA. What is job satisfaction. In: Edward EL, editor. Motivation in work organizations. Monterey: Brooks/Cole Publishing Company; 1973.

MacPhee M, Bouthillette F. Developing leadership in nurse managers: the British Columbia nursing leadership institute. Nurs Leadersh. 2008;21(3):64–75.

MacPhee M, Skelton-Green J, Bouthillette F, Suryaprakash N. An empowerment framework for nursing leadership development: supporting evidence. J Adv Nurs. 2012;68(1):159–69.

MacPhee M, Dahinten VS, Hejazi S, Laschinger H, Kazanjian A, McCutcheon A, Skelton-Green J, O'Brien-Pallas L. Testing the effects of an empowerment-based leadership development programme: part 1 - leader outcomes. J Nurs Manag. 2014;22(1):4–15.

Maslach C, Leiter MP. Early predictors of job burnout and engagement. J Appl Psychol. 2008;93(3):498–512.

Maslach C, Jackson SE, Schwab RL. Maslach burnout inventory manual. 3rd ed. Menlo Park: Mountain View; 1996.

Maslach C, Schaufeli WB, Leiter MP. Job burnout. Annu Rev Psychol. 2001;52:397–422.

Mauno S, Kinnunen U, Ruokolainen M. Job demands and resources as antecedents of work engagement: a longitudinal study. J Vocat Behav. 2007;70(1):149–71.

McClure ML, Hinshaw AS. Magnet hospitals revisited: attraction and retention of professional nurses. Kansas City: American Nurses Association; 2002.

McClure ML, Poulin MA, Sovie MD, Wandelt MA. Magnet hospitals: attraction and retention of professional nurses (the orginal study). In: McClure ML, Hinshaw AS, editors. Magnet hospitals revisited: attraction and retention of professional nurses. Kansas City: American Nurses Association; 2002. p. 1–24.

McCusker J, Dendukuri N, Cardinal L, Laplante J, Bambonye L. Nursing work environment and quality of care: differences between units at the same hospital. Int J Health Care Qual Assur Inc Leadersh Health Serv. 2004;17(6):313–22.

van Mol MM, Kompanje EJ, Benoit DD, Bakker J, Nijkamp MD. The prevalence of compassion fatigue and burnout among healthcare professionals in intensive care units: a systematic review. PLoS One. 2015;10(8):e0136955.

Needleman J, Buerhaus P, Mattke S, Stewart M, Zelevinsky K. Nurse-staffing levels and the quality of care in hospitals. N Engl J Med. 2002;346(22):1715–22.

Nelson L, Burns FL. High performance programming: a framework for transforming organizations. In: Transforming work: a collection of organizational transformation readings. Alexandria: Miles River Press; 1984.

Nowrouzi B, Lightfoot N, Larivière M, Carter L, Rukholm E, Schinke R, Belanger-Gardner D. Occupational stress management and burnout interventions in nursing and their implications for healthy work environments: a literature review. Workplace Health Saf. 2015;63(7):308–15.

Page A. Nursing: inseparable linked to patient safety. In: Committee OTWEFNAPS, Board OHCS, Institute OM, editors. Keeping patients safe: transforming the work environment of nurses. Washington, DC: National Academies Press; 2004.

Salanova M, Schaufeli WB. A cross-national study of work engagement as a mediator between job resources and proactive behavior. Int J Human Resour Manage. 2008;19(1):116–31.

Schaufeli W, Bakker A. Utrecht work engagement scale: preliminary manual. Utrecht: Utrecht University; 2003.

Schaufeli WB, Buunk BP. Burnout: an overview of 25 years of research and theorizing. In: Schabracq MJ, Winnubst JAM, Cooper CL, editors. The handbook of work and health psychology. Chichester: Wiley; 2003.

Schaufeli WB, Enzmann D. The burnout companion to study and research. a critical analysis. London: Taylor & Francis; 1998.

Schaufeli WB, Salonova M. Work engagement: on how to better catch a slippery concept. Eur J Work Organ Psy. 2011;20(1):39–46.

Schaufeli WB, Bakker AB, Salanova M. The measurement of work engagement with a short questionnaire: a cross-national study. Educ Psychol Meas. 2006;66(4):701–16.

Schaufeli WB, Bakker AB, Van Rhenen W. How changes in job demands and resources predict burnout, work engagement, and sickness absenteeism. J Organ Behav. 2009;30(7):893–917.

Schmalenberg C, Kramer M. Types of intensive care units with the healthiest, most productive work environments. Am J Crit Care. 2007;16(5):458–68; quiz 469.

Schmalenberg C, Kramer M. Essentials of a productive nurse work environment. Nurs Res. 2008;57(1):2–13.

Schubert M, Glass TR, Clarke SP, Schaffert-Witvliet B, De Geest S. Validation of the basel extent of rationing of nursing care instrument. Nurs Res. 2007;56(6):416–24.

Sermeus W, Aiken LH, Van den Heede K, Rafferty AM, Griffiths P, Moreno-Casbas MT, Busse R, Lindqvist R, Scott AP, Bruyneel L, Brzostek T, Kinnunen J, Schubert M, Schoonhoven L, Zikos D, RN4CAST Consortium. Nurse forecasting in Europe (RN4CAST): rationale, design and methodology. BMC Nurs. 2011;10:6.

Siegrist J, Starke D, Chandola T, Godin I, Marmot M, Niedhammer I, Peter R. The measurement of effort–reward imbalance at work: European comparisons. Soc Sci Med. 2004;58(8):1483–99.

Silber JH, Rosenbaum PR, Ross RN. Comparing the contributions of groups of predictors: which outcomes vary with hospital rather than patient characteristics. J Am Stat Assoc. 1995;90(429):7–18.

Silber JH, Kennedy SK, Even-Shoshan O, Chen W, Koziol LF, Showan AM, Longnecker DE. Anesthesiologist direction and patient outcomes. Anesthesiology. 2000;93(1):152–63.

Simon CE, Pryce JG, Roff LL, Klemmack D. Secondary traumatic stress and oncology social work: protecting compassion from fatigue and compromising the worker's worldview. J Psychol Oncol. 2005;23(4):1–14.

Simpson M. Engagement at work: a review of the literature. J Nurs Stud. 2009;46:1012–24.

Spreitzer GM. Psychological empowerment in the workplace: dimensions, measurement, and validation. Acad Manag J. 1995;38(5):1442–65.

Stamm BH. The concise ProQOL manual. Pocatello: ProQOL.org; 2010.

Tourangeau AE, Coghlan AL, Shamian J, Evans S. Registered nurse and registered practical nurse evaluations of their hospital practice environments and their responses to these environments. Nurs Leadersh. 2005;18(4):54–69.

Tourangeau AE, Doran DM, McGillis Hall L, O'Brien Pallas L, Pringle D, JV T, Cranley LA. Impact of hospital nursing care on 30-day mortality for acute medical patients. J Adv Nurs. 2007;57(1):32–44.

Triolo PK, Scherer EM, Floyd JM. Evaluation of the magnet recognition program. J Nurs Adm. 2006;36(1):42–8.

Upenieks VV. Assessing differences in job satisfaction of nurses in magnet and nonmagnet hospitals. J Nurs Adm. 2002;32(11):564–76.

Upenieks VV. The interrelationship of organizational characteristics of magnet hospitals, nursing leadership, and nursing job satisfaction. Health Care Manag. 2003a;22(2):83–98.

Upenieks VV. What constitutes effective leadership? Perceptions of magnet and non-magnet nurse leaders. J Nurs Adm. 2003b;33(9):456–67.

Urden LD, Monarch K. The ANCC magnet recognition program converting research findings into action. In: McClure ML, Hinshaw AS, editors. Magnet hospitals revisited: attraction and retention of professional nurses. Kansas City: American Nurses Association; 2002. p. 103–15.

Van Bogaert P. Authentic leadership influences work-life coping in new nurses. Evid Based Nurs. 2016;19(2):54.

Van Bogaert P, Clarke S, Vermeyen K, Meulemans H, Van de Heyning P. Practice environments and their associations with nurse-reported outcomes in Belgian hospitals: development and preliminary validation of a Dutch adaptation of the Revised Nursing Work Index. Int J Nurs Stud. 2009a;46(1):54–64.

Van Bogaert P, Meulemans H, Clarke S, Vermeyen K, Van de Heyning P. Hospital nurse practice environment, burnout, job outcomes and quality of care: test of a structural equation model. J Adv Nurs. 2009b;65(10):2175–85.

Van Bogaert P, Clarke S, Willems R, Mondelaers M. Nurse practice environment, workload, burnout, job outcomes, and quality of care in psychiatric hospitals: a structural equation model approach. J Adv Nurs. 2013a;69(7):1515–24.

Van Bogaert P, Clarke S, Willems R, Mondelaers M. Staff engagement as a target for managing work environments in psychiatric hospitals: implications for workforce stability and quality of care. J Clin Nurs. 2013b;22(11-12):1717–28.

Van Bogaert P, Kowalski C, Weeks SM, Van Heusden D, Clarke SP. The relationship between nurse practice environment, nurse work characteristics, burnout and job outcome and quality of nursing care: a cross-sectional survey. Int J Nurs Stud. 2013c;50(12):1667–77.

Van Bogaert P, van Heusden D, Timmermans O, Franck E. Nurse work engagement impacts job outcome and nurse-assessed quality of care: model testing with nurse practice environment and nurse work characteristics as predictors. Front Psychol. 2014;5:1261.

Van der Doef M, Maes S. The job demand-control (-support) model and physical health outcomes: a review of the strain and buffer hypotheses. Psychol Health. 1998;13(5):909–36.

Van der Doef M, Maes S. The Leiden quality of work questionnaire: its construction, factor structure, and psychometric qualities. Psychol Rep. 1999;85(3 Pt 1):954–62.

Wagner JL, Warren S, Cummings G, Smith DL, Olson JK. Resonant leadership, workplace empowerment, and "spirit at work": impact on RN job satisfaction and organizational commitment. Can J Nurs Res. 2013;45(4):108–28.

Walston SL, Burns LR, Kimberly JR. Does reengineering really work? An examination of the context and outcomes of hospital reengineering initiatives. Health Serv Res. 2000;34(6):1363.

Walumbwa FO, Avolio BJ, Gardner WL, Wernsing TS, Peterson SJ. Authentic leadership: development and validation of a theory-based measure. J Manag. 2008;34(1):89–126.

Wang S, Liu Y. Impact of professional nursing practice environment and psychological empowerment on nurses' work engagement: test of structural equation modelling. J Nurs Manag. 2015;23(3):287–96.

White M, Wells JS, Butterworth T. The impact of a large-scale quality improvement programme on work engagement: preliminary results from a national cross-sectional-survey of the 'Productive Ward'. Int J Nurs Stud. 2014;51(12):1634–43.

Wolf GA, Greenhouse PK. A road map for creating a magnet work environment. J Nurs Adm. 2006;36(10):458–62.

Wolf G, Triolo P, Ponte PR. Magnet recognition program: the next generation. J Nurs Adm. 2008;38(4):200–4.

Wong CA, Laschinger HK. Authentic leadership, performance, and job satisfaction: the mediating role of empowerment. J Adv Nurs. 2013;69(4):947–59.

Yang J, Liu Y, Huang C, Zhu L. Impact of empowerment on professional practice environments and organizational commitment among nurses: a structural equation approach. Int J Nurs Pract. 2013;19(S1):44–55.

# Organizational Predictors and Determinants of Nurses' Reported Outcomes: Evidence from a 10-Year Program of Research

**3**

Peter Van Bogaert and Sean Clarke

**Abstract**

A 10-year research program systematically examined organizational features of nurses' workplaces in relation to nurse and patient outcomes. Its major results have been published in peer-reviewed international journals and presented here with replicated analyses and largely new datasets. First, a set of measures of nurse practice environment features and nurse work characteristics such as workload, decision latitude, and social capital along with burnout and work engagement as well as nurses' self-assessed job outcomes and quality of care was developed. These were examined in various populations of nurses such as those working in acute care hospitals and in long-term facilities. Secondly, models to explain associations between these selected variables were developed and tested in samples of acute hospital nurses. Thirdly, multilevel analyses of the associations between these variables confirmed that the phenomenon of organizational influences on work experiences occurred not only at the individual level but also at the team level in various study populations and across healthcare domains. Next, a longitudinal study design was set up to investigate the impact of planned transformations in the hospital organization as well as the implementation of the Productive Ward—Releasing Time to Care™ program aimed at strengthening practice environments and outcomes in a university hospital. Finally, a phenomenological study was undertaken to examine staff nurse and nurse manager perceptions and experiences of structural empowerment and the extent to which structural empowerment supports high-quality patient care. In addition, an

P. Van Bogaert (✉)
Nursing and Midwifery Sciences, Centre for Research and Innovation in Care (CRIC),
Faculty of Medicine and Health Sciences, University of Antwerp, Antwerp, Belgium
e-mail: peter.vanbogaert@uantwerpen.be

S. Clarke
William F. Connell School of Nursing, Boston College, Chestnut Hill, MA, USA
e-mail: clarkese@bc.edu

© Springer International Publishing AG 2018
P. Van Bogaert, S. Clarke (eds.), *The Organizational Context of Nursing Practice*,
https://doi.org/10.1007/978-3-319-71042-6_3

explanatory sequential mixed methods design blended qualitative study results regarding staff nurses' experiences and perceptions of workload with prior quantitative results regarding structural empowerment to explain and interpret the findings of both models.

**Keywords**

Nurse practice environment • Quality of care • Job satisfaction • Burnout • Work engagement • Structural equation modeling • Multilevel models • Mixed methods

## 3.1 Introduction

The previous chapter provided an outline of major concepts in the study of nurses' work environments and concluded with a presentation of a testable framework tying together these concepts. This chapter presents the results of a 10-year program of research that systematically tested and refined this framework, the main findings of which were originally published in international peer-reviewed journals. Firstly, a set of nurse practice environment feature measures and nurse work characteristics such as workload, decision latitude, and social capital along with burnout and work engagement as well as nurses' assessed job outcomes and quality of care were developed and studied in various nurse populations such as acute care hospitals and long-term facilities. Secondly, models to explain associations between these selected variables were developed and tested in acute hospital population. Thirdly, multilevel analyses confirmed that associations between these variables reflected connections not just at the individual level but also at the team level in acute care and psychiatric care hospitals and at institutional level in long-term facilities. Next, a longitudinal study design was set up to investigate the impact of planned transformations in a hospital's organization alongside the implementation of Productive Ward—Releasing Time to Care™ program aiming to strengthen nursing conditions and in turn achieve better outcomes in a university hospital. Finally, a phenomenological research project was conducted to study staff nurses' perceptions and experiences regarding structural empowerment and the extent to which structural empowerment supports high-quality patient care. This work also examined nurse managers' perceptions and experiences of staff nurses' structural empowerment as an influence on nurse managers' leadership styles. In addition, an explanatory sequential study approach integrated qualitative study results regarding staff nurses' experiences and perceptions of workload as well as structural empowerment as previously studied quantitatively to explain and interpret the findings of both models.

## 3.2 Measurement Tools

To measure the nurse practice environment, the *Revised Nursing Work Index (NWI-R)* (Aiken and Patrician 2000), originally developed in the USA, was translated and adapted through exploratory factor analysis in a Dutch version and confirmed in a French version. Three dimensions or subscales have been identified in the Belgium version of the NWI-R (Van Bogaert et al. 2009a, 2013d): nurse–physician relations (3 items), nurse management at the unit level (13 items), and hospital management and organizational support (15 items). Nurses using the tool rate their agreement with various statements about the practice environment in their current positions on 4-point Likert-type scales (*strongly disagree, disagree, agree, strongly agree*).

The *Maslach Burnout Inventory—Human Services Survey* (*MBI HSS*) (Maslach et al. 1996; Schaufeli and Van Dierendonck 2000; Van Bogaert et al. 2009a) is a three-subscale measure including emotional exhaustion (eight items), reflecting one's depletion of emotional resources and diminution of energy; depersonalization (five items), reflecting one's negative attitudes and feelings as well as insensitivity and lack of compassion toward patients; and personal accomplishment (seven items) reflecting one's evaluation of their work related to their feelings of competence. On this tool, respondents rate the frequency of various job-related feelings on 7-point Likert-type scales ranging from *never* to *every day*. High scores on emotional exhaustion and depersonalization and low scores on personal accomplishment are considered suggestive of burnout.

*Work engagement* was investigated with Utrecht Work Engagement Scale (*UWES*) in a shortened nine-item version (Schaufeli and Bakker 2003; Van Bogaert et al. 2013a). The UWES yields three separate dimensions, each measured with three items: vigor, dedication, and absorption. *Vigor* is defined as high levels of energy and mental resilience at work. *Dedication* is described as strong involvement in one's work accompanied by feelings of enthusiasm and significance. *Absorption* relates to being fully engrossed in one's work and having difficulties detaching oneself from it. Respondents rate the frequencies with which they experienced various job-related feelings on a 7-point scale ranging from *never to every day*. Schaufeli and Bakker (2010) concluded that work engagement assessed by the UWES is a unitary construct that is constituted by three different yet closely related dimensions. The three-factor structure appears stable across study populations from different countries and occupational groups within slight difference in values of factor loadings and correlations. In addition, the short version scores have been found to be stable over time.

*Nurse work characteristics* (Van Bogaert et al. 2013d) were measured using three measurement scales tapping workload, decision latitude, and social capital. *Workload* was operationalized with the Intensity of Labor Scale of Richter et al. (2000), which includes statements with which respondents rated their agreement or disagreement on 4-point Likert-type scales (*strongly disagree, disagree, agree, strongly agree*). *Decision latitude* (Richter et al. 2000) was measured using a 7-item tool asking respondents to rate their agreement on the ability to make decisions, be creative, and use and develop their professional and personal skills at the workplace on 4-point Likert-type scales (*strongly disagree, disagree, agree, strongly agree*). *Social capital* was measured using a 6-item scale, asking respondents to rate shared values and perceived mutual trust within teams and organizations on 4-point Likert-type scales (*strongly disagree, disagree, agree, strongly agree*) (Pfaff et al. 2004; Ernstmann et al. 2009).

To measure *nurse reported quality of care*, nurses were asked to rate their perceived quality of care overall at their units, at the last shift, and in the hospital over the last year on 4-point Likert-type scales (*poor, fair, good, excellent*). Finally, three types of *job outcomes* were assessed: satisfaction with the current job (*very dissatisfied, dissatisfied, satisfied, and very satisfied*), intention to leave the hospital within the next year (yes, no), and intention to leave the nursing profession (*yes, no*).

All variables, with the exception of workload, were coded for analysis with higher scores indicating stronger agreement or more favorable ratings. In the case of workload, higher scores are suggestive of unfavorable perceptions or conditions. Cutoffs for high to very high mean scores for each burnout and work engagement dimension were determined based on norms described by Schaufeli and Van Dierendonck (2000) and Schaufeli and Bakker (2003), respectively.

A statistical significance level of $p < 0.05$ was set, and the Statistical Package for the Social Sciences (SPSS Inc, Chicago; IBM SPSS statistics Armonk, NY) versions 15.0 to 24.0 software were used for all the analyses reported in this chapter.

## 3.3 Descriptive Analyses of Research Datasets

Tables 3.1, 3.2 and 3.3 present descriptive findings regarding all study variables from six research datasets and provide an overview and descriptive comparison of job outcomes and nurse reported quality of care (%), burnout and engagement dimensions (%), and nurse practice environment and work characteristic dimensions (mean and standard deviation).

The proportion of nurses reporting dissatisfaction or strong dissatisfaction with one's current job ranged from 7.1% in nursing home staff to more than 10% in acute and psychiatric hospital staff nurses and nursing home staff. Intention to leave the hospital (or nursing home) ranged from 3.5% in acute care hospital nursing staff to 11.0% in nursing home staff. Intention to leave the profession ranged from 6.7% among psychiatric hospital nursing staff to 10.9% in acute hospital care nursing staff. Nurses' reported quality of care at the unit and during the last shift as poor or fair ranged from 12.8% and 9.4% in acute care hospital nursing staff to 21.9% and 16% in hospital care nursing staff and nursing home staff, respectively. Reports of quality of the care in the facility deteriorating or definitely deteriorating in the past year ranged from 29.4% in nursing home staff to 40.6% in acute hospital nursing staff.

High or very high emotional exhaustion ranged from 18.5% in psychiatric hospital nursing staff to 38.5% in acute hospital nursing staff. High depersonalization ranged from 12.3% in acute hospital nursing staff to 24.8% in nursing home staff. Low or very low personal accomplishment ranged from 5.2% in acute hospital nursing staff to 15% in psychiatric hospital nursing staff and nursing home staff.

In terms of engagement measures, high or very high vigor scores were found in 24% in nursing home staff to 58.3% in psychiatric hospital nursing staff, high or very high dedication ranged from 42.4% in nursing home staff to 70% in acute and

**Table 3.1** Job outcomes and nurse reported quality of care variables in six nurse samples

| | Facility | Published | Number | Qualification | (Very) dissatisfied with current job (%) | Intention to leave hospital (%) | Intention to leave profession (%) | Quality of care at the unit poor or fair (%) | Quality of care during the last shift poor or fair (%) | Quality hospital (definitely) deteriorated (%) |
|---|---|---|---|---|---|---|---|---|---|---|
| Dataset 1 | Acute hospital | 2009 | 401 | Staff nurses | 8.5 | 3.5 | 9.5 | 21.9 | 13.7 | 40.6 |
| Dataset 2 | Psychiatric hospital | 2013a, b | 357 | Staff nurse/other€ | 11.2 | 5.6 | 6.7 | 17.7 | 9.6 | n/a |
| Dataset 3 | Acute hospital | 2013c | 1201 | Staff nurses | 8.3 | 5.9 | 10.9 | 12.8 | 9.4 | 39.5 |
| Dataset 4 | Acute hospital | | 751 | Staff nurses | 12.0 | 5.9 | 9.2 | 13.2 | 13.5 | 35.2 |
| Dataset 5 | Nursing home | | 733 | Staff nurses/other§ | 7.1 | 11.0 | 8.0 | 17.6 | 13.5 | 29.4 |
| Dataset 6 | Nursing home | No | 739 | Staff nurses/other§ | 11.5 | 10.1 | 9.7 | 21.3 | 16.0 | n/a |

Other€, licensed practice nurses/non-registered caregivers; other§, licensed practice nurses. Job outcomes have three items: satisfaction with the current job, (1) very dissatisfied, (2) dissatisfied, (3) satisfied, and (4) very satisfied, and intention to leave the hospital and the nursing profession within a year (yes, no). Nurse-assessed quality of care has three items: at the current unit; the last shift, (1) poor, (2) fair, (3) good, and (4) excellent; and in the hospital within the last year, (1) definitely deteriorated, (2) deteriorated, (3) improved, and (4) definitely improved. n/a = not available (not measured)

**Table 3.2** Outcome variables: burnout and engagement dimensions in the six nurse samples

| | Facility | Published | Number | Qualification | (Very) high emotional exhaustion (%) | (Very) high depersonalization scores (%) | (Very) low personal accomplishment (%) | (Very) high vigor (%) | (Very) high dedication (%) | (Very) high absorption (%) |
|---|---|---|---|---|---|---|---|---|---|---|
| Dataset 1 | Acute hospital | 2009 | 401 | Staff nurses | 25.8 | 12.3 | 5.2 | 57.2 | 70.5 | 58.2 |
| Dataset 2 | Psychiatric hospital | 2013a, b | 357 | Staff nurse/other€ | 18.5 | 13.2 | 15.2 | 58.3 | 70.3 | 64 |
| Dataset 3 | Acute hospital | 2013c | 1201 | Staff nurses | 34.0 | 18.7 | 7.8 | 45 | 62 | 52 |
| Dataset 4 | Acute hospital | | 751 | Staff nurses | 38.5 | 22.4 | 5.3 | 48.7 | 70.3 | 56.8 |
| Dataset 5 | Nursing home | | 733 | Staff nurses/other$ | 19 | 18.4 | 16 | 26.6 | 44.7 | 48.6 |
| Dataset 6 | Nursing home | | 739 | Staff nurses/other$ | 26.1 | 24.8 | 15 | 24 | 42.4 | 44.1 |

Other€, licensed practice nurses/non-registered caregivers; other$, licensed practice nurses. Respondents rate their experience of various job-related feelings on a 7-point Likert scale ranging from (0) never to (6) every day. Higher scores on study measures indicate more favorable ratings, with the exception of the burnout dimensions' emotional exhaustion and depersonalization; high scores indicate unfavorable conditions

**Table 3.3** Nurse practice environment and mean scores on nurse practice environment dimensions

| | Facility | Published | Number | Qualification | Nurse–physician relations | Nurse management | Hospital management | Decision latitude | Workload | Social capital |
|---|---|---|---|---|---|---|---|---|---|---|
| Dataset 1 | Acute hospital | 2009 | 401 | Staff nurses | 2.66 (0.54) | 2.79 (0.33) | 2.50 (0.30) | n/a | n/a | n/a |
| Dataset 2 | Psychiatric hospital | 2013a, b | 357 | Staff nurse/other€ | 2.76 (0.48) | 2.88 (0.34) | 2.50 (0.34) | n/a | 2.35 (0.61) | n/a |
| Dataset 3 | Acute hospital | 2013c | 1201 | Staff nurses | 2.83 (0.53) | 2.87 (0.33) | 2.43 (0.35) | 3.01 (0.33) | 2.95 (0.51) | 2.94 (0.51) |
| Dataset 4 | Acute hospital | | 751 | Staff nurses | 2.90 (0.49) | 2.88 (0.29) | 2.56 (0.34) | 3.11 (0.33) | 3.05 (0.53) | 3.03 (0.54) |
| Dataset 5 | Nursing home | | 733 | Staff nurses/other$ | 2.84 (0.49) | 2.96 (0.40) | 2.67 (0.45) | 2.98 (0.51) | 2.80 (0.53) | 2.83 (0.63) |
| Dataset 6 | Nursing home | | 739 | Staff nurses/other$ | 2.84 (0.45) | 2.95 (0.39) | 2.69 (0.43) | 2.85 (0.39) | 2.75 (0.55) | 2.73 (0.62) |

Other€, licensed practice nurses/non-registered caregivers; other$, licensed practice nurses. Statements were rated by staff nurses on a Likert-scale from (1) strongly disagree, (2) disagree, (3) agree, to (4) strongly agree. Lake (2002) considers dimension mean score of 2.50 as a neutral point, <2.5 suggests general disagreement, >2.50 and 3.00 suggest low to moderate agreement, and >3.00 suggests general agreement with the dimension statements. All variables, with the exception of workload, were coded for analysis, whereby higher scores indicated a stronger agreement or more favorable ratings. On the latter measure, higher scores are suggestive of unfavorable perceptions or conditions. n/a = not available (not measured) psychiatric hospital nursing staff, and high or very high absorption ranged from 44.1% in nursing home staff to 64% in psychiatric hospital nursing staff.

Findings show consequently that staff nurses of acute and psychiatric hospitals as well as nursing homes were *highly dedicated* and *engaged* (e.g., vigor and absorption); that a *substantial proportion* of staff nurses experience *feelings of burnout* such as high emotional exhaustion, depersonalization, and low personal accomplishment; and that some staff nurses are dissatisfied and have intentions to leave the organization or the profession.

Staff nurses rated their agreement with statements of nurse–physician relations and nurse management at the unit level as favorable (>2.50); the former ranged, respectively, from 2.66 to 2.90 in acute hospital nursing, and the following ranged from 2.79 in acute hospital nursing staff to 2.96 in nursing home staff. Hospital management was rated less favorable in acute and psychiatric care hospitals ranging from 2.43 to 2.56. Management was rated more favorably by staff (2.67 and 2.69) in nursing homes.

Staff nurses rated their agreement with statements about engagement dimension decision latitude and social capital as favorable (>2.50); the former ranged from 2.85 in nursing home staff to 3.11 in acute hospital nursing staff and the following from 2.73 in nursing home staff to 3.03 in acute hospital nursing staff. Workload statements were rated favorable (2.35) in psychiatric hospital staff and unfavorable (3.05) in acute hospital nursing staff.

In sum, findings show *moderate* agreement of staff nurses with statements about nurse practice environments in terms of nurse–physician relations and nurse management at the unit level and *disagreement to moderate agreement* with statements about hospital management and organizational support. In addition, staff nurses show *moderate to general agreement* with nurse work characteristics such as decision latitude, social capital, and workload, the former two as favorable perceptions or conditions and the latter rather unfavorable perception or condition (Box 3.1).

---

**Box 3.1 Key Descriptive Findings**
- One out of ten staff nurses is (very) dissatisfied and has the intention to leave the hospital or the profession. More or less than one out of five staff nurses report the quality of care as poor or fair, and between one out of three and two out of five report the quality in the hospital as (definitely) deteriorating.
- Between 2 out of 10 and 2 out 5 staff nurses experience feelings of high to very high emotional exhaustion, 1 out of 10 to almost 1 out of 5 experiences feelings of high to very high depersonalization, and 1 out of 20 to almost 1 out of 6 experiences low to very low personal accomplishment.
- One out of five to more than half of staff nurses experience high to very feelings of vigor, two out of five to more than one out of three staff nurses experience high to very feelings of dedication, and more than two out five to one out of three staff nurses experience feelings of absorption.

- Staff nurses rate statements about nurse–physician relations and nurse management at the unit level as favorable (moderate agreement); instead hospital management and organizational support are rated unfavorable (disagreement to low agreement) in hospital nursing staff and favorable (moderate agreement) by nursing home staff.
- Staff nurses rate statements of nurse work characteristic dimensions' decision latitude and social capital as favorable (moderate to general agreement); instead, hospital staff nurses and nursing home staff rate workload as unfavorable (moderate to general agreement).

## 3.4 Burnout and Engagement: Mediators Between Organizational Context, Work Characteristics, and Nurses' Job Satisfaction, Turnover Intentions, and Quality of Care

### 3.4.1 Study Method

The structures of multi-item measures were thoroughly evaluated with confirmatory factor analyses and internal consistency analyses (Van Bogaert et al. 2009b, 2013a, b, d, 2014c). The confirmation of the three-factor structure of NWI-R, MBI HSS, and UWES, as well as the one-factor structure of workload, decision latitude, and social capital, was supported through various fit measures with various study populations in the first five (of six) datasets. Sufficiency of model fit was tested with comparative fit index (CFI >0.90), incremental fit index (IFI >0.90), and root mean square error of approximation (RMSEA <0.08).

All multi-item scales had Cronbach's alpha coefficients ranged from 0.65 to 0.90, with the exception of the job outcome dimension (0.32). As identified in the study populations, the inter-item correlations (an alternative measurement technique assessing internal consistency) (Briggs and Creek 1986) for the indicators of the job outcome dimension ranged from fair to moderate with values between 0.15 and 0.21.

In preparation for model testing, the data were analyzed descriptively, correlations were computed, as well as associations were determined by theoretical and empirical literature (Kanter 1993; Maslach et al. 1996; Schaufeli and Bakker 2004; Laschinger and Leiter 2006; Leiter and Laschinger 2006; Leiter and Maslach 2009; Kowalski et al. 2010). Measurement scales were used as variables to develop structural models clarifying associations between independent and mediating predictors such as practice environment dimensions and nurse work characteristic dimensions, respectively, and mediating and dependent outcome variables such as burnout dimensions (see final models Model 1 and Model 3)/work engagement dimensions (see final models Model 2 and Model 4) and nurse reported job outcomes/quality of

**Table 3.4** Observed (a) and latent variables (b) of the retested models

| | |
|---|---|
| *Nurse practice environment* | |
| Nurse–physician relationship (b) | |
| 2 | Physicians and nurses have good working relationships (a) |
| 27 | Much teamwork between nurses and doctors (a) |
| 39 | Collaboration (joint practice) between nurses and physicians (a) |
| Nurse management at the unit level (b) | |
| 33 | Working with nurses who are clinically competent (a) |
| 44 | Nurse managers consult with staff on daily problems and procedures (a) |
| 51 | Standardized policies, procedures, and ways of doing things (a) |
| Hospital management and organizational support (b) | |
| 14 | A chief nursing officer is highly visible and accessible to staff (a) |
| 36 | An administration that listens and responds to employee concerns (a) |
| 38 | Staff nurses are involved in the internal governance of the hospital (e.g., practice and policy committees) (a) |
| *Work characteristics* | |
| Workload (b) | |
| 4 | Many times I have to do a lot of work |
| 7 | Tasks that I have to solve are often very difficult |
| 13 | Normally time is short, so often I am pressed for time at work |
| Decision latitude (b) | |
| 2 | To learn continuously is necessary in my work (a)[a] |
| 8 | I can fully practice what I have learned in my training (a)[a] |
| 12 | In my work I have to take a lot of decisions independently (a) |
| Social capital (b) | |
| 2 | On our unit there is trust between nurses |
| 4 | On our unit there is favorable work climate |
| 6 | On our unit nurses share values |

[a]Superior fit measures were established by replacing two items of the decision latitude dimension and one item of the absorption dimension in Model 1 to Model 4 in dataset 4, dataset 5, and dataset 6

care, respectively. The study population of these retested models included dataset 4 to dataset 6.

In SEM, a ratio of at least five subjects for each variable, including error measurements, observed variables (indicators), and latent variables (dimensions), is recommended (Bentler and Chou 1987). A content-driven selection of observed variables (see Tables 3.4 and 3.5) was made to equalize measure weighting across indicators (Byrne 1994, 2001, 2010). For example, nurse management at the unit level included a selection of items related to the nurse manager, the clinical competence of colleagues, and the availability of nursing care plans, as well as standardized policies and procedures.

AMOS software was used to test models using the full database incorporating imputation of incomplete data, maximum likelihood estimation, and estimation of means and intercepts. To verify and improve model plausibility (Van Bogaert et al. 2009b, 2013a, b, d, 2014c), various fit measures were calculated and compared

**Table 3.5** Observed (a) and latent variables (b) of the retested model

| *Burnout* | | |
|---|---|---|
| Emotional exhaustion (b) | | |
| | 1 | I feel emotionally drained from my work (a) |
| | 2 | I feel used up at the end of the workday (a) |
| | 14 | I feel I'm working too hard on my job (a) |
| Depersonalization (b) | | |
| | 10 | I've become more callous toward people since I took this job (a) |
| | 11 | I worry that this job is hardening me emotionally (a) |
| | 22 | I feel patients blame me for some of their problems (a) |
| Personal accomplishment (b) | | |
| | 17 | I can easily create a relaxed atmosphere with my patients (a) |
| | 18 | I feel exhilarated after working closely with my patients (a) |
| | 19 | I have accomplished many worthwhile things in this job (a) |
| *Work engagement* | | |
| Vigor (b) | | |
| | 2 | At my job, I feel strong and vigorous (a) |
| | 5 | When I get up in the morning, I feel like going to work (a) |
| Dedication (b) | | |
| | 3 | I am enthusiastic about my job (a) |
| | 4 | My job inspires me (a) |
| Absorption (b) | | |
| | 6 | I feel happy when I am working intensely (a)[a] |
| | 9 | I am immersed in my work (a) |
| *Outcome variables* | | |
| Job outcomes (b) | | |
| | 1 | Job satisfaction (a) |
| | 2 | Intention to stay in the hospital (a) |
| | 3 | Intention to stay in nursing (a) |
| Nurse-assessed quality of care (b) | | |
| | 1 | At the current unit (a) |
| | 2 | At the last shift (a) |
| | 3 | In the hospital the last year (a) |

[a]Superior fit measures were established by replacing one item of the absorption dimension in Model 2 and Model 4 in dataset 4, dataset 5, and dataset 6

against accepted criterion levels (CFI and IFI ≥0.90; RMSEA <0.080). To achieve optimal model fit assessed using standard measures, pathways were included or trimmed based on the impacts on chi-square statistics through modification indices, as well as on empirical and theoretical grounds. In addition, pathways that were found not to be statistically significant were deleted. To determine whether or not to include additional parameters in the model, Byrne (2010) highlights the prime importance of the extent to which they are substantively meaningful and the model exhibits adequate fit.

New analyses with additional study population were set to confirm and/or extend previous findings. Models were retested with an acute hospital care study population (dataset 4) and two nursing home study population (datasets 5 and 6), and all models were retested without any model modifications.

### 3.4.2 Retesting Burnout and Engagement Models with Acute Hospital Study Population (One Dataset)

Retest of the burnout model (Fig. 3.1 Model 1) confirmed the previous developed burnout model (Van Bogaert et al. 2013a) describing associations between nurse–physician relations and nurse-assessed quality of care and job outcomes through

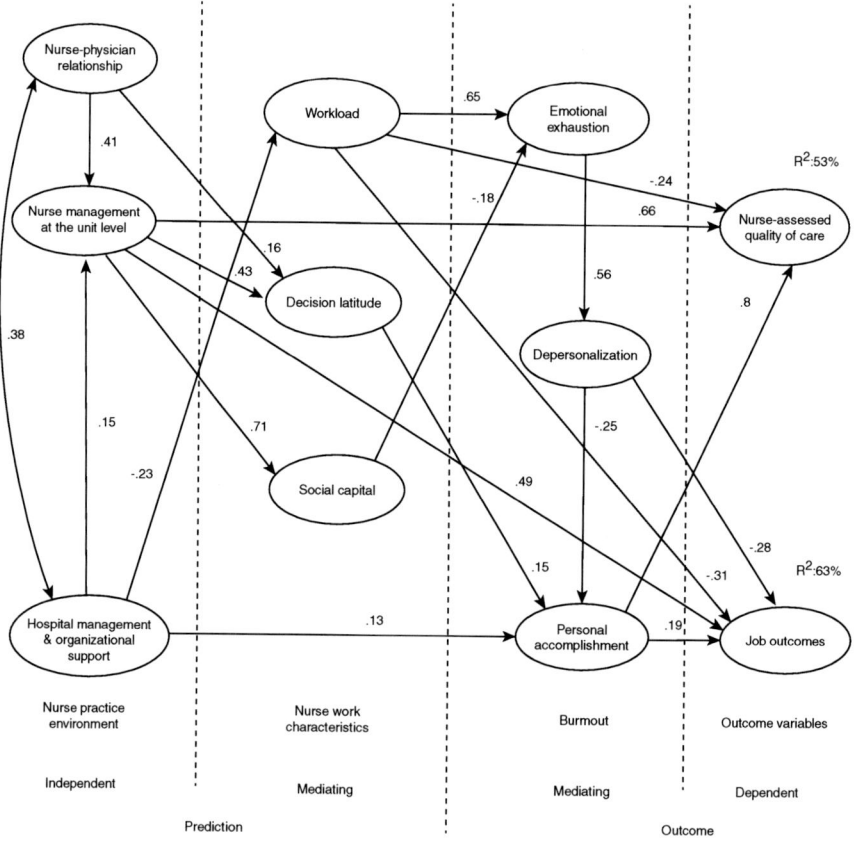

**Fig. 3.1** Model 1 burnout acute hospital dataset 4

sequentially decision latitude and personal accomplishment with explained variances 53% and 63%, respectively. Moreover, nurse management at the unit level ($R^2 = 35.7\%$), workload ($R^2 = 13\%$), and personal accomplishment ($R^2 = 4.3\%$) have a direct impact on nurse reported quality of care. Nurse management at the unit level ($R^2 = 24.3\%$), workload ($R^2 = 15.4\%$), depersonalization ($R^2 = 13.9\%$), and personal accomplishment ($R^2 = 9.4\%$) have a direct impact on job outcomes. The retest of the engagement model (Fig 3.2. Model 2) confirmed largely previous developed model (Van Bogaert et al. 2014a) and describes engagement dimensions' vigour, dedication and absorption as mirror variables of burnout dimensions' emotional exhaustion, depersonalization and personal accomplishment with explained variances $R^2$ of 53% and 59% on nurse reported quality of care and job outcomes, respectively. Nurse management at the unit level ($R^2 = 36.6\%$), workload ($R^2 = 12.4\%$) and absorption ($R$ $3.9\%$) have a direct impact on nurse reported quality of care. Moreover, nurse management at the unit level ($R^2 = 22.8\%$), workload ($R^2 = 7.9\%$) and vigour ($R^2 = 22.3\%$) have a direct impact on job outcomes. In the retest absorption had no relevant impact anymore.

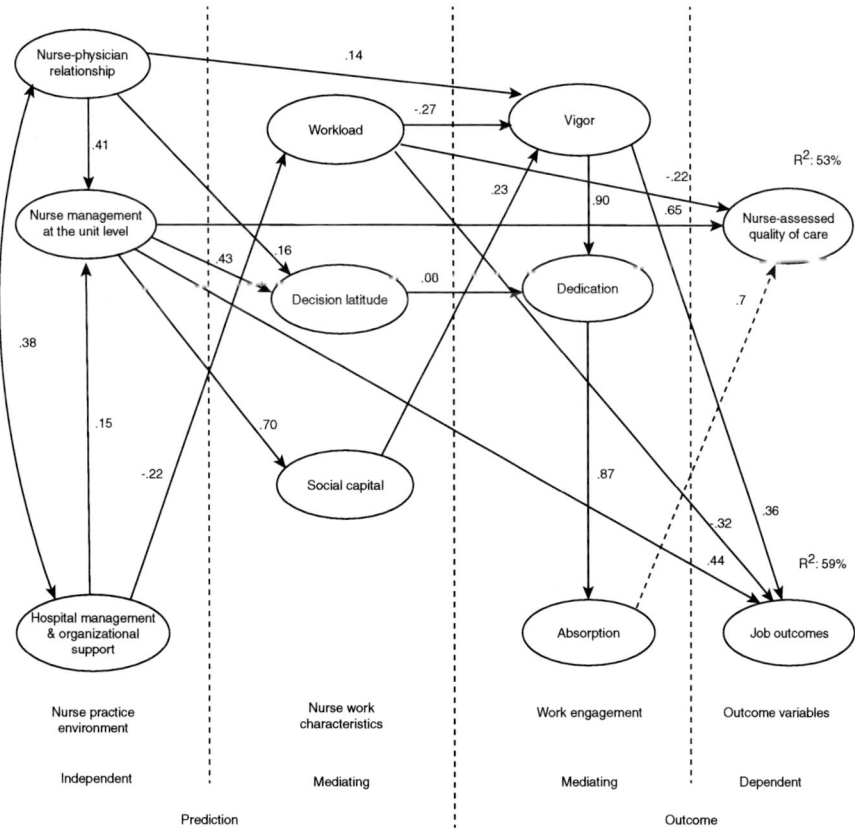

**Fig. 3.2**  Model 2 engagement acute hospital dataset 4

Findings of the final models with an additional acute hospital nursing staff population show that feelings of burnout influenced by nurse practice conditions - determined by unfavourable perceived inter-professional relations with physicians, hospital management and organizational support and the conditions within the unit (nurse management at the unit level) - as well as unfavourable nurse reported workload, decision latitude and social capital - consequently have an effect on job dissatisfaction, turnover intentions and unfavourable reported quality of care. Instead, feelings of engagement are influenced by nurse practice conditions - determined by favourable perceived inter-professional relations with physicians, hospital management and organizational support and the conditions within the unit (nurse management at the unit level) - as well as favourable nurses' reported workload, decision latitude and social capital - consequently have an effect on job satisfaction, intention to stay and favourable reported quality of care.

The retest confirmed the burnout model (Fig. 3.3 Model 3) with two nursing home datasets showing that nurse reported quality of care and job outcomes explained variances ($R^2$) of 65% and 64% in dataset 5 and 54% and 69% in dataset 6, respectively. Direct impact of nurse management at the unit level ($R^2 = 46.8\%$ and 43.6%), workload ($R^2 = 5.5\%$ and 5.5%), and personal accomplishment ($R^2 = 12.8\%$ and

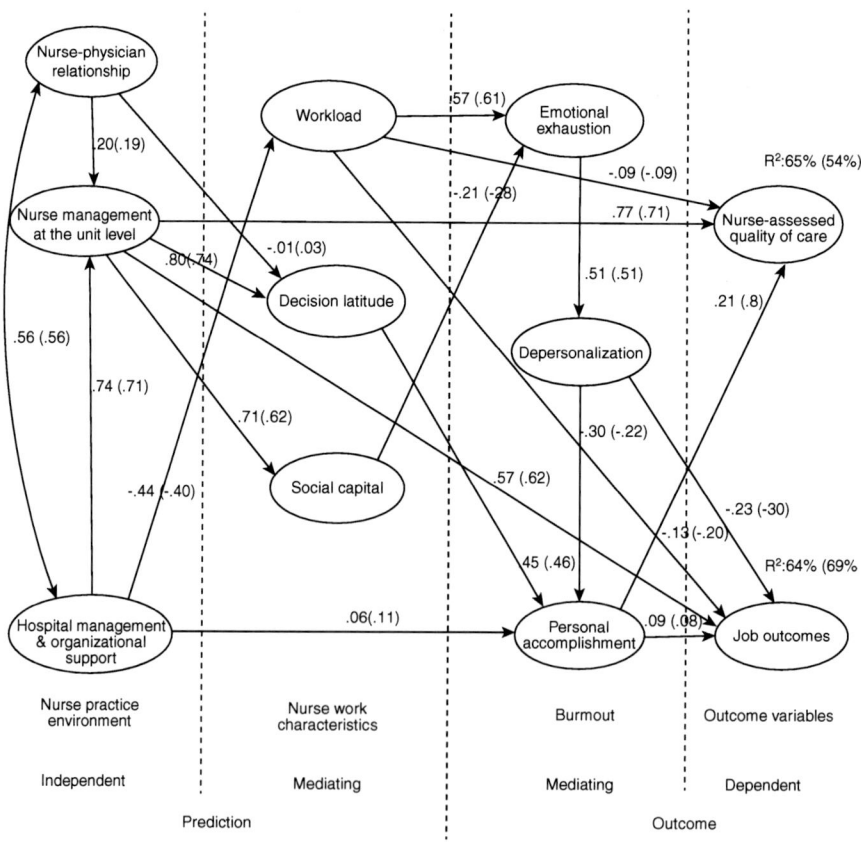

**Fig. 3.3** Model 3 burnout nursing home dataset 5 (dataset 6)

4.9%) on quality of care as well as nurse management at the unit level ($R^2 = 35.8\%$ and 35.7%), workload ($R^2 = 8.2\%$ and 11.52%), depersonalization ($R^2 = 14.4\%$ and 17.3%), and personal accomplishment ($R^2 = 5.6\%$ and 4.6%) on job outcomes is confirmed, although personal accomplishment had no significant impact anymore on quality of care in dataset 6 and on job outcomes in dataset 5 and dataset 6.

The retest confirmed the engagement model (Fig. 3.4 Model 4) and describes engagement dimensions' vigor, dedication, and absorption as mirror variables of burnout dimensions' emotional exhaustion, depersonalization, and personal accomplishment with nurse reported quality of care and job outcome explained variances ($R^2$) of 64% and 69% in dataset 5 and 54% and 70% in dataset 6, respectively. In addition, direct impact of nurse management at unit level ($R^2 = 53.2\%$ and 50.3%), workload $R^2 = (5\%$ and 0.7%), and absorption $R^2 = (5.8\%$ and 3.0%) on quality of care as well as nurse management at unit level ($R^2 = 33.8\%$ and 30.1%), workload ($R^2 = 5.3\%$ and 10.5%), and vigor ($R^2 = 29.9\%$ and 29.4%) on job outcomes is established too in nursing home datasets 5 and 6, although workload had no relevant impact anymore on quality of care as well as job outcomes in dataset 5 and along with absorption on quality of care in dataset 6 (Box 3.2).

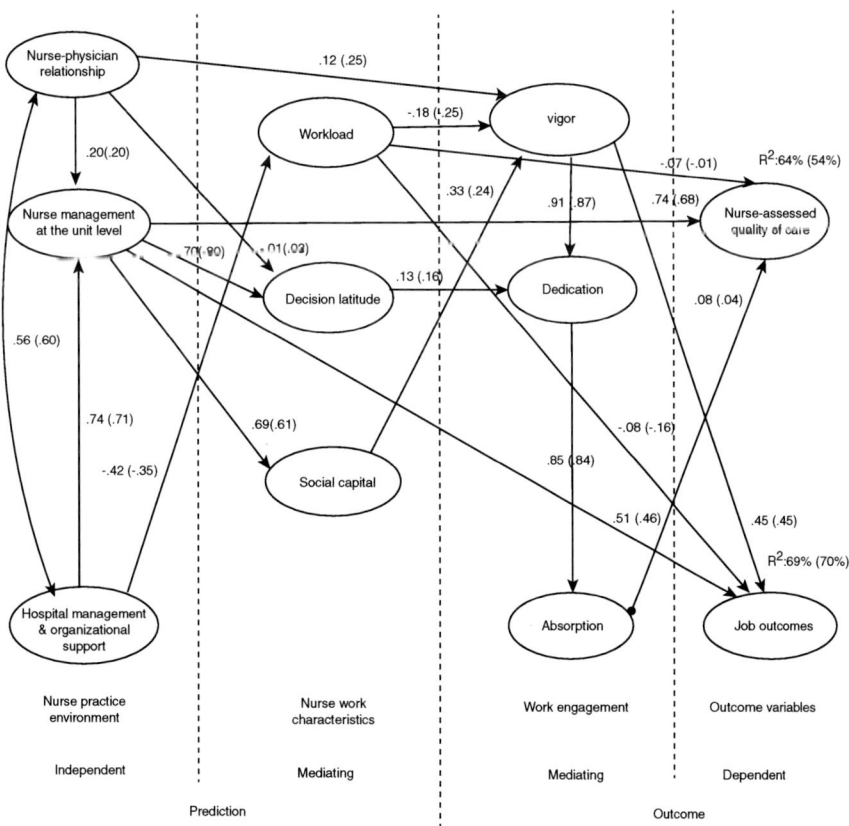

**Fig. 3.4**  Model 4 engagement nursing home dataset 5 (dataset 6)

**Box 3.2 Key Structural Equation Model or SEM Findings**
- Poor nurse work conditions identified by unfavorable perceived nurse–physician relations, hospital management and organizational support, and nurse management at the unit level predict unfavorable nurse reported job outcomes and quality of care through poor nurse work characteristics such as unfavorable perceived workload, decision latitude, and social capital and sequentially through feelings of emotional exhaustion, depersonalization, and low personal accomplishment.
- Feelings of work engagement through vigor, dedication, and absorption predict favorable reported job outcomes and quality of care determined by favorable perceived nurse work conditions such as nurse–physician relations, hospital management and organizational support, and nurse management at the unit level and sequentially by favorable perceived nurse work characteristics such as workload, decision latitude, and social capital.
- Supportive conditions through nursing management at the unit level have a strongly positive direct impact on both nurse reported quality of care at the unit, at the last shift, and in the hospital the last year and job outcomes such as job satisfaction and intention to stay and are linked to foster social capital.
- Poor perceived hospital management and organizational support is associated with unfavorable perceived workload and feelings of emotional exhaustion, sequentially.
- Social capital is potentially protective against feelings of emotional exhaustion, whereas workload has potentially deleterious influences through feelings of burnout dimensions on reported quality of care and job outcomes such as job dissatisfaction and turnover intentions.
- Decision latitude (e.g., clinical autonomy) supported by nurse–physician relations as well as nurse management at the unit level appears to have better outcomes through enhanced sense of personal accomplishment.
- In sum, poor nursing conditions are linked with poor nurse work characteristics. These conditions predict high levels of burnout and low levels of work engagement and consequently predict poor reported quality of care, job dissatisfaction, and turnover intentions.

## 3.5 Work Environment Predicts Work Characteristics and Nurse Reported Outcomes: Multilevel Analyses of Nursing Teams and Institutions

### 3.5.1 Study Method

Conventional regression analyses ignore the correlated structure of the observations on clustered data because they underestimate standard errors and increase the likelihood of a false rejection of the null hypothesis or acceptance of a relationship when in fact it does not exist (Type I error). Meanwhile, a two-level model incorporating a nested structure of staff members with nursing teams (Tables 3.6 and 3.7) or institutions (nursing homes) (Tables 3.8 and 3.9) corrects for the dependency of observations. Therefore, the effects of the independent variables on the dependent variables were tested with two-level linear mixed effects models with a random intercept. Level One involved variables related to the staff members on a given nursing unit or institution, and Level Two involved variables related to the nursing unit or the institution (Fitzmaurice et al. 2004; Van Bogaert et al. 2010, 2013c, e, 2014a).

**Table 3.6** Generalized linear mixed effects model—multiple multilevel model with random intercept: nurse reported job outcome (dependent variables) and nurse practice environment, nurse work characteristics, engagement and burnout[a] (independent variables)

| Dataset 4 (*n* = 62 units) | Unadjusted OR | Adjusted OR (f) |
|---|---|---|
| *Satisfaction with the current job (a)* | | |
| Hospital management and organizational support (e) | 4.45** [1.84; 10.8] | 4.03** [1.58; 10.25] |
| Emotional exhaustion (e) | 0.52*** [0.41; 0.67] | 0.53*** [0.40; 0.69] |
| Dedication (e) | 2.13*** [1.42; 3.18] | 2.39*** [1.56; 3.67] |
| Absorption (e) | 0.68* [0.48; 0.96] | 0.65* [0.45; 0.94] |
| *(No) intensions to leave the nursing profession (b)* | | |
| Emotional exhaustion (e) | 0.65*** [0.52; 0.81] | 0.64*** [0.50; 0.81] |
| Personal accomplishment (e) | 1.83*** [1.30; 2.59] | 1.89*** [1.31; 2.73] |
| Dedication (e) | 1.86*** [1.48; 2.33] | 2.11*** [1.64; 2.72] |

[a]Burnout and engagement dimensions were separately analyzed; ***$p$-value <0.001; **$p$-value <0.01; *$p$-value <0.05; *OR* odds ratio 95% CI [lower and upper bound]; (a) strongly satisfied or satisfied versus dissatisfied or strongly dissatisfied; (b) no, intention to leave (1), versus yes, intention to leave (0); (e) mean value; (f) adjusted for years in nursing, years on present unit, gender, bachelor of nursing science, work schedules, type of unit

**Table 3.7** Generalized linear mixed effects model—multiple multilevel model with random intercept: nurse reported quality of care (dependent variables) and nurse practice environment, nurse work characteristics, engagement, and burnout[a] (independent variables)

| Dataset 4 (*n* = 62 units) | Unadjusted OR | Adjusted OR (f) |
|---|---|---|
| *Quality of care at the unit (c)* | | |
| Nurse management at the unit level (e) | 11.03*** [3.40; 40.48] | 7.87** [1.88; 27.87] |
| Social capital (e) | 2.81** [1.48; 5.34] | 3.08** [1.55; 6.11] |
| Emotional exhaustion (e) | 0.56*** [0.42; 0.74] | 0.56*** [0.41; 0.77] |
| Personal accomplishment (e) | 1.79** [1.20; 2.68] | 1.75* [1.14; 2.69] |
| Vigor (f) | 1.26* [1.01; 1.57] | 1.33* [1.05; 1.68] |
| *Quality of care at last shift (c)* | | |
| Nurse management at the unit level (e) | 13.71*** [4.87; 38.6] | 4.63* [1.25; 17.18] |
| Workload (e) | 0.49** [0.29; 0.83] | 0.47* [0.26; 0.84] |
| Emotional exhaustion (e) | 0.61*** [0.49; 0.76] | 0.56*** [0.44; 0.72] |
| Dedication (e) | 1.30* [1.03; 1.63] | 1.41** [1.10; 1.80] |

[a]Burnout and engagement dimensions were separate analyzed; ***$p$-value <0.001; **$p$-value <0.01; *$p$-value <0.05; *OR* odds ratio 95% CI [lower and upper bound]; (c) good or excellent (1) versus poor or fair (0); (e) mean value; (f) adjusted for years in nursing, years on present unit, gender, bachelor of nursing science, work schedules, type of unit

**Table 3.8** Generalized linear mixed effects model—multiple multilevel model with random intercept: nurse reported job outcome (dependent variables) and nurse practice environment, nurse work characteristics, engagement and burnout (independent variables)

| Dataset 5 ($n = 25$) – dataset 6 ($n = 22$) | Unadjusted | Adjusted (f) |
|---|---|---|
| | OR | OR |
| *Satisfaction with the current job (a)* | | |
| Nurse–physician relations (e) | 2.09* [1.08; 4.01] | 1.81 [0.87; 3.75] (dataset 5) |
| Nurse management at the unit level (e) | 32.52*** [9.38; 12.74] | 40.38*** [10.38; 157.01] (dataset 6) |
| Nursing home management and organizational support (c) | 6.95** [2.07; 23.35] | 3.87* [10.8; 13.82] (dataset 5) |
| Workload (e) | 0.23*** [0.10; 0.51] | 0.27*** [0.12; 0.63] (dataset 6) |
| Social capital (e) | 2.28* [1.36; 3.81] | 3.62*** [2.22; 5.88] (dataset 5) |
| Decision latitude (e) | 2.52* [1.07; 5.93] | 3.75* [1.50; 9.39] (dataset 5) |
| Depersonalization (e) | 0.62* [0.43; 0.89] | 0.59* [0.41; 0.85] (dataset 5) |
| Depersonalization (e) | 0.53** [0.35; 0.80] | 0.49** [0.31; 0.76] (dataset 5) |
| Vigor (e) | 1.60** [1.05; 2.42] | 2.48* [1.47; 4.19] (dataset 5) |
| Absorption (e) | 2.33*** [1.64; 3.30] | 2.16*** [1.52; 3.08] (dataset 6) |
| *(No) intention to leave the service (b)* | | |
| Nurse management at the unit level (e) | 26.44*** [7.56; 92.43] | 41.50*** [9.41; 183.06] (dataset 6) |
| Workload | 0.45** [0.24; 0.85] | 0.36** [0.18; 0.74] (dataset 6) |
| Social capital (e) | 2.68** [1.63; 4.40] | 3.26** [1.84; 5.78] (dataset 5) |
| Emotional exhaustion (e) | 0.41*** [0.3; 0.55] | 0.36*** [0.26; 0.51] (dataset 5) |
| Emotional exhaustion (e) | 0.49*** [0.34; 0.70] | 0.49** [0.32; 0.75] (dataset 6) |
| Vigor (e) | 2.04** [1.29; 3.23] | 1.60 [0.95; 2.69] (dataset 5) |
| Dedication (e) | 1.74* [1.10; 2.76] | 2.06* [1.21; 3.53] (dataset 5) |
| Absorption (e) | 0.53* [0.32; 0.86] | 0.58* [0.34; 0.99] (dataset 5) |
| *(No) intention to leave nursing profession (b)* | | |
| Nurse management at the unit level (e) | 4.88** [1.77; 13.45] | 6.08** [1.92; 19.25] (dataset 6) |
| Decision latitude (e) | 3.65*** [1.52; 8.74] | 4.95** [1.75; 12.07] (dataset 6) |
| Emotional exhaustion (e) | 0.34*** [0.24; 0.47] | 0.41*** [0.28; 0.51] (dataset 5) |
| Emotional exhaustion (e) | 0.52*** [0.44; 0.99] | 0.50** [0.34; 0.74] (dataset 6) |
| Depersonalization (e) | 0.66* [0.37; 0.72] | 0.60* [0.39; 0.94] (dataset 6) |
| Dedication (e) | 1.79*** [1.33; 2.43] | 1.82*** [1.33; 2.50] (dataset 6) |

[a]Burnout and engagement dimensions were analyzed separately; ***$p$-value <0.001; **$p$-value <0.01; *$p$-value <0.05; *OR* odds ratio 95% CI [lower and upper bound]; (a) strongly satisfied or satisfied versus dissatisfied or strongly dissatisfied; (b) no, intention to leave (1), versus yes, intention to leave (0); (e) mean value; (f) adjusted for years in nursing, years on present unit, gender, registered nurse (RN), work schedules

Descriptive statistics and intra-class correlation coefficients (ICC) were examined. The degree of homogeneity of observations within nursing units or nursing homes of each measure was indicated by ICCs (Fitzmaurice et al. 2004; Park and Lake 2005).

Multilevel modeling was used to investigate the unit-level or nursing home-level effect of nurse practice environment, nurse work characteristics, and burnout and

**Table 3.9** Final generalized linear mixed effects model—multiple multilevel model with random intercept: nurse reported quality of care (dependent variables) and nurse practice environment, nurse work characteristics, engagement and burnout (independent variables)

| | Unadjusted | Adjusted (f) |
|---|---|---|
| | OR | OR |
| *Quality of care at the unit (c)* | | |
| Nurse management at the unit level (e) | 11.56** [3.7; 36.08] | 10.35** [3.03; 35.34] (dataset 5) |
| Nurse management at the unit level (e) | 14.73*** [5.06; 42.86] | 16.80*** [5.54; 50.99] (dataset 6) |
| Workload (e) | 0.50* [0.27; 0.93] | 0.38* [0.18; 0.78] (dataset 5) |
| Workload (e) | 0.56* [0.33; 0.96] | 0.60 [0.35; 1.02] (dataset 6) |
| Social capital (e) | 2.95** [1.61; 5.41] | 3.03** [1.53; 6.02] (dataset 5) |
| Social capital (e) | 2.88*** [1.72; 4.83] | 2.68*** [1.57; 4.58] (dataset 6) |
| Personal accomplishment (e) | 1.51* [1.01; 2.27] | 1.62 [0.99; 2.63] (dataset 5) |
| Vigor (e) | 1.61** [1.18; 2.2] | 1.56* [1.09; 2.23] (dataset 5)) |
| Vigor (e) | 1.29* [1.03; 1.63] | 1.28* [1.01; 1.62] (dataset 6) |
| *Quality of care at last shift (c)* | | |
| Nurse management at the unit level (e) | 3.15* [1.15; 8.66] | 2.90* [1.02; 8.20] (dataset 5) |
| Nurse management at the unit level (e) | 7.28** [2.44; 21.76] | 5.62** [2.02; 5.64] (dataset 6) |
| Workload (e) | | |
| Workload (e) | 0.54* [0.3; 1.0] | 0.60 [0.32; 1.11] (dataset 6) |
| Decision latitude (e) | 2.65* [1.13; 6.22] | 3.49* [1.33; 9.12] (dataset 5) |
| Social capital (e) | 2.78** [1.62; 4.76] | 2.81* [1.58; 5.00] (dataset 5) |
| Social capital (e) | 3.12** [1.69; 5.76] | 2.98** [1.60; 5.53] (dataset 6) |
| Depersonalization (e) | 0.56* [0.39; 0.81] | 0.58* [0.38; 0.87] (dataset 5) |
| Vigor (e) | 1.57** [1.22; 2.04] | 1.50** [1.14; 1.98] (dataset 6) |
| Dedication (e) | 1.45** [1.11; 1.9] | 1.55** [1.15; 2.1] (dataset 5) |

***$p$-value <0.001; **$p$-value <0.01; *$p$-value <0.05; *OR* odds ratio 95% CI [lower and upper bound]; (c) Excellent or good (1) versus fair or poor (0), (e) mean value; (f) Adjusted for years in nursing, years on present unit, gender, registered nurse (RN), work schedules

work engagement on nurse reported job outcomes and quality of care. Based on previous studies, nurse practice environment dimensions, nurse work characteristics, and burnout and work engagement dimensions were treated as independent variables (Van Bogaert et al. 2010, 2013c, e, 2014a).

Generalized linear mixed effects models were fitted analyzing first discrete dependent variables (simple multilevel models). To determine optimal predictive models, the final models were assessed with backward procedures dropping variables that did not improve goodness of fit (multiple multilevel models) (see Tables 3.6, 3.7, 3.8 and 3.9). Coefficients for all the independent measures were estimated in both unadjusted models and models adjusted for several nurse characteristics that had significant associations with at least one of the dependent variables. This was done in an attempt to adjust for potential confounders at the individual level such as age, years in nursing, years on the present unit, gender, education (dataset 4 bachelor of nursing science; dataset 5 ad 6 registered nurses RN), and work schedule as previously applied in various studies (Van Bogaert et al. 2010, 2013c, e, 2014a). In addition, adjustments were made for four types of units (dataset 4): (1) medical–surgical units, (2) ICU–medium care units, (3) OR and PACU, and (4) ER. Nursing units as well as nursing homes with sufficient response (>30%) were selected for multilevel analyses.

The Statistical Package for the Social Sciences (SPSS Inc, Chicago) version 20.0 software was used for descriptive analysis. PROC MIXED and PROC NLMIXED under SAS 9.2 (SAS Institute Inc, Cary, NC) were used to fit the multilevel models.

New analyses with additional study population of acute hospital care (dataset 4) and nursing homes (datasets 5 and 6) were set and compared with previous findings.

### 3.5.2   Multilevel Models in Acute Hospital Nursing Teams

Multilevel models show (see Tables 3.6 and 3.7) in acute hospital nursing teams that favorable assessed nurse practice environment dimensions, hospital management and organizational support predict job satisfaction with odds of 4 adjusted. In addition, emotional exhaustion predicts job dissatisfaction with odds of 47% as well as dedication and absorption predict job satisfaction with odds 2.40 adjusted. Emotional exhaustion, with odds of 36% has a negative impact, and personal accomplishment—with odds of almost 2—has a positive impact on no intention to leave the nursing profession. Moreover, dedication predicts no intention to leave the nursing profession with odds of 2.10 adjusted. We notice an unexpected *inverse* association between absorption and job satisfaction of 35% adjusted.

These results confirm largely our previous findings in acute care hospital as well as psychiatric hospital study population, although other variables were associated with job satisfaction and (no) intention to leave the hospital too such as nurse–physician relations (the latter), nurse management at the unit level (both), workload (the first), and depersonalization (the latter).

Nursing management at the unit level predicts quality of care at the unit and the last shift with odds of almost 8 and 4 adjusted, respectively. Social capital as well as engagement dimension vigor predicts quality of care at the unit with odds, respectively, of 3 and almost 1.5 adjusted. Emotional exhaustion has a negative impact on nurses' assessed quality of care (unit and last shift) with odds of 44% and 53%, respectively, and workload was negatively associated with quality of care at the last shift with odds of 53%. Personal accomplishment as well as vigor predicts quality of care at the unit with odds of almost 2 or more adjusted, and dedication predicts quality of care at the last shift with odds of almost 1.5 adjusted. These results confirm largely our previous findings in acute care hospital as well as psychiatric hospital study population, although other variables were associated with quality of care at the unit and the last shift too such as nurse–physician relations (both), hospital management and organizational support (the first), social capital (the latter), depersonalization and personal accomplishment (the latter), workload (the first), depersonalization (the latter), and dedication (the first) (Box 3.3).

---

**Box 3.3 Key Multilevel Model Findings**

- Multilevel models show that team dynamics are relevant on nurses' reported job outcomes and quality of care. Nurses' assessed practice environment and work characteristics as well as feelings of burnout and work engagement are not only individual experiences but also experiences within the team. Additional dataset of an acute hospital nursing team study population confirms largely various associations albeit certain inconsistency.

- Consistent prediction of emotional exhaustion on job dissatisfaction and nurse management at the unit level on quality of care at the unit as well as the last shift is shown in all findings, previous as well as current, adjusted for years in nursing, years on present unit, gender, bachelor of nursing science, work schedules, and type of unit.

- In previous and current findings, emotional exhaustion has an impact on intention to leave the nursing profession as well as personal accomplishment in the current findings. In current findings, emotional exhaustion has also a negative impact on quality of care at the unit and the last shift.

- Dedication has a positive impact on turnover intentions and job satisfaction in all findings, previous as well as current, and in the current findings on quality of care at the last shift along with workload. Social capital has a positive impact on nurse reported quality of care at the unit in a previous acute hospital care study population.

---

### 3.5.3  Multilevel Models: Data from Nursing Homes

Practice environment dimensions' nurse–physician relations, nurse management at the unit level, and nursing home management and organizational support (with odds of 1.8, 40.4, and 3.9, respectively) as well as nurse work characteristics' social capital and decision (with odds of 3.6 and 3.8, respectively) are associated with job satisfaction identified in one dataset. In addition, workload has a negative impact on job satisfaction with odds of 73%. Both datasets (see Tables 3.8 and 3.9) confirm association between depersonalization and low job satisfaction with odds of 41% and 51%. Work engagement dimensions vigor and absorption are associated with job satisfaction with odds of 2.50 and 2.2 adjusted.

Emotional exhaustion is associated with intention to leave the service as well as the nursing profession with odds of 64%–51% and 59%–50%, respectively, in both datasets. Nurse management at the unit level, social capital, vigor, and dedication have positive impact on (no) intention to leave the service with odds of 40, 3.3, 1.6, and 2, respectively, and workload has a negative impact with odds of 64% in one dataset. We notice an unexpected *inverse* association between absorption and (no) intention to leave the service with odds of 42% adjusted, and vigor had no relevant impact anymore adjusted. Nurse management at the unit level, decision latitude, and dedication have positive impact on (no) intention to leave the nursing profession with odds ranged from 1.8 to 6, and depersonalization has a negative impact with odds of 40% in one dataset.

Nurse management at the unit level, social capital, and vigor are positively associated with quality of care at the unit in both datasets with odds adjusted ranged from 10 to 17, 2.70 to 3, and 1.3 to 1.6, respectively. Both datasets identify an association between workload and unfavorable assessed quality of care at the unit with odds ranged from 40% to 62% although not significantly adjusted in one dataset. Personal accomplishment has a positive impact on quality of care at the unit but not significantly after adjustment in one dataset.

Nurse management at the unit level and social capital have a positive impact on nurse reported quality of care at the last shift with odds ratios of 2.9 and 5.6 in both datasets. Decision latitude and engagement dimensions' vigor and dedication are associated with favorable assessed quality of care at the last shift in one dataset with adjusted odds ratios of 3.5, 1.50, and 1.55, respectively. Workload, although not significant in adjusted models, and depersonalization are negatively associated with nurse reported quality of care on the last shift worked (Box 3.4).

---

**Box 3.4 Key Multilevel Model Findings from Nursing Homes**

- Multilevel models show that organizational dynamics are relevant on nurses' reported job outcomes and quality of care. Nurses' assessed practice environment and work characteristics as well as feelings of burnout and work engagement are not only individual experiences but also experiences within organizations. Both datasets identify some consistent results.
- Consistent predictions of depersonalization on job dissatisfaction and emotional exhaustion on intention to leave the service and nursing profession as well as nurse management at the unit level and social capital on nurse reported quality of care at the unit and the latest shift are shown in both datasets, adjusted for years in nursing, years on present unit, gender, registered nurse (RN), and work schedules.
- Vigor has a positive impact on nurse reported quality of care at the unit in both datasets and along with dedication on quality of care at the last shift in one dataset.
- Nurse practice environment dimensions, social capital, decision latitude, vigor, and absorption have a positive impact on satisfaction with the current job in one dataset.
- Nurse management at the unit level, social capital, and dedication have a positive impact on no intention to leave the nursing profession in one dataset. Unexpectedly, absorption has a negative impact on (no) intention to leave the service as well as workload in one dataset. Vigor has a positive impact on (no) intention to leave the service although not significantly adjusted in one dataset.
- Depersonalization has impact on intention to leave the nursing profession, as well as nurse management at the unit level, decision latitude, and dedication have a positive impact on no intention to leave the nursing profession in one dataset.
- Workload has a negative impact on nurse reported quality of care at the unit and the last shift although not significantly adjusted in one dataset. Personal accomplishment has a positive impact on quality of care at the unit but not significantly adjusted in one dataset.

## 3.6 Productive Ward Program™ as Part of a Long-Term Hospital Transformation Process and Changes in the Organizational Context of Nursing Practice: A Longitudinal Multilevel Study

### 3.6.1  Intervention and Study Context

In 2007, the Antwerp University Hospital's (Belgium) Chief Executive Officer (CEO) and Chief Nursing Officer (CNO) along with the hospital board decided to transform the hospital organization, guided by research findings of regarding organizational contexts of nursing practice and quality improvement processes (Van Bogaert et al. 2014b). This long-term, extensive transformation process was inspired by the principles of the ANCC Magnet Recognition Program® (ANCC 2005, 2014) to create a healthy nurse practice environment conducive to nurse professionalism, as well as retention, productivity, satisfaction of nurses, and safe and high-quality patient care. Three of the original 14 *forces of magnetism* guided a long-term organizational transformation process from a classic hierarchical and departmental form to one that was flat and interdisciplinary: (1) flat organizational structures, where unit-based decision-making prevailed, with sufficient nurse representation in the organizational committee structure; (2) a participative management style incorporating sufficient feedback from staff nurses and the presence of visible and accessible nursing leaders; and (3) positive interdisciplinary relations with mutual respect among all disciplines. Van Bogaert et al. (2014b) and the other chapters in this book (especially Chaps. 4 and 8) provide explanations and examples of changes implemented between 2007 and 2011.

In 2012 the PW program was introduced as an integral part of an internal hospital-wide governance policy to provide structural supports for nursing care and quality improvement processes (Van Bogaert et al. 2014b, 2017a, b). The Antwerp University Hospital was one of the first hospitals in Belgium to adopt and implement the Productive Ward—Releasing Time to Care™ program or PW program developed by the UK National Health Service (NHS) Institute for Innovation and Improvement, a program that was launched in 2007 (Morrow et al. 2012) (see Chap. 5). The NHS was commissioned to support the initial introduction of the program at the hospital, guided by a hospital steering committee (consisting of the CEO, CNO, HR manager, and a nursing leader) and a program management team (which included a nursing unit manager and a staff nurse).

### 3.6.2  Study Aim and Method

The aim of implementing the Productive Ward program was to support improvements in care delivery on clinical units within the structure of the long-term hospital transformation plan. The aim of the evaluation study was to investigate the impact of the quality improvement (QI) program Productive Ward—Releasing Time to Care™ using nurses' and midwives' reports of practice environment, burnout, quality of care, job outcomes (measurement periods T0 to T4), as well as workload, decision latitude, social capital, and engagement (measurement periods T1 to T4).

### 3.6.3 Study Population and Measures

Twenty-one clinical units were involved in the study: medical ($n = 7$), surgical ($n = 6$), intensive care (adult $n = 5$; neonatal $n = 1$), pediatric care ($n = 1$), and maternal care ($n = 1$). Staff nurses (all RNs) and midwives (all registered) working in these clinical units were invited by a coordinator/contact person to complete anonymous electronic questionnaires during a baseline (T0) and four measurement periods (Van Bogaert et al. 2014b, 2017a, b) with 344, 345, 377, 307, and 372 respondents, respectively: T0 (January 2006), T1 (June 2011), T2 (January 2013), T3 (October 2014), and T4 (March 2016).

Ten clinical units were early phase (Phase 1) PW adopters, followed by 11 clinical units in a second phase. Nurses and midwives on Phase 1 PW clinical units were informed about the program, implementation, and evaluation plan, followed by an invitation to complete the online survey. Rollout and learning commenced using the various PW modules and methods (between T1 and T2) with the three foundation modules at minimum, in addition to some planning and delivery modules. Nurses and midwives of Phase 2 PW clinical units were similarly informed about and enrolled in the study; however, implementation, rollout, and learning commenced using the various PW modules and methods (between T2 and T3) with at least the three foundation modules and in addition some planning and delivery modules. By T4, all modules were implemented, and it was therefore possible to evaluate the sustainability of the PW program (see Fig. 3.5).

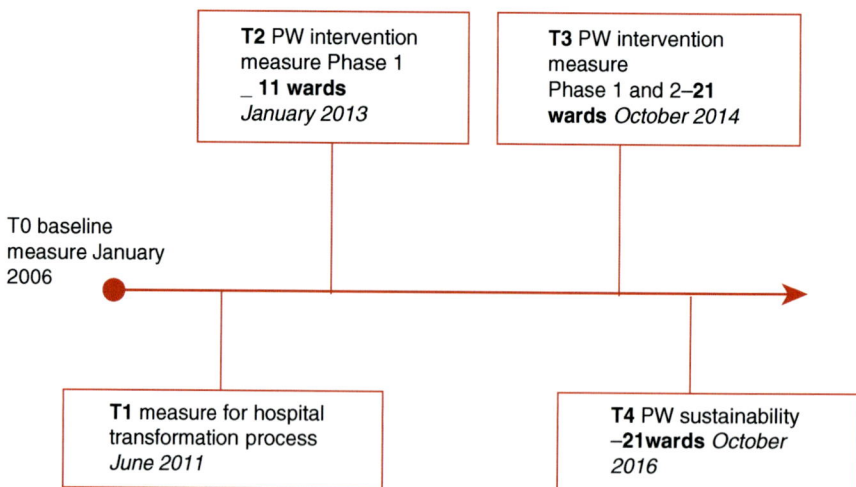

**Fig. 3.5** Intervention and study population

## 3.6.4   Data Analysis

Figures 3.6, 3.7, 3.8, 3.9, 3.10, 3.11, 3.12, 3.13 and 3.14 present the longitudinal results (means) for each variable during the study period. To investigate the effect of the PW intervention on the different outcome variables, multilevel models take into account the clustering of observations within clinical units (see Tables 3.10, 3.11, 3.12, 3.13 and 3.14). Conventional regression analysis ignores the correlation between observations coming from the same cluster, which leads to underestimate standard errors and an increased risk of Type I error. Therefore, by incorporating the nested structure of observations within nursing units, a two-level model corrects for

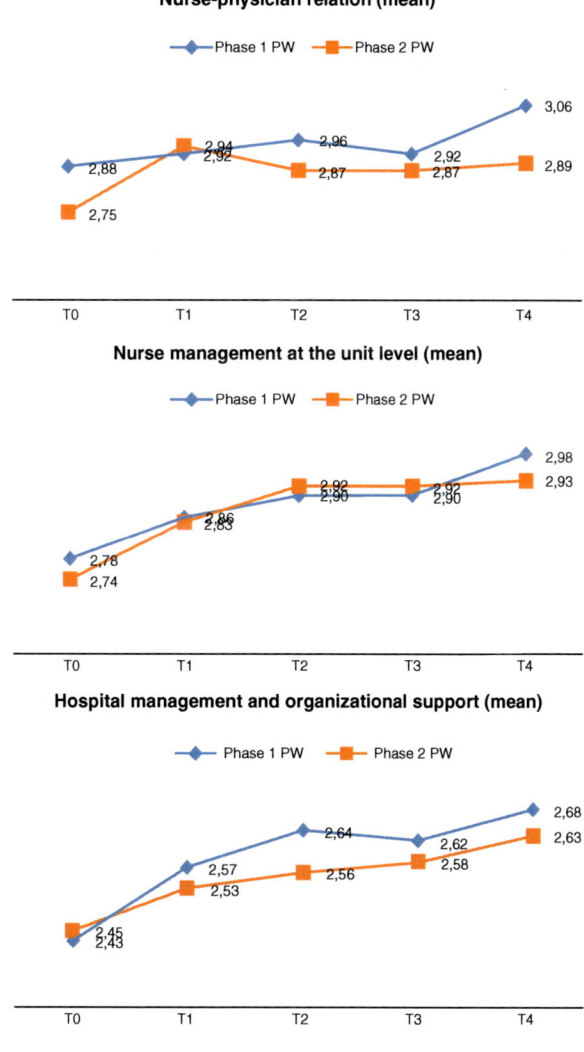

**Fig. 3.6**  Nurse practice environment dimensions

**Fig. 3.7** Nurse work
characteristics

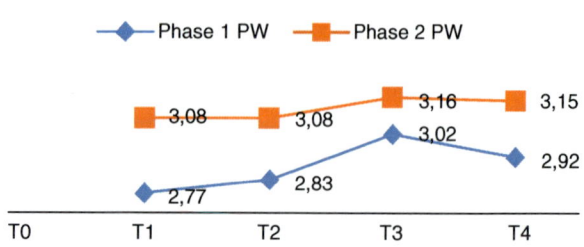

Workload (mean)

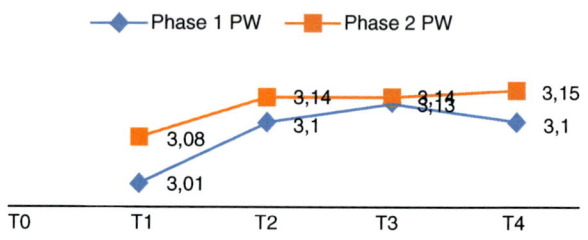

Decision latitude (mean)

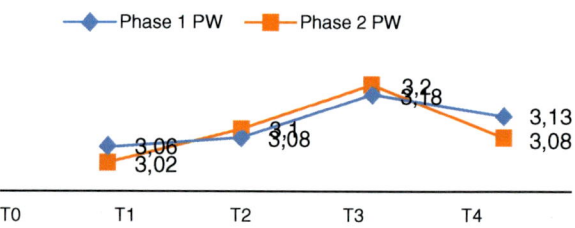

Social capital (mean)

the dependency among observations (Fitzmaurice et al. 2004; Park and Lake 2005). PROC MIXED and PROC NLMIXED under SAS 9.4 (SAS Institute Inc., Cary, NC) were used to fit multilevel models with post hoc comparisons.

Hierarchical regression analysis based on previous retested models estimated the strength of the associations with demographic characteristics (block-1), measurement period (time period T1 as indicator) (block-2), nurse practice environment dimensions (block-3), nurse work characteristics (block-4), and burnout dimensions (block-5) as explanatory variables of job satisfaction and turnover intention and quality of care as outcome variables (Tables 3.15 and 3.16) as well as demographic characteristics (block-1), measurement period (time period T1 as indicator)

**Fig. 3.8** Burnout
dimensions

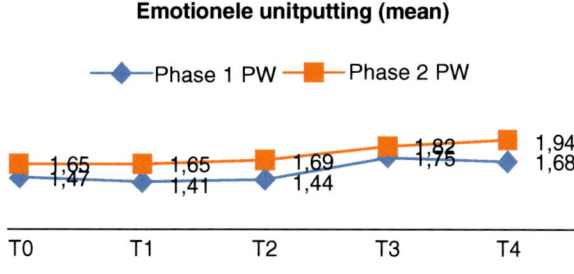

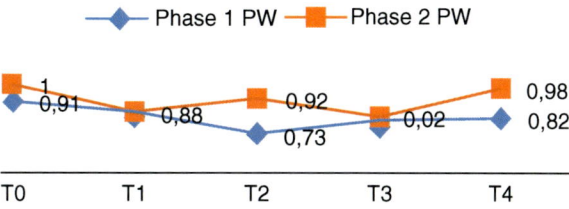

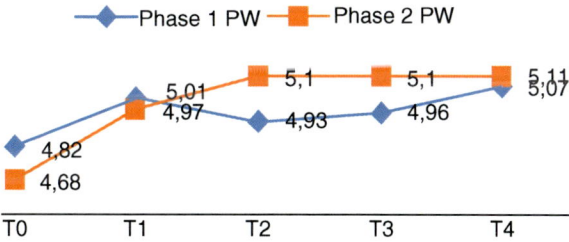

(block-2), nurse practice environment dimensions (block-3), nurse work characteristics (block-4), and engagement dimensions (block-5) as explanatory variables of job satisfaction and turnover intention and quality of care as outcome variables (Tables 3.17 and 3.18). In addition, hierarchical regression analysis estimated the strength of the associations with demographic characteristics (block-1), measurement period (time period T1 as indicator) (block-2), nurse practice environment dimensions (block-3), and nurse work characteristics (block-4) as explanatory variables of burnout risk or % high and very high on emotional exhaustion as well as depersonalization (Table 3.19).

**Fig. 3.9** Burnout risk and
high levels of burnout

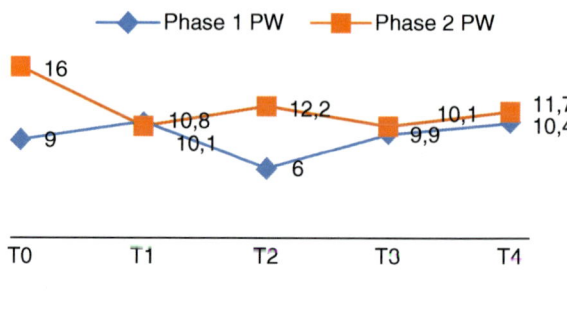

**Burnout risk %(very) hegh emotional exhaustion and
depersonalisation**

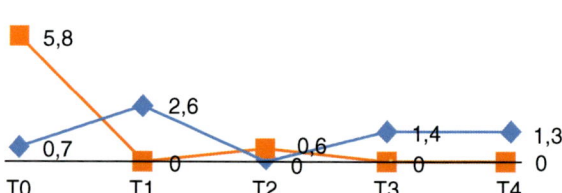

**Burnout %(very) high
on all three scales**

A generalized linear mixed effects model was fitted for the various binary variables. As the same clinical units were questioned at the different time points, clinical unit was added as a random effect to correct for this dependency. Tables 3.15, 3.16, 3.17, 3.18 and 3.19 provide the results for the final model including all the variables. Time was fitted as a categorical variable allowing difference between time points.

The percentage correctly classified for each block of variables was reported indicating the percentage of outcomes that can be predicted correctly using the model. For the outcomes' intention to leave hospital and nursing the method did not converge, hence a generalized linear model with correction for correlated structure was used. PROC GLIMMIX and GENMOD under SAS 9.4 were used to fit the models.

### 3.6.5   Study Results

Significant improvements (Van Bogaert et al. 2014a, b, c) were identified in all three nurse practice environment dimensions between measurement periods T0

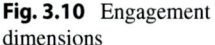

**Fig. 3.10** Engagement dimensions

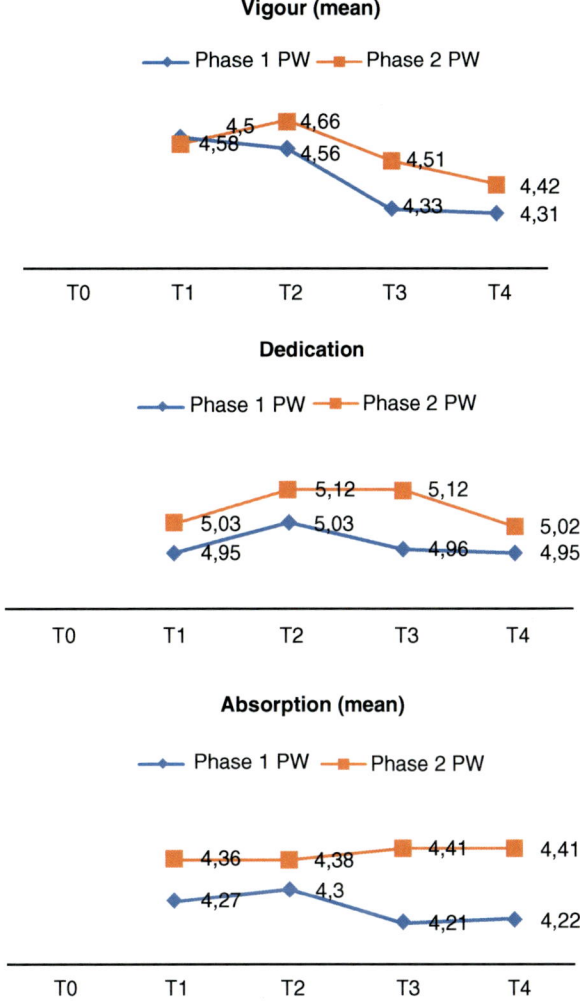

and T2 (the organizational transformation period) in Phase 1 PW as well in Phase 2 PW units, except for nurse–physician relations in Phase 1 PW units. Moreover, all dimensions increased over time during measurement periods T1 to T4 in Phase 1 PW as well as Phase 2 PW units, significantly, except for nurse–physician relations in Phase 2 PW units (see Table 3.10 and Fig. 3.6). Nurse–physician relations ranged from 2.89 to 3.06 or nurses' moderate to general agreement with the statements in T4. Agreement with nurse management at the unit-level statements was also moderate to general agreement ranging between 2.85 and 2.98. Instead nurses' assessed hospital management and organizational support was low but increased during time periods to more moderate agreements ranging from 2.53 to 2.68.

**Fig. 3.11** Job satisfaction

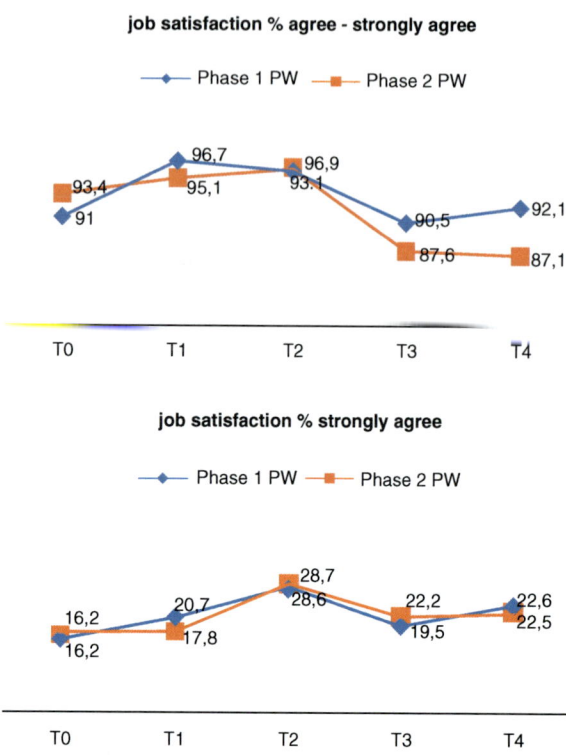

Significant improvements were noticed during the four measurement periods (T1–T4) in nurses' assessed work characteristics' decision latitude and social capital with general agreement of the statements ranging from 3.01 to 3.15 and 3.02 to 3.20, respectively, and significant for decision latitude in Phase 1 PW units (see Table 3.10 and Fig. 3.7). However, nurses' assessed workload was increased ranging from 2.77 to 3.16 and significant in Phase 1 PW units.

We found stable scores of emotional exhaustion and depersonalization during the study period for both Phase 1 PW and Phase 2 PW units; expect significant increased scores of emotional exhaustion in both PW units as well as depersonalization in Phase 2 PW units in the last two measurement periods (T3 and T4). Increased personal accomplishment scores were achieved in the organizational transformation period between T0 and T1, significant in Phase 2 PW unit, and established during the study period (see Table 3.11 and Fig. 3.8).

Burnout risk or high and very high levels of emotional exhaustion as well as depersonalization, the two primary burnout dimensions, ranged from 16% and 9% in T0 to 11.7% and 10.4% in T4 in, respectively, Phase 1 and Phase 2 PW units (see Fig. 3.9). We noticed in T2 the lowest prevalence of 6% in Phase 1 PW units. Burnout % of high and very high levels on all three burnout dimensions—staff nurses and midwives who were highly vulnerable for burnout—ranged

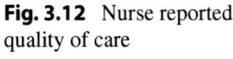

**Fig. 3.12** Nurse reported quality of care

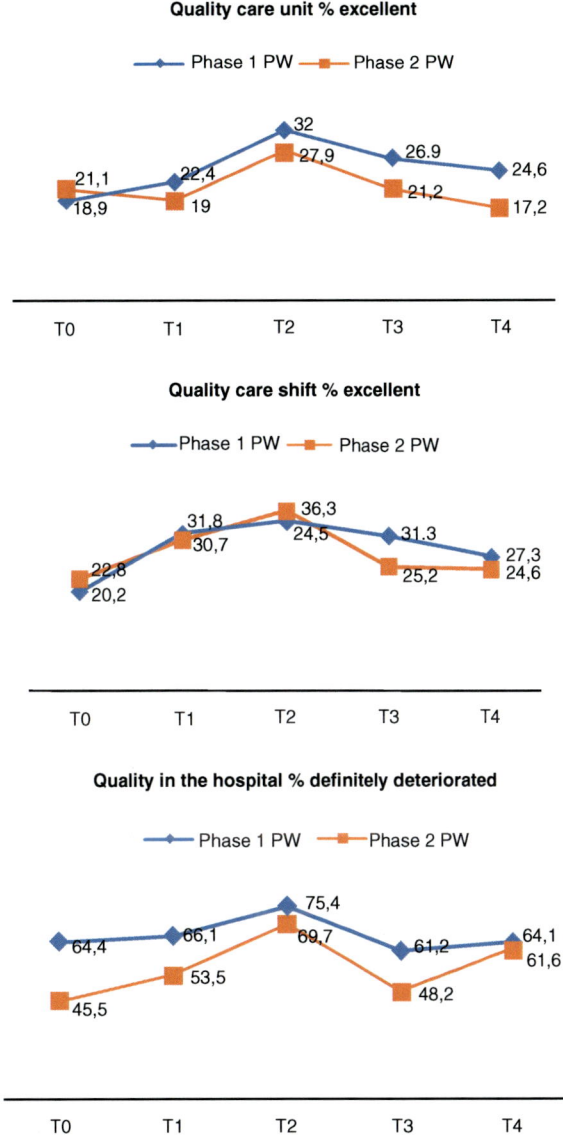

from 0.7% to 1.3% in Phase 1 PW units and 5.8% to 0% in Phase 2 PW units, respectively, in T0 and T4. We noticed prevalence of high and very high scores in all three scales in T0 of Phase 1 PW units and T1 of Phase 2 PW units, respectively.

We found also relatively stable scores of dedication and absorption during the study period for both Phase 1 PW and Phase 2 PW units. Scores of vigor

**Fig. 3.13** Staffing adequacy

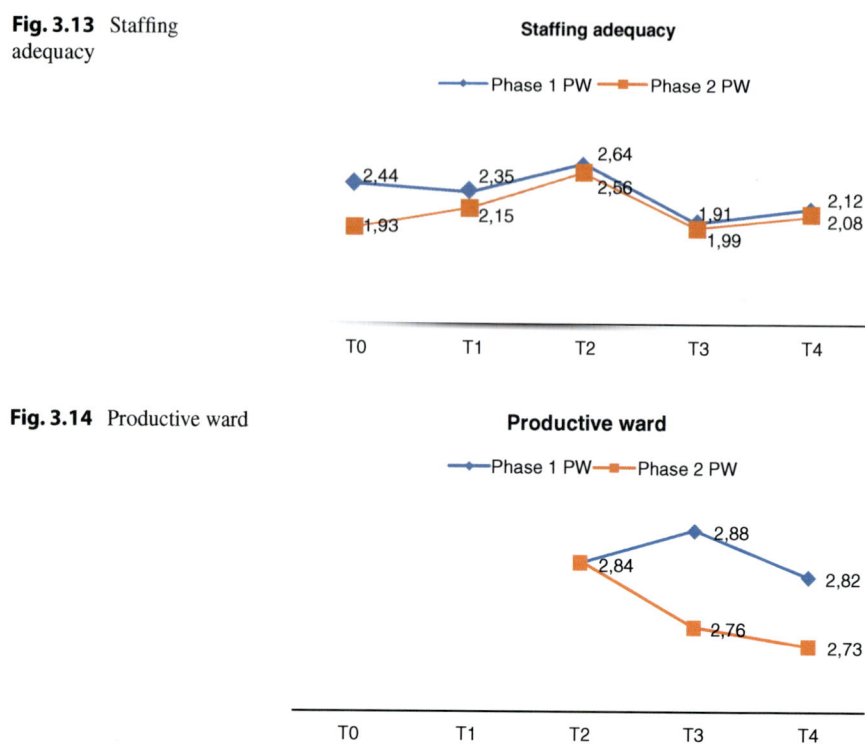

Staffing adequacy

Productive ward

**Fig. 3.14** Productive ward

decreased over the study period significantly in Phase 1 PW units (see Table 3.11 and Fig. 3.10).

In both Phase 1 PW and in Phase 2 PW units, job satisfaction evolved positively in the first three measurement periods (T0 to T2) significantly (see Van Bogaert et al. 2014a, b, c) but significant negatively in the fourth measurement period (T3) (see Van Bogaert et al. 2017a, b) with an increased number of nurses who rated (very) dissatisfied in T3 and T4, 9.5%/12.4% and 7.9% and 12.9%, respectively, in comparison with <5% in T1 and T2 (see Table 3.12 and Fig. 3.11).

In both Phase 1 PW and in Phase 2 PW units, nurse reported quality of care at the unit, the last shift, and in the hospital evolved positively in the first three measurement periods (T0–T2) significantly (see Van Bogaert et al. 2014a, b, c) but negatively in the last two measurement periods (T3 and T4) but not significant in comparison with T1 (see Table 3.12 and Fig. 3.11).

Staffing adequacy was during the study period rated as general disagreement (<2.5) with the statements "enough staff registered nurses and staff to provide quality patient care" and "enough staff to get the work done"; in Phase 1 PW units significantly decreased in T4 in comparison with T1 (see Table 3.13 and Fig. 3.13).

**Table 3.10** Descriptive measures and multilevel models of nurse practice environment and nurse characteristics

| | T1 | T3 | T4 | Estimates of mixed effects model[a] | | | |
| | | | | T4–T1 | | T4–T3 | |
| | Mean (SD) | Mean (SD) | Mean (SD) | B | SE | B | SE |
|---|---|---|---|---|---|---|---|
| *Nurse–physician relations*[b] | | | | | | | |
| Phase 1 PW | 2.92 (0.45) | 2.92 (0.55) | 3.07 (0.40) | 0.15** | 0.05 | 0.14** | 0.05** |
| Phase 2 PW | 2.94 (0.44) | 2.88 (0.46) | 2.89 (0.55) | −0.07 | 0.05 | −0.004 | 0.05 |
| *Nurse management at the unit-level*[b] | | | | | | | |
| Phase 1 PW | 2.86 (0.24) | 2.90 (0.26) | 2.98 (0.27) | 0.12*** | 0.03 | 0.03 | 0.03 |
| Phase 2 PW | 2.85 (0.36) | 2.92 (0.29) | 2.93 (0.38) | 0.06 | 0.03 | 0.002 | 0.03 |
| *Hospital management and organizational support*[b] | | | | | | | |
| Phase 1 PW | 2.57 (0.29) | 2.62 (0.32) | 2.67 (0.25) | 0.09*** | 0.03 | 0.05 | 0.03 |
| Phase 2 PW | 2.54 (0.30) | 2.58 (0.33) | 2.63 (0.35) | 0.08* | 0.03 | 0.03 | 0.03 |
| *Workload*[b] | | | | | | | |
| Phase 1 PW | 2.77 (0.44) | 3.03 (0.52) | 2.95 (0.48) | 0.18*** | 0.11 | −0.06 | 0.11 |
| Phase 2 PW | 3.08 (0.44) | 3.16 (0.51) | 3.14 (0.48) | 0.11* | 0.11 | −0.14 | 0.11 |
| *Decision latitude*[b] | | | | | | | |
| Phase 1 PW | 3.01 (0.28) | 3.13 (0.32) | 3.11 (0.27) | 0.10 | 0.03** | −0.02 | 0.03 |
| Phase 2 PW | 3.08 (0.28) | 3.14 (0.27) | 3.15 (0.31) | 0.06 | 0.03 | 0.003 | 0.03 |
| *Social capital*[b] | | | | | | | |
| Phase 1 PW | 3.06 (0.43) | 3.18 (0.50) | 3.13 (0.47) | 0.09 | 0.05 | −0.02 | 0.05 |
| Phase 2 PW | 3.02 (0.53) | 3.20 (0.53) | 3.08 (0.53) | 0.05 | 0.05 | −0.14** | 0.05 |

***$p$-value <0.001; **$p$-value <0.01; *$p$-value <0.05
[a]Linear mixed effects model with random intercept per nursing unit and fixed effects time (T1, T3, and T4), group (phase 1 PW/phase 2 PW), and interaction time × group
[b]Continuous scale ranging from 1 to 4; higher scores indicated a stronger agreement, or more favorable ratings, and workload where higher scores were indicative of a heavier burden and/or poorer conditions

A moderate agreement of the five Productive Ward statements, such as (1) I feel involved when working within the Productive Ward program; (2) I have developed required skills to work with various methodologies of the program; (3) in my unit, I

**Table 3.11** Descriptive measures and multilevel models of burnout and work engagement dimensions

| | T1 | T3 | T4 | Estimates of mixed effects model[a] | | | |
| | | | | T4–T1 | | T4–T3 | |
| | Mean (SD) | Mean (SD) | Mean (SD) | B | SE | B | SE |
|---|---|---|---|---|---|---|---|
| *Emotional exhaustion*[b] | | | | | | | |
| Phase 1 PW | 1.41 (0.97) | 1.75 (1.09) | 1.70 (1.07) | 0.26* | 0.11 | −0.06 | 0.11 |
| Phase 2 PW | 1.65 (1.00) | 1.87 (1.11) | 1.94 (1.20) | 0.037** | 0.11 | −0.14 | 0.11 |
| *Depersonalization*[b] | | | | | | | |
| Phase 1 PW | 0.84 (0.85) | 0.80 (0.70) | 0.83 (0.71) | −0.03 | 0.08 | 0.01 | 0.08 |
| Phase 2 PW | 0.85 (0.71) | 0.82 (0.71) | 0.98 (0.90) | 0.18* | 0.08 | 0.19* | 0.08 |
| *Personal accomplishment*[b] | | | | | | | |
| Phase 1 PW | 5.00 (0.78) | 4.96 (0.80) | 5.06 (0.74) | 0.08 | 0.08 | 0.12 | 0.08 |
| Phase 2 PW | 4.97 (0.77) | 5.10 (0.67) | 5.11 (0.79) | 0.12 | 0.08 | −0.01 | 0.08 |
| *Vigor*[b] | | | | | | | |
| Phase 1 PW | 4.60 (1.08) | 4.56 (1.13) | 4.31 (1.26) | −0.28* | 0.12 | 0.004 | −0.12 |
| Phase 2 PW | 4.58 (1.12) | 4.66 (1.13) | 4.42 (1.32) | −0.08 | 0.18 | −0.11 | 0.13 |
| *Dedication*[b] | | | | | | | |
| Phase 1 PW | 4.95 (1.06) | 4.96 (1.06) | 4.95 (1.06) | 0.02 | 0.11 | −0.004 | 0.11 |
| Phase 2 PW | 5.03 (0.97) | 5.12 (0.90) | 5.01 (1.09) | −0.04 | 0.11 | −0.13 | 0.11 |
| *Absorption*[b] | | | | | | | |
| Phase 1 PW | 4.27 (1.35) | 4.21 (1.38) | 4.22 (1.32) | −0.03 | 0.14 | 0.02 | 0.15 |
| Phase 2 PW | 4.38 (1.28) | 4.41 (1.12) | 4.40 (1.31) | 0.007 | 0.14 | −0.03 | 0.14 |

*PW* Productive Ward

***$p$-value <0.001; **$p$-value <0.01; *$p$-value <0.05

[a]Linear mixed effects model with random intercept per nursing unit and fixed effects time (T1, T3, and T4), group (Phase 1PW/Phase 2PW), and interaction time × group

[b]Continuous scale ranging from 0 to 6; higher scores indicated a stronger agreement, or more favorable ratings, with the exception of emotional exhaustion and depersonalization, where higher scores were indicative of a heavier burden and/or poorer conditions

**Table 3.12** Descriptive measures and multilevel models of nurse reported quality of care and job satisfaction

| | T1 (%) | T3 (%) | T4 (%) | Estimates of cumulative logit mixed model[a] | | | |
| | | | | T4–T1 | | T4–T3 | |
| | | | | OR | 95% CI | OR | 95% CI |
|---|---|---|---|---|---|---|---|
| *Quality of care at the current unit*[b] | | | | | | | |
| Phase 1 PW 1 | 0.6 | 1.3 | 1.1 | 1.08 | 0.70–1.66 | 1.13 | 0.73-1.75 |
| 2 | 8.9 | 13.8 | 10.3 | | | | |
| 3 | 68.2 | 58.1 | 64 | | | | |
| 4 | 22.4 | 26.9 | 24.6 | | | | |
| Phase 2 PW 1 | 1.2 | 0.7 | 1.6 | 0.77 | 0.50–1.21 | 0.65 | 0.42–1.03 |
| 2 | 14.1 | 12.3 | 14.2 | | | | |
| 3 | 65.6 | 65.8 | 63.5 | | | | |
| 4 | 19.0 | 21.2 | 20.7 | | | | |
| *Quality of care at the last shift*[b] | | | | | | | |
| Phase 1 PW 1 | 0.6 | 1.3 | 2.8 | 0.95 | 0.63–145 | 1.06 | 0.69–1.64 |
| 2 | 6.2 | 8.8 | 2.8 | | | | |
| 3 | 61.5 | 58.8 | 65.3 | | | | |
| 4 | 31.8 | 31.3 | 29 | | | | |
| Phase 2 PW 1 | 0.6 | 0.7 | 2.2 | 0.80 | 0.52–1.23 | 1.23 | 0.79–1.92 |
| 2 | 7.4 | 14.3 | 5.1 | | | | |
| 3 | 61.4 | 59.9 | 65.9 | | | | |
| 4 | 30.7 | 25.2 | 26.8 | | | | |
| *Quality of care in the hospital the last year*[b] | | | | | | | |
| Phase 1 PW 1 | 1.8 | 5.7 | 1.8 | 0.95 | 0.63–1.45 | 1.06 | 0.69–1.64 |
| 2 | 32.1 | 33.1 | 32.4 | | | | |
| 3 | 60.1 | 52.9 | 57.6 | | | | |
| 4 | 6.0 | 8.3 | 8.2 | | | | |
| Phase 2 PW 1 | 4.5 | 5.0 | 2.2 | 0.80 | 0.52–1.23 | 1.23 | 0.78–1.93 |
| 2 | 42.0 | 46.8 | 33.3 | | | | |
| 3 | 49.0 | 46.1 | 56.9 | | | | |
| 4 | 4.5 | 2.1 | 7.5 | | | | |
| *Job satisfaction*[c] | | | | | | | |
| Phase 1 PW 1 | 2.2 | 3.8 | 3.4 | 0.95 | 0.60–1.48 | 1.24 | 0.77–1.98 |
| 2 | 1.1 | 5.7 | 4.5 | | | | |
| 3 | 76.0 | 71.1 | 69.3 | | | | |
| 4 | 20.7 | 19.5 | 22.7 | | | | |
| Phase 2 PW 1 | 2.2 | 1.4 | 4.3 | 0.84 | 0.52–1.33 | 0.94 | 0.58–1.51 |
| 2 | 1.1 | 11.0 | 6.2 | | | | |
| 3 | 76.0 | 66.4 | 66.8 | | | | |
| 4 | 20.7 | 21.2 | 22.7 | | | | |

*PW* Productive Wards
***p*-value <0.001; **p*-value <0.01; *p*-value <0.05
[a]Cumulative logit mixed effects model with random intercept per nursing unit and fixed effects time (T1, T3, and T4), group (passive PW/active PW), and interaction time × group
[b](1) Poor, (2) fair, (3) good, (4) excellent
[c](1) very dissatisfied, (2) dissatisfied, (3) satisfied, (4) very satisfied

**Table 3.13** Descriptive measures and multilevel models of nurse practice environment staffing adequacy scale

| | T1 | T3 | T4 | Estimates of mixed effects model[a] | | | |
| | | | | T4–T1 | | T4–T3 | |
| | Mean (SD) | Mean (SD) | Mean (SD) | B | SE | B | SE |
| *Staffing adequacy scale*[b] | | | | | | | |
| Phase 1 PW | 2.44 (0.65) | 1.99 (0.69) | 2.13 (0.63) | −0.33*** | 0.06 | 0.12 | 0.06 |
| Phase 2 PW | 1.93 (0.60) | 1.91 (0.71) | 2.08 (0.73) | 0.08 | 0.06 | 0.12 | 0.07 |

*PW* Productive Wards
***$p$ value <0.001; **$p$-value <0.01; *$p$-value <0.05
[a]Linear mixed effects model with random intercept per nursing unit and fixed effects time (T1, T3, and T4), group (passive PW/active PW), and interaction time × group
[b]Continuous scale ranging from 1 to 4; higher scores indicated a stronger agreement, or more favorable ratings

**Table 3.14** Descriptive measures and multilevel models of Productive Ward scale

| | T2 | T3 | T4 | Estimates of mixed effects model[a] | | | |
| | | | | T4–T2 | | T4–T3 | |
| | Mean (SD) | Mean (SD) | Mean (SD) | B | SE | B | SE |
| *Productive Ward scale*[b] | | | | | | | |
| Phase 1 PW | 2.84 (0.42) | 2.88 (0.34) | 2.82 (0.42) | −0.008 | 0.04 | −0.042 | 0.043 |
| Phase 2 PW | | 2.76 (0.38) | 2.73 (0.46) | | | −0.023 | 0.043 |

*PW* Productive Wards
***$p$-value <0.001; **$p$-value <0.01; *$p$-value <0.05
[a]Logistic mixed effects model with random intercept per nursing unit and fixed effects time (T1, T3, and T4), group (passive PW/active PW), and interaction time × group
[b]Continuous scale ranging from 1 to 4; higher scores indicated a stronger agreement, or more favorable ratings

use learned Productive Ward methodologies; (4) in the near future, I have the intention to work further with PW methodologies; and (5) the hospital board supports the program perfectly, was assessed by the respondents ranged from 2.84 in T2 in Phase 1 PW unit to 2.82 and 2.73 in T4, respectively, in Phase 1 and Phase 2 units. For both units the following assessments were lower than the first, but not significant (see Table 3.14 and Fig. 3.14) (Box 3.5).

**Box 3.5 Key Findings of Nursing Organizational Transformation Process and Introduction Productive Ward**

- Both the hospital organizational transformation process and the introduction of the Productive Ward program appeared to have positive impact on the nurse practice environment and work characteristic dimensions with in turn significant improvements on job satisfaction as well as quality of care at the unit, the last shift, and the hospital. Burnout dimensions stayed rather stable except an improvement of personal accomplishment over the study period. Productive ward statements were assessed with moderate agreement, although staffing adequacy was rated unfavorable with a general agreement during the study period because of the Belgian hospital finance system for nursing care.
- Results in the last two measurement periods showed some discordance with increased perceived workload and feelings of emotional exhaustion and decreased feelings of vigor as well as decreased job satisfaction and nurse reported quality of care probably, among others, induced by common peculiar circumstances the hospital was going through such as an adjustment of nursing staff budget in 2014 and a Joint Commission International accreditation process in 2014 as well as in 2017.

Hierarchical regression analyses showed (see Table 3.15) nurse management at the unit level, hospital management and organizational support, and social capital were positively associated with job satisfaction (very satisfied), while the first was positively associated with no intention to leave the hospital. Emotional exhaustion and personal accomplishment were, respectively, negatively and positively associated with job satisfaction, while personal accomplishment was also negatively associated with intention to leave the hospital and nursing. However, depersonalization was positively associated with job satisfaction (very satisfied), a counterintuitive result. Relevant differences were noticed between measurement periods in job satisfaction (very satisfied), and demographic characteristics were relevant for job satisfaction (very satisfied) (women are more very satisfied), intention to leave the hospital (work schedule inverse associated), and intention to leave nursing (years in nursing and work schedule both inverse associated). The total percentage correctly classified for the proposed model with five blocks indicating the percentage job satisfaction (very satisfied), intention to leave the hospital, and intention to leave nursing that can be predicted correctly using the model were 82%, 94%, and 92%, respectively.

**Table 3.15** Hierarchical regression analyses with personal characteristics (1), measurement period (time period), (2) nurse practice environment (3) work characteristics (4) and burnout (5) (explanatory variables) and job satisfaction and turnover intentions (dependent variables)

| Independent variables | Job satisfaction (very satisfied) | | | | Intention to leave hospital (yes) | | | | Intention to leave nursing (yes) | | | |
|---|---|---|---|---|---|---|---|---|---|---|---|---|
| | Estimate | OR | 95% CI | | Estimate | OR | 95% CI | | Estimate | OR | 95% CI | |
| Intercept | −17.607 | | | | 8.073 | | | | 4.062ε | | | |
| Women | 0.641 | **1.898*** | 1.092 | 3.302 | 0.207 | 1.230 | 0.516 | 2.933 | −0.886 | 0.412 | 0.179 | 0.51 |
| Men | 0 | | | | 0 | | | | 0 | | | |
| Years in nursing | −0.003 | 0.997 | 0.969 | 1.025 | −0.003 | 0.996 | 0.944 | 1.051 | −0.052 | **0.950*** | 0.911 | 0.990 |
| Years present unit | −0.047 | **0.954**** | 0.923 | 0.986 | −0.030 | 0.970 | 0.902 | 1.043 | −0.026 | 0.975 | 0.911 | 1.043 |
| Work schedule | 0.016 | **1.016*** | 1.003 | 1.030 | −0.017 | **0.982*** | 0.970 | 0.996 | −0.026 | **0.974*** | 0.955 | 0.993 |
| Bachelor (yes) | 0.631 | 1.880 | 0.995 | 3.554 | −0.124 | 0.883 | 0.371 | 2.100 | 0.942 | 2.565 | 0.514 | 12.812 |
| Bachelor (no) | 0 | | | | 0 | | | | 0 | | | |
| T2 | 0.672 | **1.958**** | 1.191 | 3.220 | 0.360 | 1.432 | 0.660 | 3.109 | 0.169 | 1.185 | 0.551 | 2.544 |
| T3 | −0.155 | 0.857 | 0.489 | 1.502 | 0.166 | 1.180 | 0.589 | 2.365 | 0.486 | 1.625 | 0.657 | 4.022 |
| T4 | −0.019 | 0.981 | 0.587 | 1.639 | 0.533 | 1.704 | 0.919 | 3.163 | 0.246 | 1.279 | 0.661 | 2.474 |
| T1 [a] | 0 | | | | 0 | | | | 0 | | | |
| Nurse–physician relations | 0.122 | 1.129 | 0.743 | 1.717 | −0.713 | 0.490 | 0.281 | 0.855 | 0.218 | 1.243 | 0.742 | 2.085 |
| Nurse management | 2.141 | **8.511***** | 3.253 | 22.269 | −1.593 | **0.203*** | 0.062 | 0.666 | 0.168 | 1.183 | 0.320 | 4.370 |
| Hospital management | 0.962 | **2.616*** | 1.156 | 5.917 | −0.778 | 0.459 | 0.151 | 1.395 | −1.289 | 0.275 | 0.084 | 0.902 |
| Decision latitude | 0.203 | 1.225 | 0.590 | 2.545 | 1.019 | 2.770 | 1.198 | 6.405 | −0.682 | 0.506 | 0.182 | 1.404 |
| Workload | −0.326 | 0.722 | 0.46 | 1.133 | −0.716 | 0.488 | 0.194 | 1.228 | 0.259 | 1.296 | 0.642 | 2.615 |
| Social capital | 0.632 | **1.880**** | 1.181 | 2.994 | −0.060 | 0.942 | 0.502 | 1.768 | 0.277 | 1.319 | 0.662 | 2.628 |
| Emotional exhaustion | −0.861 | **0.423***** | 0.322 | 0.556 | 0.494 | 1.639 | 1.122 | 2.394 | 0.388 | **1.474*** | 1.122 | 1.938 |
| Depersonalization | 0.462 | **1.586***** | 1.178 | 2.137 | −0.082 | 0.921 | 0.681 | 1.246 | 0.065 | 1.067 | 0.785 | 1.451 |
| Personal accomplishment | 0.809 | **2.246***** | 1.625 | 3.105 | −0.558 | **0.572*** | 0.400 | 0.818 | −0.416 | **0.659*** | 0.472 | 0.920 |

*$p$-value<0.05, **$p$-value<0.01, ***$p$-value <0.001
[a]T1 as indicator

**Table 3.16** Hierarchical regression analyses with personal characteristics (1), measurement period (time period), (2) nurse practice environment (3) work characteristics (4) and burnout (5) (explanatory variables) and quality of care (dependent variables)

| Independent variables | Quality unit (good excellent) | | | | Quality last shift (good excellent) | | | | Quality hospital last year (improved certainly improved) | | | |
|---|---|---|---|---|---|---|---|---|---|---|---|---|
| | Estimate | OR | 95% CI | | Estimate | OR | 95% CI | | Estimate | OR | 95% CI | |
| Intercept | −10.128 | | | | −1.394 | | | | −7.140 | | | |
| Women | 0.331 | 1.392 | 0.772 | 2.513 | −0.549 | 0.577 | 0.259 | 1.287 | −0.024 | 0.977 | 0.615 | 1.552 |
| Men | 0 | | | | 0 | | | | 0 | | | |
| Years in nursing | −0.010 | 0.990 | 0.958 | 1.024 | −0.028 | 0.972 | 0.940 | 1.006 | −0.027 | 0.973* | 0.950 | 0.997 |
| Yearns present unit | 0.030 | 1.030 | 0.990 | 1.072 | 0.046 | 1.047* | 1.003 | 1.093 | 0.007 | 1.007 | 0.980 | 1.036 |
| Work schedule | 0.008 | 1.008 | 0.993 | 1.023 | 0.002 | 1.002 | 0.985 | 1.019 | 0.000 | 1.000 | 0.990 | 1.011 |
| Bachelor (yes) | −0.378 | 0.686 | 0.301 | 1.563 | 0.083 | 1.086 | 0.482 | 2.446 | −0.272 | 0.762 | 0.451 | 1.285 |
| Bachelor (no) | 0 | | | | 0 | | | | 0 | | | |
| T2 | −0.090 | 0.914 | 0.480 | 1.742 | 0.126 | 1.135* | 0.537 | 2.399 | 0.664 | 1.941** | 1.252 | 3.010 |
| T3 | −0.579 | 0.561 | 0.294 | 1.070 | −0.727 | 0.483 | 0.240 | 0.974 | −0.180 | 0.836 | 0.538 | 1.297 |
| T4 | −0.585 | 0.557 | 0.301 | 1.030 | 0.202 | 1.224 | 0.586 | 2.556 | 0.064 | 1.066 | 0.699 | 1.627 |
| T1[a] | 0 | | | | 0 | | | | 0 | | | |
| Nurse–physician relations | 0.089 | 1.093 | 0.679 | 1.760 | −0.532 | 0.588 | 0.332 | 1.039 | 0.336 | 1.399 | 0.966 | 2.027 |
| Nurse management | 1.006 | 2.733 | 0.953 | 7.842 | 1.282 | 3.602* | 1.127 | 11.511 | 1.621 | 5.059*** | 2.234 | 11.456 |
| Hospital management | 0.549 | 1.731 | 0.719 | 4.169 | −0.201 | 0.818 | 0.310 | 2.160 | 1.496 | 4.464*** | 2.276 | 8.756 |
| Decision latitude | 0.327 | 1.387 | 0.566 | 3.398 | 0.782 | 2.186 | 0.773 | 6.183 | −0.239 | 0.788 | 0.407 | 1.526 |
| Workload | −0.021 | 0.980 | 0.551 | 1.742 | −0.616 | 0.540 | 0.282 | 1.035 | −0.848 | 0.428*** | 0.278 | 0.659 |
| Social capital | 1.699 | 5.466*** | 3.038 | 9.833 | 0.695 | 2.003* | 1.102 | 3.643 | 0.539 | 1.713* | 1.138 | 2.580 |
| Emotional exhaustion | −0.392 | 0.676** | 0.528 | 0.865 | −0.298 | 0.742* | 0.563 | 0.978 | −0.233 | 0.792* | 0.658 | 0.954 |
| Depersonalization | 0.073 | 1.076 | 0.814 | 1.423 | −0.330 | 0.719* | 0.532 | 0.970 | 0.017 | 1.017 | 0.814 | 1.272 |
| Personal accomplishment | 0.384 | 1.468** | 1.107 | 1.947 | 0.189 | 1.208 | 0.865 | 1.687 | 0.154 | 1.167 | 0.935 | 1.456 |

*$p$-value <0.05, **$p$-value <0.01, ***$p$-value <0.001

[a]T1 as indicator

**Table 3.17** Hierarchical regression analyses with personal characteristics (1), measurement period (time period), (2) nurse practice environment (3) work characteristics (4) and engagement (5) (explanatory variables) and job satisfaction and turnover intentions (dependent variables)

| Independent variables | Job satisfaction (very satisfied) | | | | Intention to leave hospital (yes) | | | | Intention to leave nursing (yes) | | | |
|---|---|---|---|---|---|---|---|---|---|---|---|---|
| | Estimate | OR | 95% CI | | Estimate | OR | 95% CI | | Estimate | OR | 95% CI | |
| Intercept | −19.416 | | | | 6.248 | | | | 4.212 | | | |
| Women | 0.357 | 1.429 | 0.826 | 2.472 | 0.512 | 1.668 | 0.655 | 4.252 | −0.84 | 0.432 | 0.166 | 1.120 |
| Men | 0 | | | | 0 | | | | | | | |
| Years in nursing | 0.010 | 1.010 | 0.982 | 1.039 | −0.008 | 0.992 | 0.937 | 1.049 | −0.075 | 0.927* | 0.879 | 0.978 |
| Years present unit | −0.046 | 0.956** | 0.925 | 0.987 | −0.028 | 0.973 | 0.903 | 1.048 | −0.019 | 0.981 | 0.920 | 1.046 |
| Work schedule | 0.011 | 1.011 | 0.998 | 1.024 | −0.015 | 0.985 | 0.974 | 0.997 | −0.024 | 0.975* | 0.958 | 0.994 |
| Bachelor (yes) | 0.690 | 1.994* | 1.093 | 3.638 | −0.033 | 0.968 | 0.521 | 1.798 | 0.961 | 2.613 | 0.552 | 12.364 |
| Bachelor (no) | 0 | | | | 0 | | | | 0 | | | |
| T2 | 0.652 | 1.919** | 1.165 | 3.162 | 0.284 | 1.329 | 0.715 | 2.470 | 0.041 | 1.041 | 0.492 | 2.200 |
| T3 | −0.161 | 0.851 | 0.485 | 1.494 | 0.036 | 1.036 | 0.577 | 1.860 | 0.465 | 1.591 | 0.671 | 3.772 |
| T4 | 0.031 | 1.031 | 0.612 | 1.737 | 0.230 | 1.259 | 0.757 | 2.095 | 0.285 | 1.329 | 0.662 | 2.669 |
| T1[a] | 0 | | | | 0 | | | | 0 | | | |
| Nurse–physician relations | 0.085 | 1.089 | 0.703 | 1.685 | −0.631 | 0.532* | 0.324 | 0.875 | 0.385 | 1.468 | 0.835 | 2.581 |
| Nurse management | 1.861 | 6.430*** | 2.430 | 17.017 | −1.779 | 0.169* | 0.049 | 0.584 | 0.284 | 1.328 | 0.348 | 5.073 |

| | | | | | | | | | | | | |
|---|---|---|---|---|---|---|---|---|---|---|---|---|
| Hospital management | 0.625 | 1.868 | 0.813 | 4.293 | −0.471 | 0.624 | 0.206 | 1.897 | −1.211 | **0.297*** | 0.112 | 0.787 |
| Decision latitude | 0.379 | 1.461 | 0.707 | 3.018 | 0.923 | 2.516 | 0.929 | 6.818 | −0.643 | 0.525 | 0.207 | 1.334 |
| Workload | −0.835 | **0.434*****| 0.285 | 0.662 | 0.034 | 1.035 | 0.565 | 1.897 | 0.544 | **1.723*** | 1.111 | 2.672 |
| Social capital | 0.508 | **1.662*** | 1.059 | 2.607 | 0.011 | 1.011 | 0.554 | 1.844 | 0.306 | 1.357 | 0.694 | 2.654 |
| vigor | 0.240 | 1.271 | 0.958 | 1.686 | 0.045 | 0.956 | 0.774 | 1.182 | 0.035 | 1.035 | 0.775 | 1.382 |
| Dedication | 1.226 | **3.409*****| 2.170 | 5.354 | −0.875 | **0.417**** | 0.318 | 0.546 | −0.738 | **0.478**** | 0.332 | 0.686 |
| Absorption | 0.209 | 1.232 | 0.969 | 1.568 | 0.329 | **1.390*** | 1.102 | 1.752 | −0.028 | 0.972 | 0.698 | 1.352 |

*$p$-value $<0.05$, **$p$-value $<0.01$, ***$p$-value $<0.001$
[a]T1 as indicator

**Table 3.18** Hierarchical regression analyses with personal characteristics (1), measurement period (time period), (2) nurse practice environment (3) work characteristics (4) and engagement (5) (explanatory variables) and quality of care (dependent variables)

| Independent variables | Quality unit (good excellent) | | | Quality last shift (good excellent) | | | Quality hospital last year (improved certainly improved) | | |
|---|---|---|---|---|---|---|---|---|---|
| | B | OR | 95% CI | B | OR | 95% CI | Estimate | OR | 95% CI |
| Intercept | −8.796 | | | −2.115 | | | −7.368 | | |
| Women | 0.252 | 1.286 | 0.728 2.274 | −0.490 | 0.613 | 0.288 1.302 | −0.098 | 0.907 | 0.577 1.427 |
| Men | 0 | | | 0 | | | 0 | | |
| Years in nursing | −0.004 | 0.996 | 0.964 1.028 | −0.019 | 0.981 | 0.948 1.015 | −0.019 | 0.981 | 0.958 1.005 |
| Yearns present unit | 0.022 | 1.022 | 0.983 1.063 | 0.041 | 1.042 | 0.999 1.087 | 0.003 | 1.003 | 0.976 1.031 |
| Work schedule | 0.001 | 1.001 | 0.987 1.015 | −0.006 | 0.994 | 0.978 1.011 | −0.003 | 0.997 | 0.986 1.007 |
| Bachelor (yes) | −0.240 | 0.787 | 0.377 1.643 | 0.136 | 1.145 | 0.550 2.384 | −0.292 | 0.747 | 0.449 1.241 |
| Bachelor (no) | 0 | | | 0 | | | 0 | | |
| T2 | −0.059 | 0.942 | 0.514 1.727 | −0.053 | 0.949** | 0.468 1.922 | 0.673 | 1.959** | 1.275 3.011 |
| T3 | −0.536 | 0.585 | 0.317 1.080 | −0.850 | 0.428 | 0.219 0.836 | −0.215 | 0.807 | 0.523 1.246 |
| T4 | −0.483 | 0.617 | 0.341 1.115 | 0.106 | 1.112 | 0.539 2.296 | 0.104 | 1.109 | 0.727 1.694 |
| T1[a] | 0 | | | 0 | | | 0 | | |
| Nurse–physician relations | −0.045 | 0.956 | 0.603 1.513 | −0.689 | 0.502* | 0.291 0.866 | 0.241 | 1.272 | 0.886 1.828 |
| Nurse management | 1.024 | 2.783* | 1.002 7.736 | 1.087 | 2.965 | 0.950 9.255 | 1.711 | 5.534*** | 2.458 12.455 |

| | | | | | | | | | | | |
|---|---|---|---|---|---|---|---|---|---|---|---|
| Hospital management | 0.574 | 1.775 | 0.759 | 4.152 | 0.051 | 1.052 | 0.412 | 2.685 | 1.605 | **4.978***** | 2.540 | 9.754 |
| Decision latitude | 0.378 | 1.459 | 0.617 | 3.454 | 1.058 | **2.879*** | 1.041 | 7.966 | −0.233 | 0.792 | 0.412 | 1.521 |
| Workload | −0.400 | 0.670 | 0.407 | 1.103 | −1.012 | **0.364**** | 0.210 | 0.631 | −1.050 | **0.350***** | 0.238 | 0.515 |
| Social capital | 1.726 | **5.616***** | 3.189 | 9.890 | 0.705 | **2.025*** | 1.163 | 3.525 | 0.523 | **1.687*** | 1.132 | 2.513 |
| Vigor | 0.242 | **1.274*** | 1.000 | 1.622 | 0.087 | 1.091 | 0.825 | 1.444 | 0.151 | 1.163 | 0.962 | 1.406 |
| Dedication | 0.218 | 1.244 | 0.918 | 1.686 | 0.515 | **1.674**** | 1.185 | 2.366 | 0.025 | 1.026 | 0.801 | 1.313 |
| Absorption | −0.144 | 0.866 | 0.673 | 1.114 | −0.215 | 0.806 | 0.603 | 1.078 | 0.101 | 1.107 | 0.921 | 1.330 |

*$p$-value $<0.05$, **$p$-value $<0.01$, ***$p$-value $<0.001$
[a]T1 as indicator

**Table 3.19** Hierarchical regression analyses with personal characteristics (1), measurement period (time period), (2) nurse practice environment (3) work characteristics (4) (explanatory variables) and burnout risk (% high and very high levels of emotional exhaustion and depersonalization) (dependent variables)

| Independent variables | Burnout risk or % high and very high levels of emotional exhaustion and depersonalization | | | |
|---|---|---|---|---|
| | B | OR | 95% CI | |
| Intercept | −0.172 | | | |
| Women | 0.476 | 1.610 | 0.801 | 3.235 |
| Men | 0 | | | |
| Years in nursing | −0.012 | 0.988 | 0.955 | 1.022 |
| Yearns present unit | −0.012 | 0.989 | 0.948 | 1.031 |
| Work schedule | 0.006 | 1.006 | 0.990 | 1.021 |
| Bachelor (yes) | 0.246 | 1.279 | 0.616 | 2.657 |
| Bachelor (no) | 0 | | | |
| T2 | 0.011 | 1.011 | 0.547 | 1.872 |
| T3 | −0.254 | 0.776 | 0.399 | 1.508 |
| T4 | 0.145 | 1.155 | 0.637 | 2.097 |
| T1[a] | 0 | | | |
| Nurse–physician relations | 0.285 | 1.330 | 0.813 | 2.177 |
| Nurse management | −0.269 | 0.764 | 0.276 | 2.117 |
| Hospital management | −0.987 | **0.373*** | 0.159 | 0.872 |
| Decision latitude | −0.957 | **0.384*** | 0.153 | 0.963 |
| Workload | 1.616 | **5.035***** | 2.925 | 8.664 |
| Social capital | −0.817 | **0.442**** | 0.255 | 0.765 |

*p-value <0.05, **p-value <0.01, ***p-value <0.001
[a]T1 as indicator

Nurse management at the unit level was positively associated with quality of care at the last shift and the hospital, while hospital management was positively associated with the latter. Social capital was positively associated with all three quality of care variables, while workload had a negative impact on quality of care at the hospital. Emotional exhaustion was negatively associated with all three quality of care variables, while personal accomplishment and depersonalization were associated with quality of care at the unit and the hospital, respectively. Relevant differences were noticed between measurement periods in quality of care at the last shift and the hospital, and demographic characteristics were relevant for quality of care at the last shift and the hospital (the first positively associated with years on the present and the latter positively associated with years in nursing). The total percentage correctly classified for the proposed model with five blocks indicating the percentage of quality of care at the unit, the last shift, and the hospital that can be predicted correctly using the model was 70%, 72%, and 67%, respectively (see Table 3.16).

Nurse management at the unit level was positively associated with job satisfaction (very satisfied) and negatively associated with intention to leave the hospital, while nurse–physicians relations were negatively associated with intention to leave the hospital and hospital management and organizational support was negatively associated with intention to leave nursing. Social capital was positive, and workload was negatively associated with job satisfaction, while workload was positively associated with intention to leave nursing. Dedication was positively associated with job satisfaction (very satisfied) and negatively associated with both intentions to leave the hospital and nursing, while absorption was negatively associated with intention to leave the hospital. Relevant differences were noticed between measurement periods in job satisfaction (very satisfied) and intention to leave nursing, and demographic characteristics were relevant for job satisfaction (very satisfied) (inverse associated with years on present unit and positively associated with bachelor diploma) and intention to leave nursing (inverse associated with years in nursing as well as work schedule). The total percentage correctly classified for the proposed model with five blocks indicating the percentage of job satisfaction (very satisfied), intention to leave the hospital, and intention to leave nursing that can be predicted correctly using the model was 83%, 95%, and 92%, respectively (see Table 3.17).

Nurse management at the unit level was positively associated with quality of care at the unit and the hospital, while nurse–physician relations *unexpected* was negatively associated with the quality of care at the last shift, and hospital management and organizational support was positively associated with quality of care at the hospital. Social capital was positively associated with all three quality of care variables while workload with quality of care at the shift and the hospital. Vigor and dedication were positively associated with quality of care at the unit and the last shift, respectively. No differences were noticed between measurement periods, and demographic characteristics were not relevant. The total percentage correctly classified for the proposed hierarchical models with five blocks indicating the percentage of quality of care at the unit, the last shift, and the hospital that can be predicted correctly using the model was 70%, 71%, and 66%, respectively (see Table 3.18).

Hospital management, and the work characteristics decision latitude, and social capital are associated with burnout risk or high levels of emotional exhaustion as well as depersonalization with an odds ratio of 64%, 62%, and 56%, respectively. Work load is positively associated with burnout risk with an odds ratio of 5. No differences were noticed between measurement periods, and demographic characteristics were not relevant. The total percentage correctly classified for the proposed hierarchical models with four blocks indicating the percentage of burnout risk that can be predicted correctly using the model was 90% (see Table 3.19).

The hierarchical model for burnout (high and very high levels on all three burnout dimensions) did not converge (Box 3.6).

---

**Box 3.6 Key Findings of Hierarchical Analyses of Longitudinal Data in Relation to the Nursing Organizational Transformation Process and Introduction of the Productive Ward**
- Study variables analyzed based on four measurement periods in five blocks on outcome variable confirm various associations as described in retested models with percentages of outcomes that can be predicted correctly through the tested model ranged from 66% to 95%.

- In the job outcome variables—job satisfaction and intention to leave the hospital and nursing—nurse management, emotional exhaustion, personal accomplishment, and dedication are confirmed as the most relevant predictors along with relevant impact on specific job outcome variables of hospital management, workload, and absorption.
- In the quality of care variables—at the unit, the last shift, and the hospital—nurse management, social capital, and emotional exhaustion are confirmed as the most relevant predictors along with relevant impact on specific quality of care variables of nurse–physician relations, hospital management, workload, personal accomplishment, vigor, and absorption.
- Some unexpected results were identified between depersonalization and job satisfaction (positive association) and between nurse–physician relations and quality of care at the last shift (inverse association).
- Difference in measurement periods and relevant demographic characteristics are primarily noticed in both hierarchical analyses with burnout and engagement for both outcome variables such as gender (burnout) and years in nursing and present unit (engagement) and work schedule (burnout and engagement).
- The longitudinal analysis, based on four time periods, confirms workload as a risk factor and social capital as a protective factor for unfavorable outcomes along with a negative impact of emotional exhaustion and a positive impact of personal accomplishment and dedication determined by practice environment variables. Moreover, hospital management and work characteristics' decision latitude and social capital predict negative and workload predicts positive burnout risk or % high and very high on emotional exhaustion and depersonalization.

## 3.7 Predictors of Burnout, Work Engagement, and Nurse Reported Job Outcomes and Quality of Care: A Mixed Methods Explanatory Sequential Study

### 3.7.1 Study Aim and Context

The aim of the qualitative studies (Van Bogaert et al. 2015, 2016, 2017a, b) was to investigate staff nurses' and nurse managers' perceptions and experiences of staff nurses' structural empowerment in a university hospital through semi-structured interviews. Further, the studies aimed to examine the extent to which structural empowerment supports quality and safe patient care and relates to staff nurses' perceptions and experiences of workload. As described elsewhere in this chapter, the hospital had recently implemented the Productive Ward program and had engaged in an accreditation process through Joint Commission International (JCI) as a part of a larger national hospital accountability process. It is notable that the Productive Ward program supports structural empowerment in three foundational modules (see Chap. 5).

### 3.7.2 Study Method

To understand the complexity of staff nurses' work conditions, in this study, we included purposive samples with typical cases of staff nurses as well as nurse managers practicing on medical or surgical units. Assuming that medical and surgical nursing units are relatively comparable in terms of staff nurse practice environment and nurse work characteristics such as structural empowerment and workload, we might expect similar perceptions and experiences. Four study investigators invited staff nurses and nurse managers of participating units to be interviewed. Data were collected until data sufficiency was obtained on the research topics (staff nurses = 11 and 9; nurse managers = 8 and 10). The semi-structured interviews were organized in two study periods between January–March 2014 and January–March 2015 based on interview guides focused on *empowerment* and *decision-making processes* (of staff nurses); *the definition of staff nurse empowerment, how structural empowerment was being implemented in the unit, how it had impacted internal hospital governance and policy*, and *its impact on nurse unit managers' roles (nurse managers)*; as well as *the most recent personal experiences with perceived workload, aspects that influence perceived workload*, and *impact of workload* (staff nurses and nurse managers). The analysis was completed using a descriptive phenomenological approach; thematic data analysis was supported by NVivo 10 software (QRS International) (see findings Van Bogaert et al. 2014a, 2015, 2017a).

These qualitative study results assisted in explaining and interpreting the quantitative results of the final developed models—Model 1 and Model 3 burnout and Model 2 and Model 4 engagement—in a mixed methods explanatory sequential study design (Van Bogaert et al. 2017a).

### 3.7.3 Models Explaining and Interpreting Using Qualitative Study Findings

Staff nurses acknowledged their involvement in joint decision-making processes that fostered engagement, responsibility, autonomy, critical reflection, and communication. However, empowerment was not a part of their usual vocabulary, and the meaning of the term was unfamiliar to many staff nurses. Nonetheless, they recognized that leaders in *nursing management and hospital management* were initiating several strategies to improve nurse involvement in decision-making processes (*decision latitude*). Moreover, respondents reported aspects of formal and informal power sharing through their involvement in their teams' decision-making processes (*social capital*), generally on matters closely related to patients and care. Although it was not always evident, there was access to information about ongoing change initiatives to support unit decision-making processes. Certain initiatives, such as access to scientific databases and communication strategies, to guide change initiatives were noted. Nurses reported that opportunities to learn and develop personally (*personal accomplishment*) were available through training programs and workshops that were heavily supported by the hospital (*hospital management and organizational support*). Respondents reported experiencing supportive peer relationships (*social capital*) as well as support from nurse managers (*nurse management at the unit level*). Nurse managers reported perceiving various improvement projects and processes as having a positive impact on quality of care and patient safety (*quality of care*). They indicated that the majority of staff nurses were engaged and felt involved in projects such as the Productive Ward program (*vigor and dedication*). However, negative aspects of empowerment and more involvement were also reported. Staff nurses mentioned that certain top-down initiatives (*hospital management*) created confusion and misunderstandings and were contradictory to the involvement that was created by the Productive Ward program (*organizational support*). Staff nurses reported that the PW program had a strong focus on daily work and patient care in their nursing teams. Staff nurses preferred to be involved in policies related to nursing practice and patient-related care, and they were less willing to be involved in hospital internal governance and policy issues. This finding suggested that even though the hospital was in the midst of a transformation process from a classic hierarchical and departmentally based organization to one that was flat and interdisciplinary, a gap between practice and management levels was still present. However, staff nurses reported that the hierarchical approaches and structures were diminishing "little by little." Some staff nurses felt that empowerment was mandated by *hospital management* and thus experienced it as an additional demand (*workload*). Otherwise, lack of time within daily practice was generally mentioned as a threat to *high-quality direct patient care*. Staff nurses did report a desire to deliver the best possible patient care. However, the impact of empowerment on patient care quality was not clear to participants because of several concurrent change initiatives in the hospital; the effect of these initiatives was not yet known. Nurse managers also reported a number of negative aspects of empowerment, related mainly to how projects were coordinated and supported and how the nursing teams were prepared for new initiatives at the hospital (*organizational support*). In addition, both staff nurses and nurse managers were experiencing pressure as a result of direct patient care priorities, tightly scheduled projects, and miscommunication.

Study participants addressed a bundle of factors that influenced *workload* in their interviews. These factors described how daily practice was organized and certain conditions were in place (*nurse management at the unit level*) largely determined by management decisions and policies (*hospital management and organizational support*). Furthermore, study participants stated that high workloads clearly were a *risk factor* for stress in staff nurses manifested as symptoms such as fatigue, headaches, and susceptibility to illnesses (*emotional exhaustion*), for negative feelings such as frustration and negativism and behaviors such as letting go, being less accessible, and approachable (*depersonalization*) as well as thoughts of failure and ineffectiveness (*personal accomplishment*) in the face of patient needs and expectations (*quality of care*). In addition, study participants expressed their concerns about the impact of sustained severe workloads on *quality of care and patient safety* through nurses' mistakes, which often were not reported. Participants were concerned that they might overlook relevant patient vital signs and other assessment findings and neglect patients' psychological and emotional needs. Both staff nurses and nurse managers reported staff nurses' feelings of sadness and irritability (*satisfaction with the current job*).

Support from the nursing unit manager (*nurse management at the unit level*) and nursing team climate (*social capital*) were viewed as key factors in the development of empowerment and joint decision-making (*decision latitude*). Participants viewed *physicians* as not being very involved in developing nurse empowerment, although staff nurses reported open and supportive relationships with physicians. Physicians—with the exception of chief physicians—were felt to be insufficiently aware of the changes being made to foster empowerment. Findings suggested that good interdisciplinary collaboration and communication (*nurse–physician relations*) that supported nursing practice (*decision latitude*) as well as supportive collaboration between colleagues such as good teamwork and opportunities to speak up and express opinions (*social capital*) were *protective factors* for balancing workload, dealing with stressful work conditions, engaging with patients in total patient care (*vigor and dedication*), and staying in the nursing profession (*intention to stay in the profession*). However, the transition to a flatter, more interdisciplinary organizational structure was still ongoing; this meant that top-down decisions were still being made and a certain persistent degree of departmental interference was felt (Box 3.7).

---

**Box 3.7 Key Findings of the Mixed Methods Explanatory Sequential Study**
- Improvement projects initiated by administrators such as the Productive Ward initiative support staff nurses in decision-making processes within their teams and involvement in internal governance and policy mainly in relation to nursing practice and patient care. Peer and nurse manager support were seen as key in developing empowerment and meeting imperatives for quality and safety in patient care. Physicians had a less prominent role in supporting nurses' empowerment although relations are open and supportive.
- High workloads clearly are a risk factor for staff nurses' symptoms such as fatigue, headaches, and vulnerability for diseases, for negative feelings such as frustration and negativism and behaviors such as letting go, being less accessible and approachable, as well as thoughts of failure and ineffectiveness in the face of patient needs and expectations. Staff nurses were concerned that they might overlook relevant vital signs or other important patient assessment data as well as neglect patients' psychological and emotional needs; they reported feelings of sadness and irritability.
- Good interdisciplinary collaboration and communication that support nursing practice as well as supportive collaboration between colleagues such as good teamwork and opportunities to speak up and express opinions are protective factors for balancing workload, dealing with stressful work conditions, maintaining engagement in holistic patient care, and staying in the nursing profession.

## 3.8    Evidence and Quality Improvement Projects and Team-Based Interventions

The next chapters deal with topics related to the evidence presented in this chapter: Transformation to an Excellent Nursing Organisation: a Chief Nursing Officers' Vision and Experience (Chap. 4); Productive Ward—Releasing Time to Care™: A Ward-Based Quality improvement Intervention (Chap. 5); Embedding Compassionate Care: A Leadership Programme in the National Health Service in Scotland (Chap. 6); Learning and Innovation in Health Care based Teams: The Relationships between Learning, Innovative Behavior at Work and Implementation of Innovative Practices in Hospitals (Chap. 7); Project Management and PDSA-Based Projects (Chap. 8); Reporting and Learning Systems for Patient Safety (Chap. 9) and Projects that Support Professional Communication, such as Team Resource Management and Quality of Care (Chap. 10); Standardizing Care Processes Using Evidence-Based Strategy: Implementation of a Rapid Response System in Belgian Hospitals (Chap. 11); Interdisciplinary Collaboration and Communication (Chap. 12); as well as Projects Targeting Adaptation of Individual Nurses such as Stress-Resistance Strategies (Chap. 13).

## References

Aiken L, Patrician P. Measuring organizational traits of hospitals: the revised nursing working index. Nurs Res. 2000;49(3):146–53.

American Nurses Credentialing Center (ANCC). (2005). The Magnet Recognition Program. Recognizing Excellence in Nursing Service. Application manual. Maryland.

American Nurses Credentialing Center (ANCC). (2014). The Magnet Recognition Program. Recognizing Excellence in Nursing Service. Application manual. Maryland.

Bentler P, Chou C. Practical issues in structural equation modeling. Sociol Methods Res. 1987;16:78–117.

Briggs SR, Creek JM. The role of factor analysis in the development and evaluation of personality scales. J Pers. 1986;54:106–48.

Byrne B. Burnout: testing for the validity, replication, and invariance of causal structure across elementary, intermediate, secondary teachers. Am Educ Res J. 1994;31:645–73.

Byrne B. Structural equation modeling with Amos. Basic concepts, applications and programming. London: Lawrence Erlbaum Associates; 2001.

Byrne B. Structural equation modeling with Amos. Basic concepts, applications and programming. 2nd ed. London: Lawrence Erlbaum Associates; 2010.

Ernstmann N, Ommen O, Driller E, Kowalski C, Neumann M, Bartholomeyczik S, Pfaff H. Social capital and risk management in nursing. J Nurs Care Qual. 2009;24(4):340–7.

Fitzmaurice G, Laird N, Ware J. Applied longitudinal analysis. Hoboken: Wiley; 2004.

Kanter RM. Men and women of the corporation. 2nd ed. Basis Books: New York; 1993.

Kowalski C, Ommen O, Driller E, Ernstmann N, Wirtz MA, Köhler T, Pfaff H. Burnout in nurses - the relationship between social capital in hospitals and emotional exhaustion. J Clin Nurs. 2010;19(11-12):1654–63.

Lake E. Development of practice environment scale of the nursing work index. Res Nurs Health. 2002;25:176–88.

Laschinger HK, Leiter P. The impact of nursing work environments on patient safety outcomes: the mediating role of burnout engagement. J Nurs Adm. 2006;36(5):259–67.

Leiter MP, Laschinger HK. Relationships of work and practice environment to professional burnout: testing a causal model. Nurs Res. 2006;55(2):137–46.

Leiter MP, Maslach C. Nurse turnover: the mediating role of burnout. J Nurs Manag. 2009;17(3):331–9.

Maslach C, Jackson SE, Leiter MP. Maslach burnout inventory manual. 3rd ed. Mountain View: CPP, Inc; 1996.

Morrow E, Robert G, Maben J, Griffiths P. Implementing large-scale quality improvement: lessons from The Productive Ward: Releasing Time to Care. Int J Health Care Qual Assur. 2012;25(4):237–53.

Park S, Lake ET. Multilevel modeling of a clustered continuous outcome: nurses' work hours and burnout. Nurs Res. 2005;54(6):406–13.

Pfaff H, Lutticke J, Badura B, Piekarski C, Richter P. Weiche' kennzahlen fur das strategische krankenhausmanagement. Stakeholderdinteressen zielgerichtet erkennen und einbeziehen. Hans Huber Bern. 2004.

Richter P, Hemmann E, Merboth H, Fritz S, Hänsgen C, Rudolf M. Das Erleben von Arbeitsintensität und Tätigkeitsspielraum—Entwicklung und Validierung eines Fragebogens zur orientierenden Analyse (FIT). Zeitschrift für Arbeits-und Organisationspsychologie. 2000.

Schaufeli W, Bakker A. Utrecht work engagement scale: preliminary manual. Utrecht: University of Utrecht; 2003.

Schaufeli WB, Bakker AB. Job demands, job resources, and their relationship with burnout and engagement: a multi-sample study. J Organ Behav. 2004;25(3):293–315.

Schaufeli W, Bakker A. Defining and measuring work engagement: bringing clarity to the concept. In: Bakker AB, Leiter MP, editors. Work engagement: a handbook of essential theory and research. New York: Psychology Press; 2010. p. 10–24.

Schaufeli WB, Van Dierendonck D. UBOS Utrechtse Burnout Schaal (UBOS): Manual (Duch). Lisse: Swets Test Publishers; 2000.

Van Bogaert P, Clarke S, Vermeyen K, Meulemans H, Van de Heyning P. Practice environments and their associations with nurse-reported outcomes in Belgian hospitals: development and preliminary validation of a Dutch adaptation of the Revised Nursing Work Index. Int J Nurs Stud. 2009a;46(1):54–64.

Van Bogaert P, Meulemans H, Clarke S, Vermeyen K, Van de Heyning P. Hospital nurse practice environment, burnout, job outcomes and quality of care: test of a structural equation model. J Adv Nurs. 2009b;65(10):2175–85.

Van Bogaert P, Clarke S, Roelant E, Meulemans H, Van de Heyning P. Impacts of unit-level nurse practice environment and burnout on nurse-reported outcomes: a multilevel modelling approach. J Clin Nurs. 2010;19(11–12):1664–74.

Van Bogaert P, Clarke S, Willems R, Mondelaers M. Nurse practice environment, workload, burnout, job outcomes, and quality of care in psychiatric hospitals: a structural equation model approach. J Adv Nurs. 2013a;69(7):1515–24.

Van Bogaert P, Clarke S, Willems R, Mondelaers M. Staff engagement as a target for managing work environments in psychiatric hospitals: implications for workforce stability and quality of care. J Clin Nurs. 2013b;22(11-12):1717–28.

Van Bogaert P, Clarke S, Wouters K, Franck E, Willems R, Mondelaers M. Impacts of unit-level nurse practice environment, workload and burnout on nurse-reported outcomes in psychiatric hospitals: a multilevel modelling approach. Int J Nurs Stud. 2013c;50(3):357–65.

Van Bogaert P, Kowalski C, Weeks SM, Van Heusden D, Clarke SP. The relationship between nurse practice environment, nurse work characteristics, burnout and job outcome and quality of nursing care: a cross-sectional survey. Int J Nurs Stud. 2013d;50(12):1667–77.

Van Bogaert P, Wouters K, Willems R, Mondelaers M, Clarke S. Work engagement supports nurse workforce stability and quality of care: nursing team-level analysis in psychiatric hospitals. J Psychiatr Ment Health Nurs. 2013e;20(8):679–86.

Van Bogaert P, Timmermans O, Weeks SM, van Heusden D, Wouters K, Franck E. Nursing unit teams matter: impact of unit-level nurse practice environment, nurse work characteristics, and burnout on nurse reported job outcomes, and quality of care, and patient adverse events—a cross-sectional survey. Int J Nurs Stud. 2014a;51(8):1123–34.

Van Bogaert P, Van heusden D, Somers A, Tegenbos M, Wouters K, Van der Straeten J, Van Aken P, Havens DS. The Productive Ward program™: a longitudinal multilevel study of nurse perceived practice environment, burnout, and nurse-reported quality of care and job outcomes. J Nurs Adm. 2014b;44(9):452–61.

Van Bogaert P, van Heusden D, Timmermans O, Franck E. Nurse work engagement impacts job outcome and nurse-assessed quality of care: model testing with nurse practice environment and nurse work characteristics as predictors. Front Psychol. 2014c;5:1261.

Van Bogaert P, Peremans L, de Wit M, Van Heusden D, Franck E, Timmermans O, Havens DS. Nurse managers' perceptions and experiences regarding staff nurse empowerment: a qualitative study. Front Psychol. 2015;6:1383.

Van Bogaert P, Peremans L, Diltour N, Van heusden D, Dilles T, Van Rompaey B, Havens DS. Staff nurses' perceptions and experiences about structural empowerment: a qualitative phenomenological study. PLoS One. 2016;11(4):e0152654.

Van Bogaert P, Peremans L, Van Heusden D, Verspuy M, Kureckova V, Van de Cruys Z, Franck E. Predictors of burnout, work engagement and nurse reported job outcomes and quality of care: a mixed method study. BMC Nurs. 2017a;16:5.

Van Bogaert P, Van heusden D, Verspuy M, Wouters K, Slootmans S, Van der Straeten J, Van Aken P, White M. The Productive Ward Program™: a two-year implementation impact review using a longitudinal multilevel study. Can J Nurs Res. 2017b;49(1):28–38.

## Part II

## Large-Scale Quality Improvement Projects and Team-Based Interventions

# Transformation to an Excellent Nursing Organization: A Chief Nursing Officer's Vision and Experience

4

Paul Van Aken

**Abstract**

This chapter takes a pragmatic approach, inspired by current evidence and scientific insights, to the journey of nursing services in health-care organizations aspiring to excellence. Here, excellence is used as in Jim Collins' definition of a good company in his book *Good to Great*: "Good is not good enough." The focus is on sustainability of the results obtained, supported by leadership and the organizational culture. Excellence seems to be a problem or challenge rather than a status or reality. It is indeed important to build organizations that are able to continuously improve their results. However, health care involves people-intensive organizations, which means that results depend on the actions or behavior of people rather than on making the right machine settings. People are the determinants of variations in care. Consequently, it is important for an organization whose goal is to maintain and improve health, that is, any hospital, to have its own approach for achieving excellence. With this in mind, guided by principles of leadership and good governance, excellence will be discussed in terms of four components: strategy and leadership, structure, process, and outcome.

**Keywords**

Nursing leadership • Nursing excellence • Health-care management • Value-based healthcare • Magnet hospitals • Productive Ward

P. Van Aken
Nursing Department, Antwerp University Hospital, Edegem, Belgium
e-mail: paul.vanaken@uza.be

## 4.1    Introduction

This chapter takes a pragmatic approach, inspired by current evidence and scientific insights, to the journey of nursing services in health-care organizations aspiring to excellence. Here, excellence is used in the sense of Jim Collins' (2001) definition of a good company in his book *Good to Great*: "Good is not good enough." The focus is on sustainable results, supported by leadership and organizational culture.

Excellence seems to be a problem or challenge rather than a status or a reality. Thinking about nosocomial infections and the effects of a measure as simple as hand hygiene, we know from research that nurses tend to reach only 48% compliance in implementing this simple measure (Erasmus 2010). Similar findings apply to other aspects of care. For example, Australian research shows that nurse compliance with patient identification before administration of medication is at a meager 52% (Westbrook et al. 2011). The annual cost of preventable catheter-associated urinary tract infections (CAUTI) in the USA has been estimated at $367 million (Schmier et al. 2016), despite clear indications that this complication can be greatly reduced through simple measures. It is indeed a paradox that preventable hospital-acquired conditions remain so common. Excellent nursing organizations are able to break through this paradox by aiming at and succeeding in establishing best-in-class performance and the highest conceivable standards as norms.

It is indeed important to build organizations that are able to continuously improve their outcomes. However, health care involves people-intensive organizations. This means that results depend on the actions or behavior of people rather than on the correct machine settings. People are the determinants of variations in care. Consequently, it is important for an organization whose goal is to maintain and improve health, that is, any hospital, to have its own approach for achieving excellence. With this in mind, guided by principles of leadership and good governance, excellence will be discussed in terms of four components: strategy and leadership, structure, process, and outcome.

## 4.2    Strategy and Leadership

The first but still valid and frequently used definition of strategy is that of Chandler (1962): "Strategy is the determination of the basic long term goals and objectives of an enterprise, and the adoption of courses of action and the allocation of resources necessary for carrying out these goals." Strategy is doing the right things and consequently boils down to making the right choices. The process starts with the mission of the organization and ends with the appreciation of this mission by the customer or patient. Kaplan and Norton (2008) state that strategy is not a stand-alone management process. Establishing a mission and vision focusing on values and guiding principles is a prerequisite to strategy.

Strategy is based on a clear understanding of the context in which the organization wants to achieve its objectives. Today's contexts for hospital environments and in particular nursing departments are complex, to say the least. The following elements are among the most important:

1. Nursing shortage is probably one of the most important factors to consider in terms of challenging contexts. Depending on the type of health-care organization, two issues are more or less decisive in terms of the adequacy of labor supply to meet needs. First, there is the local or regional labor market. Even in a small country such as Belgium, there are regional differences in the availability of nurses on the labor market. It is important to be aware of these differences, because they may be critical to the strategy an organization adopts. Trend analyses show that the labor market for nurses and other care professionals is subject to the economic cycle. Nursing is still seen as a line of work ensuring a stable income; it is widely believed in the general public that nurses will always be needed. However the supply of nurses over time seems to be linked to economic cycles. Second, there is also a demographic element to supply. The evolution of 15–18-year-old age group must be taken into account—indeed, in Belgium the size of this age group heavily influences the number of potential entrants to nursing schools. However, obviously, this is a variable not under the control of health-care organizations. Through a number of initiatives and campaigns, the Flemish government managed to increase the attractiveness of nursing education, resulting in an increased inflow. Government agencies and professional organizations track information about trends and produce promotional materials and media to stimulate interest in nursing. However, hospitals also have a part to play in encouraging young people to choose nursing. From a strategic perspective, there may not be an immediate return on investments in recruitment into the profession, but we believe that the sector's commitment to sustaining long-term supply is important.

2. Account must also be taken of workforce attrition (turnover) from the organization. It's our organization's practice to hold exit interviews with staff members leaving the organization, to understand the reasons they are leaving. From these interviews, it has become clear that commuting time is the main reason nurses leave. This was confirmed in an unpublished study we conducted in 2014 surveying third-year nursing bachelor students about the determinants of their choice of employer—in other words, how do they decide what hospital they want to work at. In addition to the practice environment factors already known to be important to nurses (the Magnet® forces), more than 35 min of commuting time between the nurse's home and the employing hospital of employment was among the top 5 determinants of selecting an employer. Concretely, this means that a recruitment strategy needs to clearly focus on retaining nurses who live close by, since initiatives to encourage nurses to move closer to the hospital have proven less successful. Demographic realities in the evolving workforce pose further strategic challenges. Currently there are not only diversity issues to be addressed in terms of national origins, especially in the members of interdisciplinary teams, but we are facing important challenges in finding the right way to approach age diversity. Generation manage-

ment is becoming one of the most important challenges in the context in which the strategy is aligned and implemented. The age pyramid of Antwerp University Hospital's staff shows a large share of younger nurses (average age 32) as well as of older nurses aged around 57. Generation X nurses (born between 1965 and 1980) are sandwiched between the baby boomers (born between 1949 and 1964) and Generation Y nurses (born between 1981 and 1996). These generations appear to have distinctive perceptions of social realities and particularly of management and leadership. It has been argued that Generation X nurses believe that trust in and loyalty to an organization are not automatically given by workers as the automatic result of employment and tenure, but are earned (Carver et al. 2011). This has critical implications for recruitment, talent development, and training. Workforce management and engagement will be required to optimize our most valuable resource: nurses. Leaders will play a crucial role in this. An old adage applies here: "When you take care of the people, the people will take care of the business."

3. Uncertainty surrounding hospital funding seems to be common to most countries. Both federal and regional initiatives impose limitations on resources that determine which elements of strategy can be implemented. Because in Belgium the government divided resources based on similar parameters for all agencies, health-care facilities are unable to create competitive advantages relative to each other. It is certain that there will be a shift from linear funding to funding through value creation for patients and the community. Recently the Belgian government announced the introduction of pay-for-quality (P4Q), a funding system that uses measureable indicators focused on patient value or some "form of value creation" for patients. Currently the program is focused solely on the prevention of hospital-acquired conditions. More broadly, we are seeing increased interest in patient-reported outcomes and experiences, and hospital leaders with an orientation to the future are well advised to begin thinking about strategy to optimize these as well.

4. The pressure to reduce costs will remain central to management strategies and needs to be tackled on several levels. On a macro level, the governments are introducing models to discourage overconsumption and control costs, for example, through price negotiations with the pharmaceutical sector. The above components are linked together in the Triple Aim concept (Berwick et al. 2008), a care model suited to chronic illness care: lower health-care costs per capita, improved health status, and a better experience in the patient-provider encounter. The goal is to address the elements of the above triad simultaneously, and it would be logical to make the translation of this more abstract care model at the local level an element of the strategic plan for departments of nursing. In the words of Charles Kenney, "The Triple Aim is a frame and a destination. It gives clarity about what you need to do" (Bisognano and Kenney 2012).

5. The customer is king. Health-care providers are increasingly aware of patients being increasingly articulate and critical, to the point of being more demanding, and may not always be happy about this. There are two realities:

- We must empower patients by allowing them to take part in their care journey, from diagnosis through treatment.
- Patients' rights to be assertive are inherent to the patient-health-care worker relationship.

Because the nurse-patient relationship is in evolution, nursing departments must need to teach their nurses how to deal with relevant changes.

To be sure, increased assertiveness is not the only shift in the patients we work with. Demographic trends point clearly to an aging population presenting for treatment who are more likely than ever to have multiple concurrent conditions. Today, 80-year-olds undergo procedures that at one time had age caps of 60. Knowledge not only of various diseases common to older adults (such as diabetes and cardiovascular disorders) but of current evidence-based treatments for them, including pharmacological therapy, is a challenge for nurses (as well as the organizations in which they work). Implementing treatments safely is often very stressful for nurses and frequently creates training needs. Skills like critical thinking and understanding how multiple co-occurring conditions are managed are important challenges for nurse educators as well as nurse leaders in practice settings. Patient outcomes (among them, unnecessary deaths) and patient survival will undeniably remain dependent on the nurses' ability to detect and remedy complications in an early stage. Organizational leaders need to remain sure that nurses are capable of providing the best possible care to inpatients.

6. Ubiquitous and continuous monitoring technologies are creating new opportunities in care, most recently with mobile technology applications and sensor technology. Currently, health care of the future has been described as virtual clinic visits, bedless hospitals, and oversight and monitoring of patient care wirelessly and from afar. Arguably, the day is coming when a computer crunching billions of pieces of data from patient records, medical literature, and analyses of patient DNA will be able to pinpoint the cancer treatments most apt to be effective for a particular patient presentation (Howard 2016). Consequently, it is extremely important for an organization to keep abreast of developments in information technology that could affect decision-making in the present. Nurses in the Mercy Virtual Care Center already participate in care delivery by interdisciplinary teams to patients of 38 hospitals in seven states across the USA; in this model of care, sometimes, patient care problems are being identified and resolved through the use of telemonitoring and other methods before they even manifest themselves.

7. Finally, the accessibility of the care system also plays a role in defining the context in which the strategy of the nursing department is developed. This problem extends in two opposite directions: On the one hand, there is the problem of overconsumption and the unnecessary use of resources. The use of EDs is a clear example. On the other hand, it is difficult for some populations to get access to the system, and because of this they do not get the necessary care in time. Optimized transmural cooperation between primary and secondary care providers may be the answer to this problem.

Together, these seven elements above can be thought of as disruptive forces that are currently greatly impacting strategy for hospitals and departments of nursing more specifically. Every chief nurse officer must assess these elements within their hospital's operating contexts when establishing a strategic plan for their nursing departments. Answering the question of what to address first in the hospital's strategy must begin with a consideration context and can be done from different perspectives. At Antwerp University Hospital, we wanted to develop the characteristics of a Magnet® Hospital within the organization, because the main emphasis in our institution has been and still is on shortage of nurses. Indeed, because the Magnet® Recognition Program is based on scientific research regarding nurse retention, it was easier to justify the decision to implement it in the environment of a university hospital. From a question of ongoing operations, dealing with nurse shortages is the main priority. However reducing costs is also crucial. Frequently in the search to reduce costs, labor expenses, the biggest chunk of which lies with nursing departments, emerge quickly (and erroneously) as a target. This is often overly simplistic thinking. Lorenz curves drawn from internal data will quickly reveal which activities or patients are associated with the highest costs. Data of the national health insurance show that nationally the top 5% of health-care consumers in the population generates 53% of health-care costs. It is also very important to clearly distinguish between goals (what we want to achieve), indicators (when do we know if a change is also an improvement), and interventions (which changes are improvements in the hospital) when defining strategy.

A reactive approach, fighting crisis after crisis, can be adopted. Many leaders in the sector perceived this as the dominant way of organizing hospitals. It is more difficult but potentially more fruitful to become able to deal with continuous changes. To that end, structure, and particularly the decision-making structure, needs to be adapted to enable staff members to continuously participate in the change process, keeping in mind that staff members want to change but do not want to be changed. Workers in adaptive organizations retain change-oriented mind-set continuously, and holding onto the status quo is perceived as a step backward.

## 4.3    Structures

Structures are the components of an organization enabling working environments to support the professional practice of nurses in a context of continuous change. Here, continuous change is understood as adaptation to internal and external changes in the organization's operating environment. Well-designed structures should also create space to promote innovations, development, and improved results.

The main leadership challenge with regards to structure is how to create a culture supporting continuous adaptation, resilience and improvement. Leaders face struggles in achieving four key elements:

- *Alignment*: Alignment is the extent to which services and staff members all work together toward a common goal. Proactive system thinking determines how operations are performed. In a context of leadership, this demands close collaboration between staff members and across services. Skills like listening and show-ing respect and support are called for to achieve alignment, because commitment to achieving a common goal is rarely possible through a top-down approach.

- *Transformation*: Constantly rethinking and redesigning services (what we do) and systems (how we do it) in order to thoroughly improve performance and to more effectively meet the mission and purpose of the organization to build a culture of resilience.
- *Excellence*: The organization positions itself as a company with a zero-tolerance policy for average results. Remember: "Good is not good enough." Ambitious goals such as "journey to zero (complications)" should not be shied away from, but rather embraced.
- *Engagement*: Staff members who are not only motivated but also passionate about their work and are aware of their meaningful contribution to the organiza-tion and to health care and as such are strongly engaged in the success of the organization. Structures can ensure that engagement in the organization is devel-oped and cultivated.

Traditional hierarchical organization forms and the leadership styles associated with them appear poorly suited to achieve these. In our organization we are strongly focused on developing the above four elements of a culture of agility and resilience. In doing so, we have focused on two aspects: the engagement of the frontline nurse and the development of the role of the nurse manager.

The introduction of the NHS Productive Ward™: Releasing Time to Care (PW) program has laid the foundations for culture change. PW is an approach based largely on Lean principles related to patient value. To improve patient value, a bot-tom-up approach is needed since change is impossible without engaging staff. Indeed, staff members know very well how to perform certain processes and where opportunities for improvement exist. The PW program offers a whole series of tools to introduce and enhance staff engagement and breaks with the tradition that employee engagement is obtained through extensive, time-consuming team meet-ings that result in longer lead times for initiating necessary change.

PW starts by defining a shared vision. Alignment with the organization's mission is key here. The potential pitfall of a "bottom-up" approach is that teams may develop separate visions that are not aligned with the objectives of the organization. Another problem that we noticed is that different teams develop diverse solutions for the very same problem, resulting in wasted resources and creating difficulties in achieving the degree of standardization critical to a large organization. Therefore, finding the correct right balance between "bottom up" and "top down" is essential and very much a challenge. Top down (leadership) should lead the way with regard to the "what" part and the possibilities of alignment with the mission and vision of the organization. Also, a clear definition of excellence needs to be established at the top. Bottom up is the best route to define the "how" and with which means the goal is to be reached. A team is best placed to break down an organizational goal into priorities and determine what steps for their team are the most relevant to assist in reaching the organization's goal. This is best illustrated using a short example:

Let's say that a general goal relating to pressure ulcer prevalence on a department level reads as follows: "Over three quarters, pressure ulcer prevalence will be reduced by 2%." Subsequently, teams can align this goal to their own activities and scope. This may mean rethinking nutritional assessment and counseling in case of malnutrition problems, for instance. Teams then start working and follow up on the progress for this subgoal after a few weeks. Subsequently the team might decide to address risk factors related to mobility assessment and decide on an action plan for follow-up. Daily (or weekly) huddles are very well suited to this type of follow-up. Presumably, all elements can eventually be covered in the way the team itself chooses. Important in this is to define "nonnegotiable," i.e., aspects of the standard that must not/cannot be deviated from (e.g., "reducing pressure ulcer prevalence by 2% over three quarters"). For other aspects the team can decide itself how it want to achieve their goals and subgoals.

During our Magnet® journey (our process of self-assessment and preparation for review for possible designation), we were faced with the professional standard of having peer review at all levels. When we wanted to introduce this method, it appeared as if no hospital in Belgium had implemented this type of peer review method. Traditional peer review—where one colleague gives feedback on the professional (observable) behavior of another nurse on a number of parameters—met with huge resistance from nurses. All this has to do with the fact that giving professional feedback was not part of nursing education until a few years ago. As expected, the unions representing the nurses rejected the introduction of behavior-oriented peer review. As an alternative, we decided to link (align) peer review with the clinical objectives. For each nurse-sensitive outcome, good practice checklists were developed for use in the peer review process. In this process one nurse checks the extent to which a colleague followed adopted clinical processes (e.g., pressure injury/ulcer screening and prevention) correctly and completely. At the end of shift, the observing nurse gives this feedback to the nurse who performed the clinical process. This model is described by LeClair-Smith and colleagues and has demonstrated favorable effects on outcomes relevant to the areas touched upon by peer-to-peer feedback (LeClair-Smith et al. 2016).

Combining different approaches to boost accountability of frontline nurses was based on involving nurses in decisions and aligning objectives. The nurse manager plays a crucial role in engagement in this. In a triple-layered organization, communication lead time is very slow, and there is a risk that messages will be distorted or interpreted differently at each layer. Middle-management nurse leaders may get frustrated because they feel they are mere go-betweens between the chief nursing officer and the nurse managers. However, the chief nursing officer always has indirect information about what is happening on the front line because this information passes through the middle managers. This phenomenon is sometimes described as the middle management being the "clay layer": the chief nurse officer only receives the information from the middle managers that they think the chief nurse officer wants to hear; any other information gets filtered out. The nurse managers on the front line receive selective information selectively to hide bad news or in efforts to maintain hierarchical positions.

We addressed this in the Antwerp University Hospital structure by revisiting the position of the nurse manager. Communication between chief nurse officer and nurse managers has intensified. The general meeting with all nurse managers (there are over 35) has been supplemented with regular meetings of the chief nursing officer with smaller groups of nurse managers (on average 10). The nurse leaders actively participate in these meetings, where decisions are reviewed and support for them is checked out. In addition, a council of charge nurses was set up within the shared governance structure to represent the interests of charge nurses and, for instance, to make suggestions regarding how nurse managers can be supported by the organization. One of the achievements of this council was achievement of a professional peer review structure for charge nurses in the organization. Clarifying the direct relationship between chief nurse officer and nurse manager also resulted in optimized communication lines. Currently, the nurse managers receive a monthly communication letter, giving clear information to everyone in the organization at the same time. We also try to include most communication regarding ancillary services in this communication letter. The color of each section's title tells the nurse manager what to do with the information obtained:

- A title in red means take action; what kind of action is expected is also indicated.
- A title in green means share information with the members of the team (this information is also repeated in the newsletters to all nurses).
- A title in black reflects "nice to know" news.

Additionally, the contents of the nurse manager communication letter are shared with physicians. Specifically, the chief medical officer posts reports on relevant topics in the physician newsletter and vice versa. Nurse managers indicate that communication in the organization has been greatly improved and collaboration has been enhanced through this process.

Nurse leaders in middle management positions are currently more involved in coaching and supporting nurse managers and coordinating hospital-wide improvement projects. In this sense, they are now much closely connected with the chief nurse officer's position, and one of their core activities is to strategically align organization-wide objectives with team-specific ones.

It can be said that we undertook the abovementioned actions in the departmental structure with the aim of developing a shared governance structure. Although the focus was on the positioning of the hierarchical layers above the frontline employees, frontline nurses are involved through a system of nurse champions throughout the institution (staff nurses with experience, expertise, and interests in particular domains of care). At the Antwerp University Hospital, there are several such groups of nurse champions. Each of these groups has a different focus on care practice and/or on the nurse work environment. The main groups are those of the mentoring coaches, the nurse champions for patient safety and infection control, the nurses responsible for nursing excellence, and the nurses responsible for pain, palliative care, and ethical issues. Each nursing unit has at least one of these nurse champions in their team. Nurse champions receive training at least two times a year. Their task is to verify (along with the nurse manager) what is new within their scope of practice, where the desired situation differs from current conditions on their units and how they intend to any gaps. Nurse champions make important contributions to their teams' meetings.

For each focus area of nurse champions, there is a delegation of about five to seven nurses. They constitute a nursing council. The nursing council autonomously decides on the topics to discuss and the practices to develop in the organization. For example, the patient safety and infection nursing council was responsible for implementing SBAR communication and bedside handover. It is considered the responsibility of the chief nursing officer and nurse leaders to support the work of these nursing councils.

In the framework of the Magnet® leadership model, this is called structural empowerment: various ways in which transformational leaders develop, direct, enable, and reward frontline nurses to perform at their highest level of practice and achieve autonomy in patient care. These leaders generally create flat management structures that facilitate vertical communication and maximize involvement of the point-of-care staff (Drenkard et al. 2011). In this context the element of professional development of the nurse is inescapable in the structures of the department of nursing. Possibilities for professional development are still one of the top three reasons why nurses want to work at a hospital. Consequently, professional development is of considerable strategic importance given our need to balance the supply of and our need for registered nurses.

We offer both internal and external professional development opportunities. Education to promote career advancement, for instance, from nurses' aid to nurse, from technically trained to bachelor's-prepared nurse, and from bachelor's-prepared nurse to holding a master's in nursing and midwifery, is encouraged and supported by the organization. In addition, a lot of attention is paid to the onboarding process for nurses and nurse managers in order to develop nurse autonomy and accountability. Given the strategic importance of this component, we cannot overemphasize the importance of professional development within the departmental structure. Obviously this process will be aligned with human resources to avoid redundant collection of data and fragmented use of resources.

## 4.4 Processes

Processes are developed to reach a goal or outcome. That is why formulating goals is inherent to initiating a process. As has already been said, it is extremely important to manage the tension between top-down versus bottom-up processes. First of all, it is important to have clear goals. Personally, we are not in favor of rigid adherence to formulating all goals in SMART format, but it is important to have a clear target audience in mind and that goals need to be formulated with a specific patient or organization outcome in mind whenever possible.

Outside pressures and influences are major problems when initiating processes with achievement of an outcome in mind. Nurse managers sometimes feel that new standards or accreditation guidelines are generated in a black box, and because they do not understand the underlying rationale for new standards, so they are unable to successfully communicate their importance or means of achieving them to frontline nurses. This results in an atmosphere where everybody has questions about the change processes to be initiated, yet everyone is afraid of asking voicing their questions and concerns. Also, nurse managers are often overwhelmed by competing priorities. In other words, it is important to remove the barriers preventing good communication about the processes to be implemented. Nurse managers need to find or build support from various angles to develop the frontline commitment and accountability that are fundamental to high reliability and excellent outcomes. It is notable that using champion nurses and nurse councils as described in the previous section can be an excellent method for supporting nursing managers.

A recurring mistake when implementing processes is to give so much priority to adherence to processes completely and without reflection, including any problems or flaws that may be inherent in them. We can easily fall into the trap of formulating a worthy goal and then immediately implementing the process and interventions needed to achieve it. We tend to overlook the step of consulting the literature and, especially, of contacting a network to verify whether anyone has had prior experience with this process or intervention in other organizations. The latter is a form of peer support inside and outside institutional walls. At any rate, any process or intervention must be explored and verified as much as possible in terms of available evidence and experience in other organizations. A process that can be demonstrated to be evidence-based is more readily accepted by the nurses who will need to carry it out.

A second pitfall in terms of initiating processes is the so-called "all or nothing" mind-set. Because of internal and external pressures, standards tend to be implemented through organization-wide processes. As a result, all departments experience the "teething pain" associated with implementation at the same time. We would therefore argue that it is better for the processes to be tested on a smaller scale among a pilot group of clinical areas in order to discover problems before they become organization-wide challenges. A process can be tested in a simulated environment or on a smaller set of nursing units that have been given clear instructions to detect errors in the process. In this way, nurses are much more inclined to apply their professional judgment to the implementation and offer informed opinions about the process, increasing the buy-in for properly implementing the process. Later on, nurses working on units where processes have been piloted can be used as early adopters to help their peers elsewhere in the organization. Nurses who can speak about a process from experience have more credibility among their fellow nurses than managers (their own or those from other areas of the organization). We have successfully used this method for the introduction of bedside handover. A similar positive experience involved nurses who developed their own video clip about a process and who used this video to train other nurses. It is important not to underestimate the power of peer-to-peer relationships in change processes; these relationships should therefore be carefully leveraged in organizational change processes.

When implementing processes, but especially when designing processes within the nursing unit, ensuring continuous buy-in from frontline nurses is pivotal. Hospital-wide process improvements are important, but unit-based process improvements that do not involve waiting for other nursing units are almost just as valuable. The reason is that the buy-in of frontline staff into change processes is felt most strongly when staff has greater autonomy over implementation. In this way, a team becomes an incubator for continuous process improvement and a culture of resilience is created. This happened under the PW program: PW looks inward to the ward level to understand the impact of change on other departments (NHS Institute for Innovation and Improvement 2008). To manage the change process, the PW philosophy uses elements from the care process (prepare, assess, diagnose, plan, treat, evaluate) rather than the industry terms of "plan," "do," "check," and "act." This brings change methodology closer to frontline nurses, improving acceptance. Throughout this process, a "Sustain" Milestone Checklist was used, which consists of using a standardized checklist for efficient teamwork consisting of five simple questions:

1. Did all of the team participate?
2. Was the discussion open?
3. Were the "hard" questions discussed?
4. Did the team remain focused on the task?
5. Did the team focus on the area/process, rather than the individual?

The rationale for this checklist was to continuously monitor the team's commitment to change processes. Our experience tells us that it is better to give the teams more time to create general buy-in for the process improvement than to apply top-down pressure. After all, pressure from the top tends to generate more resistance and result in incomplete process implementation and questionable results.

A method that is equally successful and used during the onboarding process is that of single ownership. Clearly assigning responsibility for a process or procedure to a single nurse in the team can greatly improve the efficiency with which this process is taught and applied. Various nursing managers have assigned a process to a nurse who is then responsible for making sure that the process or procedure is correctly passed on to a new nurse in the team or to the pool of nurses. This methodology ensures that the process is taught and/or copied by a new colleague in a standardized way. The nursing process owner also makes sure that the process or procedure for which he or she is responsible is always up-to-date.

We have also come to see that peer coaching for nursing managers and leadership processes is a very productive activity. We developed a peer review model for nurse managers where managers as a group developed a pick list of processes about which they might wish to get feedback from a colleague. A nurse manager then selected a process from the list and identifies himself or herself as interested in feedback about their performance on it. Next, pairs of peers were created consisting of nurse managers seeking feedback about a process and peer nurse manager willing to provide that feedback. After these feedback meetings, 26 out of 29 head nurses stated that this approach had provided them with useful insights into how they could better manage leadership-related processes. We are currently determining how this feedback can be adapted for the entire organization, allowing more nursing managers to benefit from this method.

## 4.5    Outcome

Outcomes are obviously very important, and so it is vital to use outcomes to depict the contribution of nurses to a health-care organization or to health care more broadly. We can also think in terms of the concept of value creation: what value do nurses add to the care provision in improving the health and well-being of patients? The importance of outcomes has come under close scrutiny following the 1999 publication of *To Err is Human: Building a Safer Health System* (the US Institute of Medicine). This book and the discussions that followed its appearance favored greater transparency regarding tracking and reporting on safety. In the IOM's subsequent publication, *Crossing the Quality Chasm: A New Health System for the 21st Century*, the focus was on quality indicators to ensure care was provided according to the best available scientific evidence. The Magnet® recognition program came to embrace this emphasis, and program leaders progressively increased attention to so-called empirical outcomes.

Magnet® organizations are expected to create structures and implement and sustain evidence-based processes that lead to improved outcomes for patients, the nursing workforce, organizations, and communities (Drenkard et al. 2011). Any organization now applying for Magnet® recognition needs to provide more than 30 sources of evidence, presenting outcome data regarding patients, the broader organization, and health care in general.

Excellence means continuously improving structures and processes, preferably at a level better than relevant industry benchmarks, recalling the Good to Great motto from the beginning of this chapter, "Good is not good enough." A Magnet® organization is one that takes a leading role in terms of value-based health care: there is a strong convergence between the foundation that was provided by the IOM and the selection of sources of evidence required by the Magnet® model, both of which speak to six well-known characteristics of high-quality care: safety, effectiveness, patient-centeredness, timeliness, efficiency, and equity.

A major problem for most European countries is accessing benchmarks regarding outcomes. Many organizations have data about structural and process indicators but fall short when it comes to outcomes. However, more and more countries are moving toward a system of pay-for-quality or pay-for-performance funding, where reporting of outcomes is linked to reimbursement. Some countries have moved even further and now withhold payments to cover treatment of certain preventable complications, such as hospital-acquired pressure ulcers. As we noted in an earlier section, it has always been our strategy to anticipate movement toward this type of funding by tracking and improving nursing-sensitive outcomes (contextual element 3 in Sect. 4.2 Strategy and Leadership).

Based on our experience with the introduction of Lean methods on our organization's front lines, we decided to use Lean methods to visualize our outcomes; an important precondition is having a well-functioning model for promoting excellence. Each of our nursing units now has an improvement bulletin board showing their outcomes in relation to hospital and team objectives. For each objective, the outcomes are presented visually. We are currently in a phase where we present outcomes using statistical process control methods.

Every team-related objective that focuses on either a patient-focused or organization-focused outcome is put into a standard layout. We use the A3 method for this. The A3 method is a structured method for problem solving. We have developed a strict template to guide improvement efforts through the plan-do-check-act cycle. The title of the A3 corresponds with the objective formulated. As part of our Journey to Magnet®, we included the template for visualizing data as required by the Magnet® Application Manual in the A3 template (American Nurses Credentialing Center 2014). This way, our nurses and nursing manages are familiarized with both the A3 method and the requirements for publishing data as part of developing the written documentation required for the Magnet® Hospital application, while simultaneously meeting one of the Lean principles: working smarter, not harder.

Improving outcomes is also part of the performance evaluation of nursing managers and nursing leaders. On the one hand, this highlights the importance of improved outcomes, but at the same time, it supports supervisors in achieving their own objectives aimed at improving outcomes. The organizational aspect is supported by a biannual measure of the nurses' working environment and psychosocial risks caused by, for example, disruptive behavior through surveys open to all staff with results fed back to teams for improvement purposes. The surveys have had response rates greater than 50%.

Improving outcomes depends on providing high-quality feedback to the frontline nurses. Our experiences have taught us that visualizing results using graphics is insufficient for providing frontline nurses with information about unsatisfactory outcomes. That is why the infection control department shares the stories of patients experiencing hospital-acquired infections while receiving immediate reports of cases of CAUTI or central line-associated bloodstream infections (CLABSI) at the time of diagnosis. The aim of sharing stories is to provide insights behind the statistics and help nurses better understand their contributions to the prevention of hospital-acquired conditions—over the last few years, we have noticed the power of storytelling when presenting outcomes. We are currently attempting to apply this principle to the performance evaluation of nurses more broadly, by having them reflect on their roles in the outcomes achieved by their teams with the aim of encouraging frontline accountability related to outcomes. This is just one further example of the role of transformational leadership in using measurement to continuously improving outcomes. In the case of hospital-acquired conditions, it is the foundation for the so-called "journey to zero."

Underlying the above approach to structure, process, and outcome is a single theme: the relationship between the quality of the working environment and quality of care. A great place to work tends to be a great place to provide care and vice versa. This idea also allows us to focus on key values and guiding principles that are important both for the health-care team and for the patient. We developed the professional practice model (PPM) in this context and decided to use the metaphor of the nursing's DNA. DNA is of course a macromolecule that acts as the main carrier of hereditary information. The two long strands of nucleotides symbolize the team (and its working environment) and the patient. The connecting base pairs symbolize values and guiding principles important to both the team and the patient. From the onboarding stage onward, we attempt to explain this notion of our discipline's DNA at our hospital in terms of the vision and values of the organization and where the Antwerp University Hospital nurse can make a difference. It is not easy to get everyone to agree to the same principles in matters such as patient care and teamwork. Including the metaphor of the DNA of nursing in our professional practice model has been a very useful tool in this. Nurse managers also use the DNA model for performance evaluation during the onboarding of new staff. Our experience with implementation of the PPM has been very positive, specifically because it has helped develop a shared vision among our nurses regarding care and relationships with colleagues and supervisors. We are taking this one step beyond professionally oriented development to personal development and health, for instance, by offering fitness programs and yoga classes to hospital staff. This also helps develop staff commitment to the organization, which promotes employee retention. It is the duty of supervisors to develop the Antwerp University Hospital as a community where members have a sense of belonging and are happy in their place in the organization—all of these elements go hand-in-hand and cannot be considered low-priority or "soft" considerations. They are underlying, firm preconditions for developing the health-care organization of the future where nurses will play a leading role in contributing to outcomes.

## Conclusion

In our quest for continuous improvement of outcomes while aspiring to excellence, we found that we needed to turn to the essential components of an organizational context for nursing practice that would support this work. Health care is delivered in organizations that involve extensive human resource inputs, and outcome results depend on the actions or behavior of workers. Until fairly recently, shortages of nurses' drive were the main driver of research and reflective practice to improve nurse work environments. Insights gained from this earlier work are still relevant today, but now challenges also relate to broader issues in hospital policy and governance such as hospital funding, pressures to reduce costs, the focus on patients as whole people and as customers having choices, accessibility of services, and the need for successful introduction of new technologies and opportunities in care. This chapter has presented a number of key structural elements that favor a culture supporting continuous adaptation, resilience, and improvement. As discussed broadly throughout this book, a culture of improvement and excellence begins with staff member alignment toward common goals. In our organization the introduction of the NHS Productive Ward™: Releasing Time to Care (PW) program was a powerful driver of our journey toward better outcomes and more engaged staff. Arguably, promoting ownership of carefully designed processes by unit-level nursing teams and steady introduction of small-scale changes with a focus on developing commitment are preferable to organization-wide implementation of change with a single-minded focus on adherence and compliance. Given the move afoot toward pay-for-quality or pay-for-performance funding of hospitals, improving outcomes that are benchmarked nationally and internationally will likely become imperative. We were strongly inspired by the commitment of Magnet® organizations to take a leading role in developing value-based health care through strong engagement of clinical nurses and leveraging of nursing management and governance structures. Together, all of the various projects and initiatives we undertook gave us the courage to pursue our own Magnet® recognition journey, which was to our knowledge, one of the very first in Europe. We hope others will be inspired to join us on this path to excellence.

## References

American Nurses Credentialing Center. 2014 MAGNET® application manual. Silver Springs: American Nurses Credentialing Center; 2014.

Berwick DM, et al. The triple aim: care, health, and cost. Health Aff. 2008;27(3):759–69.

Bisognano M, Kenney C. Pursuing the triple aim: seven innovators show the way to better care, better health, and lower costs. San Francisco: Jossey-Bass Publishers; 2012.

Carver L, Candela L, Gutierrez A. Survey of generational aspects of nurse faculty organizational commitment. Nurs Outlook. 2011;59(3):137–48.

Chandler A. Strategy and structure: chapters in the history of the industrial enterprise. Cambridge: MIT Press; 1962.

Collins J. Good to great. New York: HarperCollins Publishers; 2001.

Drenkard K, Wolf G, Morgan S. Magnet®: the next generation-nurses making the difference. 1 red. Silver Spring: American Nurses Credentialing Center; 2011.

Erasmus V. Systematic review of studies of compliance with hand hygiene guidelines in hospital care. Infect Control Hosp Epidemiol. 2010;31(3):283–94.

Howard B. The 21st century hospital: are virtual care clinics the wave for the future? US News & World Report: Best Hospitals 2017 edition; 2016.

Kaplan R, Norton D. Mastering the management system. Harv Bus Rev. 2008:57–62.

LeClair-Smith C, Branum B, Bryant L, Cornell B. Peer-to-peer feedback: a novel approach to nursing quality, collaboration, and peer review. JONA. 2016;46(6):321–8.

NHS Institute for Innovation and Improvement. Releasing time to care: the Productive Ward- executive leaders guide. Coventry: National Health Service; 2008.

Schmier JK, et al. Estimated hospital costs associated with preventable healthcare-associated infections if if health care antiseptic products were unavailable. Clinicoecon Outcomes Res. 2016;8:197–205.

Westbrook J, et al. Errors in the administration of intravenous medication in hospital and the role of correct procedures and nurse experience. BMJ. 2011;20(12):1027–34.

# Productive Ward: Releasing Time to Care™ (A Ward-Based QI Intervention)

Mark White

**Abstract**

The Productive Ward: Releasing Time to Care™ initiative has most arguably been the largest scale quality improvement initiative involving nurses and ward-based teams in the UK and Europe in recent years. One of its main aims is to increase the proportion of time nurses spend in direct patient care. Reports of the initiative and its influences have been well described. Robust, systematic evaluations of the initiative and its impact continue but remain sparse. This chapter comprehensively reviews 36 peer-reviewed papers and 9 evaluation reports in terms of outputs, outcomes and impacts. It discusses achievements of Productive Ward: Releasing Time to Care™, some of the unintended consequences that have been reported, the role of context and conditions that influence implementation and indications of how the initiative can be sustained. As quality improvement initiatives go, Productive Ward: Releasing Time to Care™ is now relatively mature (more than 12 years of experience), and its popularity and appeal may well have peaked. The future of Productive Ward: Releasing Time to Care™ will depend on the intentions of its current licensor and decisions at the many sites that commenced the initiative and/or adapted it into their larger quality improvement programmes.

**Keywords**

Productive Ward: Releasing Time to Care • Quality improvement • Implementation Impact review • Ward teams

M. White
Nursing and Midwifery Planning and Development Unit, HSE South, Kilkenny, Ireland

School of Health Sciences, Waterford Institute of Technology, Waterford, Ireland

Faculty of Nursing, Royal College of Surgeons, Dublin, Ireland
e-mail: mark.white@hse.ie

© Springer International Publishing AG 2018
P. Van Bogaert, S. Clarke (eds.), *The Organizational Context of Nursing Practice*,
https://doi.org/10.1007/978-3-319-71042-6_5

## 5.1    Introduction

In recent years, healthcare organisations throughout the world have been focusing their efforts on improving quality and controlling costs. Whilst the focus of many healthcare management teams in the past has tended to be costly, more recently, considerable attention is now being directed towards service quality, care outcomes and process improvement. Over the last decade, quality improvement (QI) interventions have grown, matured and gained higher profile in healthcare systems around the world —they have taken a variety of forms and guises, including Lean, Six Sigma, Total Quality Management and the Model for Improvement.

There are many motivations and drivers for improving quality in healthcare. The pressures associated with growing populations to be served, changing healthcare needs and increasing healthcare costs, in addition to concerns about patient safety and reducing harm, are amongst some of the most compelling. In addition, poor patient experiences with healthcare and negative media images and portrayals have combined with the trends just mentioned to provide many of the ingredients for a 'perfect storm' in terms of crises in healthcare. This has led to an international call to 'rescue' the provision of healthcare with a particular renewed focus on healthcare QI (Ovretveit 2013; Ferlie and Shortell 2001).

Although there is a well-established imperative for healthcare organisations to improve whilst trying to master what works well, and why, there is in fact a limited understanding amongst many clinicians and managers of the workings and impacts of interventions designed to improve healthcare quality. This lack of understanding has motivated many healthcare professionals to seek guidance in carrying out successful healthcare QI projects in their clinical settings (Gill et al. 2012).

Whilst the current practices in implementing healthcare quality innovations and improvements have a foundation in Pressman and Wildavsky (1973) study of policy implementation and Havelock (1973) change agent studies in education, there appears to be broad agreement in the literature that the implementation of healthcare QI is decidedly more complex and demanding, and has many more variables, than previously assumed (Fixsen et al. 2005; Ovretveit 2011).

Improvement science has evolved to fill a void left by descriptive theories of innovation, implementation and change related to other important components required for effective implementation of QI interventions and strategies. These include the contextual variables, circumstances, behaviours and interactions that result in improvements in healthcare quality. Even though many of these components are reflected in the process work of Deming (1986), and the root cause analysis work of Juran and Gryna (1988), improvement science continues to grow and develop as a general loose term, to refer to the field of study devoted to capturing meaning, detecting relationships between components and developing the practice and science of implementation. Implementation science focuses on systematically and rigorously exploring 'what works' and the best ways to capture, measure and disseminate best practices to engage clinicians and influence positive change (The Health Foundation 2011).

In the past, QI initiatives have typically faltered or failed to engage healthcare professionals and many studies report apathy and resistance from clinicians (Davies et al. 2007; Taitz et al. 2012). Getting individuals to think and behave in different ways is not straightforward, especially healthcare professionals who may not be convinced of the value and merits of improvement methods tools or programmes (Gollop et al. 2004). It is becoming widely acknowledged that engaging clinicians (regardless of setting or discipline) is one of the many preconditions for QI success (Siriwardena 2009; Dixon-Woods et al. 2012).

In trying to find recipes for successful QI, healthcare organisations worldwide have adopted new improvement programmes and work systems originating in sectors such as manufacturing and industry. Many healthcare organisations have attempted to replicate touted improvement successes in these industries, yet only a handful have succeeded. It could be argued that failures result from competing logics in healthcare, with a drive by clinicians towards the quality and patient safety aspects of QI (a professional logic) and healthcare administrators and management generally preoccupied by cost elements in QI and prospects for doing more with fewer resources (a business logic) (van Os et al. 2015; Reay and Hinings 2009; van den Broek et al. 2013).

Healthcare QI programmes inspired by industrial models have taken a variety of forms, including 'Lean' which has its origins in the Toyota production system (Graban 2012; Burgess and Radnor 2013; Mazzocato et al. 2010); 'Six Sigma', which was developed by engineers working at Motorola (Charles et al. 2012; Kenett 2011); 'Total Quality Management' which is thought to have originated in the quality control movement in Japan (Feigenbaum 1983); and the 'Model for Improvement', which has its basis in the process improvement movement (Langley et al. 2009). Many of these programmes have been remodelled, adapted and mutated in attempts to make them applicable to healthcare settings. In contrast, Productive Ward: Releasing Time to care™ (PW) is a programme that has been specifically designed to meet the many healthcare QI requirements, more specifically, those of acute hospital settings and nurses.

## 5.2    What Is Productive Ward: Releasing Time to Care?

Relative to other nursing programmes, the PW programme remains a new QI initiative. It is best described as a nurse-led, ward-based 'improvement' programme designed and licensed by the NHS Institute for Innovation and Improvement (NHSI) to healthcare organisations outside the NHS. It was created to help nurses and ward-based teams redesign and streamline the way they work, releasing more time to care for patients and empowering nurses to improve the safety, quality and delivery of care. It was originally developed by the UK's NHSI in 2005 and aims to:

- Increase the proportion of time nurses spend in direct patient care
- Improve experience for staff and for patients
- Make structural changes to the use of ward spaces to improve efficiency in terms of time, effort and money (NHS Institute and NNRU 2010b)

The PW programme utilises some of the principles and tools of 'lean' or 'lean thinking', a concept popularised by Womack et al. (1990). Using some of the improvement techniques from 'Lean', the intrinsic motivators of social movement theory and the front-line engagement theories of large-scale change, the PW encourages nurses to look at how their ward is organised and to make improvements that will 'Release Time to Care' (NHS Institute and NNRU 2010b) .

When the PW initiative was launched and marketed, it promised many team, patient and improvement deliverables. The initiative gained a reputation within the nursing and healthcare press for being the panacea or 'silver bullet' for all woes in nursing clinical environments. As an improvement initiative, it certainly made headlines, attracting both the attention and the financial backing of the UK Health Secretary in 2008 and the UK Prime Minister in 2012 (Nursing Standard 2012). However, a lot has happened in the years that followed. The main driving force and implementation support for the PW initiative (both in the UK and internationally) was its creator, the NHSI. However, since 2015, interest in and uptake of the PW initiative appear to have declined. This has manifested itself in a reduced number of reviews and reports in the nursing and healthcare press. The opposite, however, can be said in relation to academic interest and studies, which have increased in recent years (White et al. 2014a), making it difficult to gauge if the initiative is flourishing or not, or just a time delay between evidence gathering and publication.

## 5.3  The Component Parts of Productive Ward: Releasing Time to Care

After early testing in 2006 by the UK NHSI in four sites (the Royal Liverpool and Broadgreen University Hospitals NHS Trust, the Basingstoke and North Hampshire NHS Foundation Trust, the Barnsley Hospital NHS Foundation Trust and the Luton and Dunstable NHS Foundation Trust), the tagline 'Releasing Time to Care' was added, in response to feedback from the test sites indicating that Lean and improvement language and methods were not appealing to front-line clinical staff. The language and focus of the tools were amended and softened to emphasise the 'Releasing Time to Care' element, and PW was formally launched in the UK by the Chief Nursing Officer for England, Dame Christine Beasley, at the Royal College of Nursing Conference in 2007. Early phase implementation sites, also called 'learning partner sites', were recruited by the NHSI later in 2007 and widespread NHS implementation commenced.

PW is a self-directed improvement programme. The programme comprises 11 modules which provide tools and guidance to help nurses make required changes to their ward environment and work processes.

The modules are arranged in a framework (and depicted diagrammatically) known as the 'Productive Ward House': foundation modules provide a base of QI activity and process modules build on the QI capacity the foundation modules create. All modules and specific project role guidance are included in the PW box set that is provided under licence that contains 14 booklets that include all the tools.

The booklets serve as a reference guide and can be utilised over the life of the programme. Included with the 11 modules listed below are *The Executive Leader's Guide, The Project Leader's Guide* and *The Ward Leader's guide* information booklets. The three foundation modules are as follows:

1. *Knowing how we are doing*—introduces measurement systems that help understanding/benchmarking the ward's performance and subsequently how to make decisions on what to do to improve performance.
2. *Patient status at a glance*—focuses on the use of visual management to show important patient information so that it can be updated regularly, seen at a glance and used more effectively.
3. *Well-organised ward*—aims to increase the proportion of time spent providing direct care to patients and improve patient and staff experience. This module also gives guidance for an approach to simplify the workplace and reduce waste by having everything in the right place, at the right time, ready to go.

Once the foundation modules are complete, the ward team then progress through the following eight process modules:

1. *Meals*—Reduce the time the team spends physically delivering meals and allow more time for the team to assist with feeding and ensure proactive nutritional assessment for the patients in their care
2. *Medicines*—Ensure medicine rounds do not clash with other ward processes. Reduce interruptions on staff and ensures everything is ready for delivery of medicines
3. *Admission and planned discharge*—Remove the rush of admission and discharge through process planning. Ensure the team and support functions launch early to aid discharge at the correct point in the patient journey
4. *Shift handovers*—Reduce the time the team spends on handovers, whilst making the information handed over more appropriate, easier to remember and easier to understand
5. *Patient hygiene*—Ensures the dignity of patients by delivering safe, clean and responsive care
6. *Patient observations*—Increase the standard of patient observations being carried out. Ensure they are accurate and that appropriate action is taken on the results
7. *Nursing procedures*—Improve the supporting processes for nursing procedures so they are consistent, provide a better patient experience and achieve the standards the organisation aspires to
8. *Ward rounds*—Ensure clarity of outcome and clear planning from ward rounds whilst making the ward round quicker and consistent (NHS Institute and NNRU 2010a)

Although concern was raised from an internationalisation perspective in relation to the branding, the content and the language, it has been translated into other languages with only slight modifications to address cultural and contextual differences in some countries (Moore et al. 2013; Health Quality Council 2011). The modular design with practical, pictorial examples aims to assist with international application.

## 5.4 Reviewing Impacts and Outcomes of the Productive Ward: Releasing Time to Care

An updated review of the literature from a previous study (White and Waldron 2014) was performed and identified research papers, case-study reports and evaluations related to the PW or its implementation, and that reported impact, outcomes or outputs. The review was limited to material published between January 2006 and May 2017 and covers the period during which the PW was being both developed and implemented in the UK and internationally. The search methods, databases used and selection criteria were identical to a bibliometric analysis performed previously (White et al. 2014a). However, on this occasion the 'grey literature' (news reports, cover stories, commissioned reports and updates in professional journals) was excluded (with the exception of government papers, evaluations or independent reports), and 49 published peer-reviewed articles and evaluation reports (within the agreed inclusion criteria) were examined. Four NHSI-commissioned evaluation reports were removed on further analysis as a previous study has highlighted that these reports were commissioned and that there was a potential bias (Wright and McSherry 2013a). In total, 45 documents (36 peer-reviewed papers and 9 evaluation reports) were examined and the reported impacts, outcomes and outputs from the abstracts and conclusions recorded (see Table 5.1).

### 5.4.1 Does the PW Initiative Deliver Improvement?

The results of this update confirm and expand the findings from the previous review (White and Waldron 2014), highlighting that the PW is reported to deliver improvement in a multitude of ways, specifically impacting and benefiting participants. The initiative has been reported as being generally successful, with ample accounts of very positive impacts, outcomes and outputs, although one must always be cautious of both reporting and publishing bias. The majority of scholarly papers and research reports available suggest that PW has influenced a wide range of improvements in healthcare quality and patient safety. Unintended consequences (outcomes that were not explicitly targeted) from implementation of PW continue to be reported with positive impacts on empowerment, leadership, engagement, improved teamwork and staff morale remaining amongst the most commonly cited. A small number of papers identify negative aspects of impact, outcome and output and are highlighted in italics in Table 5.1.

Some studies report that PW creates a 'culture' and an 'appetite' for improvement reportedly absent from nursing of late, although it could be argued that there

**Table 5.1** Current peer-reviewed papers and evaluation reports

| Name | Reference No. | Year of publication | Peer-reviewed publication | Evaluation or Report within agreed criteria | Main reported outcomes/findings |
|---|---|---|---|---|---|
| Allsopp et al. | Allsopp et al. (2009) | 2009 | Nursing Times | – | Increased patient care times, ward improvements |
| Armitage and Hingham | Armitage and Hingham (2011) | 2011 | Nursing Mgmt. | – | |
| Avis | Avis (2009) | 2009 | – | √ | Ward improvements, positive staff attitudes, engagement |
| Avis | Avis (2011) | 2011 | – | √ | Staff engagement, stronger patient focus, increased use of measurement |
| Blakemore | Blakemore (2009) | 2009 | Nursing Mgmt | – | Empowerment, improved leadership |
| Bloodworth | Bloodworth (2009) | 2009 | Nursing Times | – | Gives control back to staff, involves the whole organisation |
| Bloodworth | Bloodworth (2011) | 2011 | JPOP | – | Culture change for improvement, increased direct patient care times |
| Brunoro-Kadash and Kadash | Brunoro-Kadash and Kadash (2013) | 2014 | Lead Health Serv | – | Improved patient safety, staff engagement, leadership opportunities, affirmative organisational cultural shift |
| Burston et al. | Burston et al. (2011) | 2011 | JAN | – | *Converging different strategies should be considered* |
| Coutts | Coutts (2010) | 2010 | Healthcare Quarterly | – | Positive change management, *poor corporate leadership* |
| Clarke and Marks-Maran | Clarke and Marks-Maran (2014) | 2014 | Br J Nur | | Improved patient safety, impact on leadership |
| Davis and Adams | Davis and Adams (2012) | 2012 | JNM | – | Positive impact on staff attitudes, morale, development |

(continued)

**Table 5.1** (continued)

| Name | Reference No. | Year of publication | Peer-reviewed publication | Evaluation or Report within agreed criteria | Main reported outcomes/findings |
|---|---|---|---|---|---|
| Foley and Cox | Foley and Cox (2013) | 2013 | – | √ | Improved performance, patient safety, measurements, organisational culture |
| Foster et al. | Foster et al. (2009) | 2009 | Nursing Times | – | Increased patient care times, reduced infection rates |
| Grant | Grant (2008) | 2008 | IJCL | – | *Lack of medical colleague involvement,* engagement |
| Gribben et al. | Gribben et al. (2009) | 2009 | – | √ | Valuable tools, improved communication and values |
| Hamilton et al. | Hamilton et al. (2014) | 2014 | | | Increases QI capacity, Improved engagement, leadership, teamwork |
| Health Quality Council | Health Quality Council (2011) | 2011 | – | √ | Ward improvements, engaged motivated staff, *more improvement and measurement training needed* |
| Kemp and Merchant | Kemp and Merchant (2011) | 2011 | Men Heal Prac | – | Improved patient care times |
| Lennard | Lennard (2012) | 2012 | Men Heal Prac | – | Improved teamwork |
| Lennard | Lennard (2014) | 2014 | JPMHN | – | Improved teamwork, communication and patient flow |
| Moore et al. | Moore et al. (2013) | 2013 | – | √ | Improved patient care times, better organised clinical environments, clear vision, improved ward documentation and standardised processes |

**Table 5.1** (continued)

| Name | Reference No. | Year of publication | Peer-reviewed publication | Evaluation or Report within agreed criteria | Main reported outcomes/findings |
|---|---|---|---|---|---|
| Morrow et al. | Morrow et al. (2012) | 2012 | IJHCQA | – | Positive leadership, improved social and work environment |
| Morrow et al. | Morrow and Robert (2014) | 2014 | J of HO&M | – | Develops leadership skills |
| NHS Scotland | NHS Scotland (2008) | 2008 | – | √ | Increased patient care times, improved morale |
| NHS Scotland | Scotland (2013) | 2013 | – | √ | Increased patient care times, efficiency savings, ward improvements |
| QIPP-NHS Evidence | QIPP-NHS Evidence (2009) | 2009 | – | √ | Increased patient care times, efficiencies, time saved, reduced falls, reduced waste, ward improvements |
| Robert | Robert (2011) | 2011 | Nursing Times | – | Lessons for spread, communication, champions |
| Robert et al | Robert et al. (2011) | 2011 | JCN | - | Improved teamwork, staff experience, leadership |
| Rudge | Rudge (2013) | 2013 | Nursing Phil | – | *Creates productivity as a desired state* |
| Smith and Rudd | Smith and Rudd (2010) | 2010 | Nursing Stand | – | Improved absenteeism, reduced complaints, ward organised |
| Van den Broek | van den Broek et al. (2013) | 2013 | Pub Man Review | – | *Confusing communication, poor long-term engagement* |
| Van Bogaert et al. | Van Bogaert et al. (2014) | 2014 | JONA | – | Improved teamwork, quality of care and job outcomes |

(continued)

**Table 5.1** (continued)

| Name | Reference No. | Year of publication | Peer-reviewed publication | Evaluation or Report within agreed criteria | Main reported outcomes/findings |
|------|--------------|--------------------|--------------------------|--------------------------------------------|---------------------------------|
| Van Bogaert et al. | Van Bogaert et al. (2017) | 2017 | CJNR | – | Practice environment, decision latitude, social capital *perceived workload, emotional exhaustion and vigour quality of care and job satisfaction* |
| White et al. | White et al. (2014c) | 2013 | JNM | – | Seven key characteristics for implementation identified |
| White et al. | White et al. (2013) | 2013 | IJLPS | – | Leadership, empowerment, engagement |
| White et al. | White et al. (2014a) | 2014 | JCN | – | Reducing bibliometric interest in the initiative |
| White et al. | White et al. (2014b) | 2014 | IJNS | – | Positive work engagement (vigour, absorption, dedication) |
| White and Waldron | White and Waldron (2014) | 2014 | BJN | – | Empowerment, leadership, engagement |
| White | White (2015) | 2015 | Nursing Times | – | Improved patient care times, ward improvements, staff engagement, improved teamwork, leadership development, empowerment, change management |
| White et al. | White et al. (2017b) | 2017 | JNR | – | Work engagement (vigour, absorption, dedication) capacity for compassion |
| Wilson | Wilson (2009) | 2009 | JNM | – | Positive patient satisfaction, patient care times, safety |

**Table 5.1** (continued)

| Name | Reference No. | Year of publication | Peer-reviewed publication | Evaluation or Report within agreed criteria | Main reported outcomes/findings |
|------|---------------|---------------------|---------------------------|---------------------------------------------|--------------------------------|
| Wright and McSherry | Wright and McSherry (2013a) | 2013 | JCN | – | Improved patient safety, patient care times, patient/staff experience and financial savings |
| Wright and McSherry | Wright and McSherry (2013b) | 2013 | Nursing Times | – | Patient care times |
| Wright and McSherry | Wright and McSherry (2014) | 2014 | JCN | – | Enthusiasm, empowerment, improved teamwork, increase morale, patient care times |

is rarely an instinctive appetite for QI amongst healthcare professionals (Siriwardena 2009; Dixon-Woods et al. 2012). Like all QI methods and initiatives, PW requires considered planning, implementation and reporting. The evidence provided from examples the literature reviewed suggest that many of the organisations that have actively managed planning, implementation and reporting have benefitted the most in terms of reported achievements and improvements.

A small number of the papers reviewed highlighted the lack of impact data, empirical evidence and evaluative research to substantiate the marketing claims of PW (Wright and McSherry 2013a; Gribben et al. 2009; Moore et al. 2013; Foley and Cox 2013). Because the number of peer-reviewed, scholarly publications identified in Table 5.1 is relatively small (less than 35 over a 9-year period), it is clear that the research and evidence base in relation to PW is still expanding which therefore makes detailing substantive claims in relation to the impact of PW difficult. However, the results from this review draw attention to the point that the majority of reports on the initiative are generally positive and that improvements (in multiple forms) are delivered.

## 5.4.2 Tailoring PW Implementation to Local Contexts

When it comes to improving quality in healthcare, context is defined as all factors that are external to the QI intervention (Ovretveit 2011). There are a number of 'lessons' available in the PW literature that clearly identify good context conditions which influence the chances of success. In a recent report of PW participant's experiences (White et al. 2017b), the most frequently noted theme (in terms of the number of references/citations) related to how the initiative was implemented and managed. The prominence of this theme is not surprising considering the prescriptive methods outlined in the module guides and the programmatic approach that is encouraged to be applied. However, PW is no different than any other QI intervention, in that it is a complex social intervention (Ovretveit 2011), and requires the right climate, conditions and context in order to be implemented successfully and in a sustainable manner and produced sustained improvements. Whilst the structured programmatic approach does appear to provide guidance in terms of governance, clarity, timelines, roles and responsibilities, this mode may not suit every ward team, environment or context.

Several studies highlight that how PW is implemented and managed is key to its success (Allsopp et al. 2009; Robert et al. 2011) and 'one size does not necessarily fit all' when it comes to implementation (Hamilton et al. 2014). The experience of implementing the PW initiative in Canada (Hamilton et al. 2014) emphasises the roles of organisational context, environment, positive culture and emotional and structural aspects in the successful implementation of PW. Experiences in Ireland and Canada demonstrate how existing (pre-PW) factors like QI capacity, capability, attitude and ward leadership all influence the effectiveness of implementation. The Irish and the Canadian studies therefore suggest the use of a pre-PW assessment, like the *Organizing for Quality framework* (Bate et al. 2008), {Bate 2008, Organizing for Quality: The Improvement Journeys of Leading Hospitals in Europe and the United States} for assessing the various context domains (structural, political, cultural, educational, emotional, physical and technical) that are associated with QI success and sustainability.

Although designed to facilitate the successful implementation of research and evidence into practice, there are some reports that support the use of an implementation framework (e.g. Consolidated Framework for Implementation Research (CFIR), Promoting Action on Research Implementation in Health Service (PARIHS)), prior to implementing QI interventions like PW (Damschroder et al. 2009; Harvey and Kitson 2016). Although the PW guidance/modules and the 'readiness assessment tool' provided by NHSI do pay some attention and diligence to assessing context and facilitation requirements for pre-PW implementation, it is fair to say that it is not to the same extent that either the PARIHS or the CFIR frameworks do. As the 'readiness assessment tool' is now no longer available with the PW licence, using well-tested context assessment models and frameworks (like PARIHS, CFIR or the Organising for Quality framework) would be advantageous prior to implementation to enhance and would influence the likeliness of success.

A number of the themes and key determinants that support the successful implementation of PW which were highlighted in a previous literature review (White et al. 2014c) were also observed in the latest 2017 Irish study (White et al. 2017b). Project management roles, good communication, appropriate training and corporate/management support all played a substantial part in the participant's experiences and perceptions of successful PW implementation and should be given prudent consideration when pre-planning PW.

For many PW participants, applying a 'programmatic' approach in busy clinical environments greatly impacts and regularly impedes progress of the initiative. The QI activities and efforts associated with PW can rarely be prioritised over the everyday activities associated with busy acute and non-acute clinical environments. For many participating sites, competing demands and conflicting logics become one of the main reasons for falling behind on implementation schedules (van den Broek et al. 2013; White et al. 2017b; Morrow et al. 2012). Previous reports and studies suggest a crucial role for project leads or quality facilitators in managing momentum and schedules. However; in the main, most studies observing the implementation of PW suggest that even with structured QI facilitation and resources, ward-based teams working in busy clinical environments really struggle to support the many QI activities and modules associated with a large-scale programme like PW (Morrow et al. 2012; Hamilton et al. 2014; Davis and Adams 2012). Factoring flexible timelines into project plans should be considered in the pre-planning phase of PW.

It is important to learn from implementations that go well and not so well (Pressman and Wildavsky 1973). There are a number of references in the literature highlighting how PW implementation was hampered by aspects of organisational context, particularly departmental structure, governance and culture (Wright and McSherry 2014; White et al. 2017b; Davis and Adams 2012; Morrow et al. 2012). For many participants and sites, successful implementation hinges on the extent (or not) that each ward manager (ward lead) invests in, facilitates and interacts with the initiative and participants. Leadership style, the ability to empower and enable (or disable) members of the ward team, appears to affect the pace, progress and interest of PW implementation (Morrow and Robert 2014; White et al. 2013). Poor or less-engaged leadership can lead to frustration and discontent within the implementing ward teams and has the potential to affect the momentum of the initiative (White et al. 2017a; Davis and Adams 2012).

It is most probable that varying leadership styles and 'how' ward managers invest in, interact with and implement PW have a relatively large part to play in the very mixed results that the initiative has had demonstrating if it has actually 'released time to care' (White et al. 2017c; Wright and McSherry 2014; Gribben et al. 2009). For those considering future implementation of PW, it would be worth considering ensuring that ward managers/PW leads embrace 'enabling' and 'empowering' leadership styles and positive, flexible, adaptive 'can do' approaches to effectively introduce and manage the initiative for the organisational context in which it is being introduced. It is unlikely that any 'one approach' will 'fit all' and maximise the potential of the QI tools and activities and release the benefits (Hamilton et al. 2014).

### 5.4.3   Sustaining the PW Initiative and Ownership

One crucial question pertaining to all 'QI' relates to how QI interventions and improvements are sustained (Glasgow et al. 2012). When it comes to assessing whether PW as an initiative will be sustained, it is important to ask, or at least get a sense of, whether PW is alive and well in many of the organisations that have adopted it. Without available data from the licence provider (NHS Improvement) or any national reporting system, this is impossible to gauge. Experience in Ireland indicates that it is a complex matter deciding whether a PW site is mid-implementation or has stalled (White 2015). Particularly in light of the competing clinical contexts outlined earlier, a number of the studies reviewed suggest that many implementing sites and wards take an 'à la carte' (piecemeal or selective) approach to fully applying PW modules (Moore et al. 2013; Wright and McSherry 2014). Many decide to just use some of the tools and to 'park' aspects or elements of modules which may not suit the context or clinical environment at that moment in time (Morrow et al. 2012; Davis and Adams 2012).

QI initiatives (like PW) are complex social interventions (Ovretveit 2011), and much of the literature in relation to the implementation of PW to date demonstrates that the momentum of PW and the associated QI activity ebbs and flows in accordance with the hustle and bustle of busy clinical environments (White et al. 2017b; Davis and Adams 2012; Hamilton et al. 2014). PW activities regularly get temporarily 'suspended' to deal with the various crises and competing priorities that routinely impact clinical environments (Davis and Adams 2012; Wright and McSherry 2014), making it almost impossible to precisely gauge how many sites that have commenced PW are still using it or where dissemination of the initiative sits nationally or internationally.

Participants in a recent study of PW identified that the sustainability of both the QI interventions and the initiative as a whole relied heavily on how the ward teams adopt, develop and incorporate PW as a way of working (White et al. 2017b). Introducing the initiative and assigning 'champions' in a well thought-out, open and transparent manner enhanced the chances of applicability and interest whilst reducing the risk of team members feeling isolated or excluded. Whilst adoption and front-line ownership have previously been cited as key components of QI success (Dixon-Woods et al. 2012; Mountford and Shojania 2012), participants implementing PW were able to recognise the relationship of their 'ownership' of PW to the momentum and sustainability of the initiative (Hamilton et al. 2014; White et al. 2017b; Davis and Adams 2012), specifically, the negative impact that nonparticipation and lack of engagement within the team can have on both the culture of innovation and improvement and the future or sustainability of PW (Hamilton et al. 2014; White et al. 2017b).

It is apparent that as the academic literature develops around QI initiatives like PW and their implementation, so will our understandings of the conditions that might support or detract from the success and the sustainability of these types of complex social interventions.

## 5.4.4   The Future of Productive Ward: Releasing Time to Care

The creator, and national and international sponsor of PW, the NHSI, became one of the many casualties of the UK government's focus on reducing 'quangos' (quasi-autonomous non-governmental organisations) and was abolished on the 31st March 2013. However, the PW continues to be supported internationally and in the UK through various consultancy-based 'partners' and a licensed e-learning package. There is little doubt that the closure of the NHSI, the PW's creator and sponsor in 2013, has had consequences on the pace and scale of roll-out and of this quality improvement initiative. Much of the resources, expertise and intellectual capital previously provided by the NHSI for implementing sites have evaporated. One could argue that it was the resources, the promotion, the marketing and the desirability that were behind much of the initiative's uptake and documented successes. Efforts to sustain this initiative as a viable national and international QI initiative now precariously lie with NHS Improvement, which promotes a range of QI interventions and offerings. Whether PW remains current and relevant, is renewed and refreshed or becomes another 'QI fad' will very much depend on how much NHS Improvement invests and continues to market and support the initiative. It will also depend on the QI intentions and adaptability of the many organisations that have already adopted it and are at various stages of implementation.

Results from the National Institute for Health Research (NIHR) study (13/157/44) https://njl-admin.nihr.ac.uk/document/download/2007807, which aims to explore if PW has had a sustained impact at the clinical microsystem level in English NHS acute trusts, are due in 2018. This study is designed to specifically examine QI initiatives like the PW as specific examples of initiatives where there has been 'no systematic evaluation of impact'. It is only when the 'hard' evidence is available from studies like these large-scale, independent impact evaluations that we will be in a position to judge the future of PW in its entirety. In the meantime, however, there are some signs internationally, and within some NHS Trusts, that PW has served its purpose as a QI 'aperitif' and that it has paved the way for larger system/organisation-wide 'Lean' or QI initiatives to be implemented and more readily accepted by front-line clinical teams (Avis 2011; Scotland 2013).

## Conclusion

This chapter has presented an overview of the PW initiative, its background, design, modular content and a general but comprehensive, up-to-date review of the peer-reviewed literature which highlights that the reported experiences of PW are overwhelmingly positive. The evidence in the literature suggests that 'one size does not fit all' when it comes to how the initiative is implemented and managed and that assessing context (environment, readiness, leadership capability, QI capacity and other conditions) greatly influences the success of implementation and the degree that it is sustained. Utilising existing implementation and quality frameworks will go some way to help identify specific context requirements and allow implementation and the programme to be tailored accordingly.

A number of studies reviewed highlight the difficulties that ward-based teams working in busy clinical environments experience as many of the QI activities and modules associated with PW compete with everyday clinical demands and priorities. Aspects that did not go so well during the implementation and management of PW provide the greatest opportunity for insight, learning and understanding the conditions for success, and the literature reviewed highlights the pivotal role that ward managers/PW have 'enabling' and 'empowering' a culture of improvement. Utilising some of the emerging implementation and quality frameworks outlined in this paper to assess context and determine unit/ward readiness more comprehensively will go some way to addressing the individual needs of clinical environments and teams prior to implementing PW and will influence its success.

A more pertinent question in relation to the future of PW remains, however. It appears, on the face of it, that interest in PW may well have peaked and that it is less 'en vogue' than many of the QI programmes, initiatives and collaboratives being marketed by its international competitor, the Institute for Healthcare Improvement (IHI). NHS Improvement now markets and promotes other more contemporary QI tools and interventions ahead of PW. As a former flagship QI programme for NHS Improvement, it is no longer openly visible amongst the organisation's web-based offerings. What is less obvious to gauge is the level of interest from existing or new 'start-up' PW sites either in the UK or elsewhere because this information is not readily available from NHS Improvement. If support for PW dwindles in the coming years, it will be very important to recognise and remember that the PW initiative has served or in some instance is still serving as an appetiser or stimulant for other large-scale organisation-wide QI programmes.

# References

Allsopp P, Faruqi J, Gascoigne L, Tennyson R. Productive Ward 2: practical advice to facilitators implementing the programme. Nurs Times. 2009;105(25):19–21.

Armitage C, Hingham P. The Productive Ward: encouraging teambuilding and innovation. Nurs Manag. 2011;18(1):28–31.

Avis K. Releasing time to care in Saskatchewan: promising signs that programme engages clinicians. Saskatoon: Health Quality Council; 2009.

Avis K. Looking Back Thinking forward; Insight and recommendations from health region leadership on creating a culture of continuous performance in Saskatchewan. Saskatoon: Health Quality Council. 2011.

Bate P, Mendel P, Robert GB. Organizing for quality: the improvement journeys of leading hospitals in Europe and the United States. Oxford: Radcliffe Publishing. 2008.

Blakemore S. How Productive Wards can improve patient care. Nurs Manag. 2009;16(5):14–8.

Bloodworth K. Productive Ward. 1: implementing the initiative across a large university teaching hospital. Nurs Times. 2009;105(24):22–5.

Bloodworth K. The Productive Ward and the productive operating theatre. J Perioper Pract. 2011;21(3):97–103.

Brunoro-Kadash C, Kadash N. Time to care: a patient-centered quality improvement strategy. Leadersh Health Serv. 2013;26(3):220–31.

Burgess N, Radnor Z. Evaluating lean in healthcare. Int J Health Care Qual Assur. 2013;26(3):220–35.

Burston S, Chaboyer W, Wallis M, Stanfield J. A discussion of approaches to transforming care: contemporary strategies to improve patient safety. J Adv Nurs. 2011;67(11):2488–95.

Charles RG, Kathleen LM, Sriranjita S. Contrasting continuous quality improvement, Six Sigma, and lean management for enhanced outcomes in US hospitals. Am J Bus. 2012;27(2):133–53.

Clarke U, Marks-Maran D. Nurse leadership in sustaining programmes of change. Br J Nurs. 2014;23(4):219–24.

Coutts J. Releasing time to care. Healthc Q. 2010;13(2):21–3.

Damschroder LJ, Aron DC, Keith RE, Kirsh SR, Alexander JA, Lowery JC. Fostering implementation of health services research findings into practice: a consolidated framework for advancing implementation science. Implement Sci. 2009;4(1):50.

Davies H, Powell A, Rushmer R. Why don't clinicians engage with quality improvement? J Health Serv Res Policy. 2007;12(3):129–30.

Davis J, Adams J. The 'releasing time to care - the Productive Ward' programme: participants' perspectives. J Nurs Manag. 2012;20(3):354–60.

Deming WE. Out of the crisis: quality, productivity and competitive position. Cambridge: Cambridge University Press; 1986.

Dixon-Woods M, McNicol S, Martin G. Ten challenges in improving quality in healthcare: lessons from the Health Foundation's programme evaluations and relevant literature. BMJ Qual Saf. 2012;21(10):876–84.

Feigenbaum AV. Total quality control. New York: McGraw-Hill; 1983.

Ferlie EB, Shortell SM. Improving the quality of health care in the United Kingdom and the United States: a framework for change. Milbank Q. 2001;79(2):281–315.

Fixsen DL, Naoom SF, Blase KA, Fiedman RM, Wallace F. Implementation research: a synthesis of the literature. Tampa: University of South Florida, Louis de la Parte Florida Mental Health Institute; 2005.

Foley B, Cox A. Work organisation and innovation: case study: Nottingham University Hospitals NHS Trust, UK. Dublin: European Foundation for the Improvement of Living and Working Conditions; 2013.

Foster S, Gordon P, McSherry W. Rolling out Productive Ward foundation modules across a hospital trust. Nurs Times. 2009;105(30-31):28–30.

Gill D, Mountford J, Arasaratnam R. What is a quality improvement project? Br J Hosp Med. 2012;73(5):252–6.

Glasgow JM, Davies ML, Kaboli PJ. Findings from a national improvement collaborative: are improvements sustained? BMJ Qual Saf. 2012;21(8):663–9.

Gollop R, Whitby E, Buchanan D, Ketley D. Influencing sceptical staff to become supporters of service improvement: a qualitative study of doctors' and managers' views. Qual Saf Health Care. 2004;13(2):108–14.

Graban M. Lean hospitals; improving quality, patient safety, and employee engagement. 2nd ed. New York: CRC Press; 2012.

Grant P. The Productive Ward round: a critical analysis of organisational change. Int J Clin Leadership. 2008;16(4):193–201.

Gribben B, McCance T, Slater P. Belfast health and social care trust, Productive Ward-releasing time to care evaluation report. Belfast: BHSCT; 2009.

Hamilton J, Verrall T, Maben J, Griffiths P, Avis K, Baker GR, Teare G. One size does not fit all: a qualitative content analysis of the importance of existing quality improvement capacity in the implementation of releasing time to care: the Productive Ward™ in Saskatchewan, Canada. BMC Health Serv Res. 2014;14(1):1–14.

Harvey G, Kitson A. PARIHS revisited: from heuristic to integrated framework for the successful implementation of knowledge into practice. Implement Sci. 2016;11(1):33.

Havelock RG. The change agent's guide to innovation in education. Englewood Cliffs: Educational Technology Publications; 1973.

Health Quality Council. Releasing time to care: the Productive Ward long-term care pilot project report. Saskatoon: Health Quality Council; 2011.

Juran JM, Gryna FM. Juran's quality control handbook. London: McGraw-Hill; 1988.

Kemp P, Merchant S. How to turn innovations into everyday practice. Ment Health Pract. 2011;15(2):20–4.

Kenett RS. Lean six sigma for hospitals: strategic steps to fast, affordable. Flawless Healthcare. 2011;44(11):62–3.

Langley G, Nolan K, Norman C, Provost L, Nolan T. The improvement guide: a practical approach to enhancing organizational performance. 2nd ed. San Francisco: Jossey-Bass; 2009.

Lennard C. How the Productive Ward scheme gives staff more time to care: implementation of a work efficiency initiative in an acute mental health adult ward is improving nurses' welfare while providing a more effective service to clients. Ment Health Pract. 2012;15(5):30.

Lennard C. Productive Ward initiative promotes better communication between mental health teams and ensures timely discharge for patients. J Psychiatr Ment Health Nurs. 2014;21(1):4.

Mazzocato P, Savage C, Brommels M, Aronsson H, Thor J. Lean thinking in healthcare: a realist review of the literature. Qual Saf Health Care. 2010;19(5):376–82.

Moore D, Blick G, Leggott J, Bloodworth K. Assessment of the implementation of the Productive Ward and Productive Operating Theatre programmes in New Zealand. Wellington: Sapere Research Group; 2013.

Morrow E, Robert G. Exploring the nature and impact of leadership on the local implementation of the Productive Ward releasing time to care. J Health Organ Manag. 2014;28(2):154–76.

Morrow E, Robert G, Maben J, Griffiths P. Implementing large-scale quality improvement: lessons from The Productive Ward: Releasing Time to Care. Int J Health Care Qual Assur. 2012;25(4):237–53.

Mountford J, Shojania KG. Refocusing quality measurement to best support quality improvement: local ownership of quality measurement by clinicians. BMJ Qual Saf. 2012;21(6):519–23.

NHS Institute and NNRU. Improving healthcare quality at scale and pace, lessons for the Productive Ward: Releasing Time to Care programme. Warwick: NHS Institute; 2010a.

NHS Institute and NNRU. The Productive Ward: Releasing Time to Care learning and impact review. Warwick: NHS Institute; 2010b.

NHS Scotland. NHS Scotland, releasing time to care evaluation. Edinburgh: NHS Scotland; 2008.

Nursing Standard. Full roll-out for Productive Wards by 2013. Nurs Stand. 2012;26(19):7.

Ovretveit J. Understanding the conditions for improvement: research to discover which context influences affect improvement success. BMJ Qual Saf. 2011;20(Supplement 1):i18–23.

Ovretveit J. Contemporary quality improvement. Cad Saude Publica. 2013;29(3):424–6.

Pressman JL, Wildavsky AB. Implementation: how great expectation in Washington are dashed in Oakland; or, why it's amazing that federal programs work at all, this being a saga of the economic development administration as told by two sympathetic observers who seek to build morals on a foundation. Berkeley: University California Press; 1973.

QIPP-NHS Evidence. The Productive Ward - quality and productivity example; 2009.

Reay T, Hinings CR. Managing the rivalry of competing institutional logics. Organ Stud. 2009;30(6):629–52.

Robert G. Progress of the Productive Ward. Nurs Times. 2011;107(7):18–9.

Robert G, Morrow E, Maben J, Griffiths P, Callard L. The adoption, local implementation and assimilation into routine nursing practice of a national quality improvement programme: the Productive Ward in England. J Clin Nurs. 2011;20(7-8):1196–207.

Rudge T. Desiring productivity: nary a wasted moment, never a missed step. Nurs Philos. 2013;14(3):201–11.

Scotland N. Releasing time to care: making our priorities possible—final report. Edinburgh: NHS; 2013.

Siriwardena AN. Engaging clinicians in quality improvement initiatives: art or science? Qual Prim Care. 2009;17(5):303–5.

Smith J, Rudd C. Implementing the Productive Ward Management programme. Nurs Stand. 2010;24(31):45–8.

Taitz JM, Lee TH, Sequist TD. A framework for engaging physicians in quality and safety. BMJ Qual Saf. 2012;21(9):722–8.

The Health Foundation. Evidence scan: improvement science. London: The Health Foundation; 2011.

Van Bogaert P, Van heusden D, Somers A, Tegenbos M, Wouters K, Van der Straeten J, Van Aken P, Havens DS. The Productive Ward Program™: a longitudinal multilevel study of nurse perceived practice environment, burnout, and nurse-reported quality of care and job outcomes. JONA. 2014;44(9):452–61.

Van Bogaert P, Van heusden D, Verspuy M, Wouters K, Slootmans S, Van der Straeten J, Van Aken P, White M. The Productive Ward Program™: a two-year implementation impact review using a longitudinal multilevel study. Can J Nurs Res. 2017;49:28–38.

van den Broek J, Boselie P, Paauwe J. Multiple institutional logics in health care: Productive Ward: 'releasing time to care'. Public Manage Rev. 2013;16(1):1–20.

van Os A, de Gilder D, van Dyck C, Groenewegen P. Responses to professional identity threat. J Health Organ Manag. 2015;29(7):1011–28.

White M. How effective is Productive Ward. Nurs Times. 2015;111(11):12–4.

White M, Butterworth T, Wells JS. Healthcare quality improvement and 'work engagement'; concluding results from a national, longitudinal, cross-sectional study of the 'Productive Ward-Releasing time to care' programme. BMC Health Serv Res. 2017a;17(510):1–11.

White M, Butterworth T, Wells JSG. Reported implementation lessons from a national quality improvement initiative; Productive Ward: Releasing Time to Care™. A qualitative, ward-based team perspective. J Nurs Manag. 2017b;25(7):519–30. https://doi.org/10.1111/jonm.12489.

White M, Butterworth T, Wells JSG. Productive Ward: Releasing Time to Care, or capacity for compassion: results from a longitudinal study of the quality improvement initiative. J Res Nurs. 2017c;22(1/2):91–109.

White M, Waldron M. Effects and impacts of Productive Ward from a nursing perspective. Br J Nurs. 2014;23(8):419–26.

White M, Wells JGS, Butterworth T. Leadership, a key element of quality improvement in healthcare. Results from a literature review of 'Lean-Healthcare' and the Productive-Ward: Releasing-Time-to-Care Initiative. Int J Leadership Public Serv. 2013;9(3/4):1–22.

White M, Wells JS, Butterworth T. The transition of a large-scale quality improvement initiative: a bibliometric analysis of the Productive Ward: Releasing Time to Care programme. J Clin Nurs. 2014a;23(17–18):2414–23.

White M, Wells JSG, Butterworth T. The impact of a large-scale quality improvement programme on work engagement: preliminary results from a national cross-sectional-survey of the 'Productive Ward'. Int J Nurs Stud. 2014b;51(12):1634–43.

White M, Wells JSG, Butterworth T. The Productive Ward: Releasing Time to Care™ – what we can learn from the literature for implementation. J Nurs Manag. 2014c;22(7):914–23. https://doi.org/10.1111/jonm.12069.

Wilson G. Implementation of releasing time to care – the Productive Ward. J Nurs Manag. 2009;17(5):647–54.

Womack JP, Jones DT, Roos D, Massachusetts Institute of Technology. The machine that changed the world: based on the Massachusetts Institute of Technology 5-million dollar 5-year study on the future of the automobile. New York: Rawson Associates; 1990.

Wright S, McSherry W. A systematic literature review of Releasing Time to Care: The Productive Ward. J Clin Nurs. 2013a;22(9-10):1361–71.

Wright S, McSherry W. How much time do nurses spend on patient care? Nurs Times. 2013b;109.

Wright S, McSherry W. Evaluating the Productive Ward at an acute NHS trust: experiences and implications of releasing time to care. J Clin Nurs. 2014;23(13–14):1866–76.

# Embedding Compassionate Care: A Leadership Programme in the National Health Service in Scotland

Juliet MacArthur

**Abstract**

This chapter presents the findings from a 3-year research study examining the impact of the Leadership in Compassionate Care (LCC) Programme undertaken in Scotland. The study led to the development of a conceptual model for strengthening organisational capacity for the delivery of compassionate care. This model recognises compassionate care as focussing on meeting the needs of patients, relatives *and* staff. The study revealed that embedding and sustaining compassionate care were strongly influenced by work environment and organisational context; these two elements are examined in terms of their impact on the sustained adoption of the LCC Programme's aims. Findings suggest that establishing a sustained culture of compassionate care demands strategic vision and investment in a local infrastructure that supports relationship-centred care, practice development and effective leadership at all levels. The most influential aspects of organisational context were strategic buy-in, leadership style, support from charge nurses and clinical nurse managers and an appreciative facilitation approach by the LCC Programme team.

**Keywords**

Compassion • Relationships • Practice development • Realist evaluation • Context
NHS • In-patient

J. MacArthur
Chief Nurse Research and Development, NHS Lothian, University of Edinburgh,
Edinburgh, Scotland
e-mail: juliet.macarthur@nhs.net

© Springer International Publishing AG 2018
P. Van Bogaert, S. Clarke (eds.), *The Organizational Context of Nursing Practice*,
https://doi.org/10.1007/978-3-319-71042-6_6

## 6.1    Introduction

> Patient-centred compassionate care will never be fully realised until patients are woven into
> the fabric of healthcare organisational structures and functions.
>     (Frampton and Goodrich 2014, p. 203)

Despite the public's strong endorsement of the National Health Service (NHS) in
the UK, there has been long-standing concern about the delivery of compassionate
care, particularly in hospital settings. In recent years this has created a level of
debate voiced by the public, media, politicians and healthcare professionals that
resonates with McMahon and White (2017) depiction of a 'deficit' of compassion at
a societal, organisational, professional and individual level. In the UK compassion
is now put forward as a central tenant of healthcare policy and educational standards
and is at the heart of nursing professional practice within *The Code*, where nurses
are required to 'treat people with kindness, respect and compassion' (Nursing and
Midwifery Council (NMC) 2015, p. 4). The Scottish Government's (2017) health
and social care standards identify compassion as one of five underpinning principles,[1]
with compassion embodied in warm, nurturing care and support that is provided by
professionals and workers who understand and are sensitive to an individual's needs
and wishes (p. 5). As Cornwell and Goodrich (2009) highlight, from the patient's
perspective, it is often the 'little things' (such as making family members a cup of
tea or remembering significant events going on in the patient's life) and the presence
or absence of compassion that mark lasting memories of healthcare.

Whilst the UK is not unique in expressions of concern about healthcare provision, the scandal of poor care in Mid Staffordshire NHS Foundation Trust from
2005 to 2009 (Francis 2010, 2013) is widely recognised as having been a major
catalyst in bringing the issue of organisational culture and compassionate nursing
practice into sharp focus. The Independent Inquiry into the care provided by the
Trust made specific reference to poor nursing practice, identifying failures in bladder and bowel care and inadequate attention to patient modesty leading to loss of
dignity (Francis 2010). Lord Francis emphasised that the organisational culture was
not conducive to good patient care or a supportive working environment for staff
and that concerns had been voiced repeatedly about 'the lack of compassion and
uncaring attitude exhibited towards vulnerable patients and the marked indifference
they showed to visitors' (p. 15). A later publication listed 290 recommendations
(Francis 2013), which included the need for clear and robust accountability, openness and transparency, effective regulation and intentional development of a culture
of caring. Recommendation 185 made strong reference to preconditions for compassionate nursing care including careful management of recruitment, training,
leadership and care delivery (p. 105). What was clearly absent in Mid Staffordshire
Foundation NHS Trust was an organisational culture that recognised the importance

---

[1] The five principles are dignity; respect; compassion, being included; responsive care and support;
and well-being (Scottish Government 2017).

of the context of care delivery and the centrality of caregiver-patient relationships to the functioning of the NHS.

This chapter reviews the evidence for work environment as a key factor in embedding compassionate care in healthcare settings. Furthermore, it discusses the role of relationship-centred care (Nolan et al. 2006) as a means to enable valuable communication and effective teamwork, not only between healthcare professionals but also between healthcare staff and patients and their family members. Whilst work environment and relationships are relevant to most analyses of the organisational context of nursing, here it is analysed through the lens of the concept of *compassion*. We describe research carried out in Scotland critically examining an organisational-wide programme aimed at embedding compassionate care in nursing practice and education.

The Leadership in Compassionate Care (LCC) Programme was a joint initiative undertaken in 2008–2011 between Edinburgh Napier University and NHS Lothian[2] (Adamson et al. 2011). The longitudinal qualitative research study reported here adopted a realist evaluation design (Pawson and Tilley 1997) and yielded insights regarding how best to recognise and support existing good practice and achieve sustainable improvements in the delivery of compassionate care. Data collection was conducted over 3 years and led to the development of a conceptual model for strengthening organisational capacity for the delivery of compassionate care (MacArthur et al. 2017). This model which depicts a 'compassionate core' focussed on the needs of patients, of relatives *and* of staff. The study findings revealed that embedding and sustaining compassionate care is strongly influenced by organisational context. Meaningful progress in establishing compassionate care demands both strategic vision and investment in a local infrastructure that supports relationship-centred care, practice development and effective leadership at all levels.

### 6.1.1 Compassionate Care

Two landmark papers presenting conceptual analyses of the term 'compassionate care' centred on the question of 'how important is compassion to nursing?', with Schantz (2007, p. 48) describing compassion as being nursing's 'most effective strength' and its 'most precious asset' (von Dietze and Orb 2000; Schantz 2007). There are numerous definitions of compassionate care, many of which share the key elements outlined by Lown et al. (2017): understanding another's pain or suffering and a commitment to doing something about that pain. Atkins and Parker (2012) suggest that compassion has four components: attending, understanding, empathising and helping, all of which convey a sense of purposeful action. In a systematic

---

[2] NHS Lothian is one of 14 regional Health Boards in Scotland. It provides a comprehensive range of primary, community-based and acute hospital services for the populations of Edinburgh, Midlothian, East Lothian and West Lothian, serving the second largest residential population in Scotland—circa 850,000 people. It employs approximately 24,000 staff of whom around 16,000 are nurses and midwives.

review of 24 studies reporting interventions for compassionate nursing care, Bloomberg et al. (2016), p. 139 synthesised four key components of what they termed 'the narrative' of compassion (my italics):

> The *moral attributes* of a 'compassionate' nurse includes empathy, the nurse's *situational awareness of vulnerability and suffering*, the nurse's *responsive action* aimed at relieving suffering and ensuring dignity and the nurse's *relational capacity*.

The emphasis on the nurse's situational awareness here is on both the personal situation of the patient and the context in which care is being delivered.

Bloomberg et al. (2016) narrative echoes the findings of a critical review of the nursing literature undertaken by McCaffery and McConnell (2015) which identified three interrelated themes: (1) compassion as a practice, (2) its position as a moral virtue and (3) the implications of institutional environments in facilitating or limiting expressions of compassionate care. The latter theme is a clear reference to the organisational context of nursing practice.

## 6.1.2   Organisational Context of Nursing in the UK

There is recognition that the context and nature of the UK NHS have shifted in recent years towards a more market-driven and bureaucratic culture, which some argue is dominated by achieving targets and efficiencies (Bradshaw 2009; Crawford et al. 2013). Such depictions are set alongside the well-recognised backdrop (that has international equivalence) of an ageing population, pressures on public finance, higher patient acuity and reductions in length of hospital stay leading to an increase in the pace and complexity of the working environment in healthcare settings (Patterson et al. 2010; Scottish Government 2013; NHS England 2014).

These changes are believed to have influenced professional working relationships as well as relationships between healthcare workers and patients/families (Firth-Cozens and Cornwell 2009; Patterson et al. 2010). Furthermore, concerns have been raised regarding the impact of difficult working environments on staff health and well-being and ultimately on the quality of patient care (Boorman 2009). Within nursing there is evidence of specific challenges for newly qualified nurses (Maben 2014), along with high proportions of experienced nurses reporting burnout and intentions to leave their jobs (Aiken et al. 2012). All these observations echo the findings of West et al. (2013) research into the prevailing culture and behaviours in the NHS which documented high levels of stress and burnout which could impact on individual performance, patient experience and outcomes. Their recommendations included the need for strategies and effective management to promote staff health and well-being, positive work environments and effective teamwork.

There is also growing evidence about the prerequisites for fostering a high-quality environment for care (Nolan et al. 2006; West et al. 2017). In a review of her own programme of research with newly qualified (Maben et al. 2007) and newly appointed nurses and an examination of the potential link between staff experiences of work and their psychological well-being and patient experiences

**Table 6.1** Factors influencing positive environments of care (based on Maben 2014, p. 129)

| Leadership | Support structures | Operational issues | Relationships |
|---|---|---|---|
| Good role models | Support for staff including mentorship and preceptorship | Adequate staff and good skill mix | Motivated and receptive colleagues |
| Ideas welcomed and change encouraged | Staff feel valued and receive feedback | Staff performance well managed | Supportive co-workers (idea of family at work) |
| Philosophy supporting compassionate care | Space and opportunity to 'process' work challenges with colleagues | Low demand, high control over work | |
| Staff feel heard and voice 'counts' | | | |
| Excellent team leadership | | | |

(Maben et al. 2012a, b), Maben (2014) developed a comprehensive framework of factors influencing positive environments of care. These can be related to organisational context in terms of leadership, support structures, operational issues and relationships (summarised in Table 6.1).

Given the growing recognition of the links between work environment, staff well-being and patient experience, it is important to understand potential organisational interventions aimed at strengthening capacity for compassionate care. The LCC Programme was one of the earliest UK examples of such an intervention.

### 6.1.3 Leadership in Compassionate Care Programme

The LCC Programme was funded by a benefactor and aimed 'to embed compassionate care as an integral aspect of all nursing practice and education' (Adamson et al. 2011, p. 14) and included establishing 'Beacon Wards,' 'Development Sites' and 'Development Units' to showcase excellence in compassionate care. It originated with the findings of an internal inquiry into specific episodes in two hospitals that identified a lack of respect from caregivers that had adverse effects on the personal dignity of older patients (NHS Lothian 2006). The developers recognised the need for a range of initiatives, largely focussed on organisational values and leadership, that would refocus attention on care delivery and the patient's experience of care. The term 'compassion' was chosen as a focus for this work at a time when the concept was not in common use in healthcare policy and practice; instead dignity and person-centred care were the main foci of nursing projects and research studies (Baillie and Gallagher 2010; McCormack and McCance 2006, 2010). The originators of the LCC Programme recognised that the patient experience of healthcare was a vital dimension of service delivery along with compassion towards staff (Adamson et al. 2011). They felt research was needed to support this agenda to determine what constitutes compassionate care and how it could be recognised and assessed appropriately. Furthermore, they recognised the importance of examining team and

---

**Phase 1 Beacon Wards 2008**
- Acute medicine of older people (Ward A)
- Older people with enduring mental health conditions (Ward B)
- Acute medical specialty (Ward C)
- Acute and long term medical specialty (Ward D)

**Phase 2 Development Sites 2009**
- Rehabilitation in mental health (Ward E)
- Older people and palliative care (Ward F)
- Acute assessment (Ward G)
- National rehabilitation specialty (Ward H)

**Phase 3 Development Units 2010**
- Maternity services (3 areas, 2 sites) (Unit I)
- Surgical wards (3 areas, 1 site) (Unit J)
- Inpatient community (5 services, 3 sites) (Unit K)
- Discharge lounges (3) and medical day care (3 sites) (Unit L)
- Regional medical and surgical specialty (3 areas, 1 site) (Unit M)

**Fig. 6.1** Phases of the LCC Programme and specialties involved

organisational influences that contribute to compassionate care and determining how these could be strengthened in the everyday realities of healthcare delivery.

The LCC Programme was conducted as a 3-year action research study (Meyer 2000) undertaken by a team of four LCC Senior Nurses and one Lead Nurse who worked with a total of 33 wards across the Health Board in three phases (Fig. 6.1). It explored the delivery of compassionate care in these in-patient settings with a view to understanding its meaning and expression from the perspective of healthcare practitioners, patients and relatives and to fostering methods of embedding compassion in practice. The findings from the study reported in this chapter, which was separate from the LCC Programme action research, focussed on the Beacon Wards (A–D) and Development Sites (E–H). The purpose and selection methods for both groups of units are outlined in Box 6.1.

---

**Box 6.1 Purpose and Selection of Beacon Wards and Development Sites (MacArthur et al. 2017)**

*Beacon Wards*

Expected to demonstrate excellence in compassionate caring, with a view to sharing and spreading effective practice to other areas. Wards selected through evidence and demonstration of (1) caring environment, (2) collaborative and effective team working and (3) staff development.

*Development Sites*

The purpose was to test methods and processes understood from the Beacon phase and to develop relationship-centred, compassionate care practice. Wards were required to demonstrate a commitment to support change and develop practice at a senior level and within the multidisciplinary team.

The theoretical principles of relationship-centred care (Nolan et al. 2006) and appreciative inquiry (Cooperrider et al. 2008) underpinned the LCC Programme. Beach and Inui (2006, p. 53) define relationship-centred care as 'care in which all participants appreciate the importance of their relationships with one another', and in this respect the LCC Programme was strongly influenced by Nolan et al. (2006) Senses Framework where the focus on relationships is based on six senses[3] that have been linked to 'enriched' environments of care and learning (Brown et al. 2008).

Appreciative inquiry focuses on the positive elements of both individuals and the organisation and is based on a 4-D Cycle involving 'Discovery' (what is), 'Dream' (what might be), 'Design' (what could be) and 'Destiny' (what can be). The Senior Nurses acted, therefore, as action researchers with an appreciative stance. Dewar and Mackay (2010) reported that this meant working with staff, patients and families to understand compassionate care in the clinical areas by systematically discovering what was happening through active curiosity and affirmation of different points of view.

During each phase, the LCC team worked with staff in each ward/unit for 7–9 months, conducting the action research and facilitating a range of innovative practice development approaches, including:

- Emotional touchpoints (Dewar et al. 2011)—a method of eliciting stories based on an individual's (patient, family, staff or student) emotional experience of a number of 'touchpoints' during their care, work or learning.
- Beliefs and values clarification (Adamson et al. 2011, p. 38)—this involved facilitation of staff groups to develop a common shared purpose/vision and understand how purpose and vision influence compassionate practice and culture.
- Photo elicitation (Dewar 2012)—using photographs to prompt discussions with all patients, family members, staff and students about the meaning of compassionate care, with statements subsequently being displayed and discussed as 'positive care practices'.

The outcome of the action research undertaken by the LCC team was an analytic framework that included six themes for person-centred compassionate care (Box 6.2) (Adamson et al. 2011, p. 159–161).

---

**Box 6.2 Leadership in Compassionate Care Themes for Person-Centred Compassionate Care (Adamson et al. 2011, p. 26)**
*Caring conversations*: Discussing, sharing, debating and learning how care is provided, amongst staff, patients and relatives, and the way in which caring practice is talked about.

---

[3] The six senses are sense of security, sense of belonging, sense of purpose, sense of continuity, sense of achievement and sense of significance (Nolan et al. 2006).

*Flexible, person-centred risk taking*: Making and justifying decisions about care in respect of context and working creatively with patient choice, staff experience and best practice.

*Feedback*: Staff, patients and families giving and receiving specific feedback about their experience of care.

*Knowing me, knowing you*: Developing mutual relationships and knowing the person's priorities, to enable negotiation in the way 'things are done around here'.

*Involving, valuing and transparency*: Creating an environment throughout the organisation where staff, patients and families actively influence and participate in the way things are done around here.

*Creating spaces that work: the environment*: Need to consider the wider environment and where necessary be flexible and adapt the environment to provide compassionate care.

## 6.2 Realist Evaluation of the LCC Programme

The study that forms the basis of this chapter is reported in full elsewhere (MacArthur 2014; MacArthur et al. 2017). Here, the focus is on a critical examination of the impact of the context (at macro, meso and micro levels[4]) in which implementation took place and affected programme outcomes. The specific research questions relating to this component were:

1. What are the views, experiences and perceptions of the participating stakeholders of the impact of the LCC Programme?
2. How is context seen to influence the outcomes of the LCC Programme in different clinical settings?

The study design was based on Pawson and Tilley (1997) theory-driven realistic evaluation approach that places emphasis on understanding context. Rather than seeking to determine whether a programme or intervention has 'worked' (or not), realistic evaluation is designed to provide detailed answers to the question of 'why a programme works, for whom and in what circumstances'. The theoretical underpinning of this approach was what Pawson and Tilley (1997) describe as CMO configurations: the link between the context (C) within which the programme is being delivered and the ideas and opportunities known as mechanisms (M) that the programme brings, which in turn lead to programme outcomes (O).

---

[4] In this context macro is defined as Health Board level where the focus is on strategic decision-making, meso is 'directorate' level which represents a group of wards/departments focussed on related specialties and micro is individual ward or department level.

Pawson and Tilley (1997) discuss the initial identification of what they describe as 'folk theories' as a fundamental element of their theory-based approach; this includes what it is about the programme under investigation that might generate change and in what sort of settings, and under what sort of conditions. Most of the 'folk theories' identified at the outset of the study had strong links to the organisational context of nursing at macro, meso and micro level. They included:

- Impact of workplace demands (Ramunujam et al. 2008; Patterson et al. 2010)
- Organisational culture (Kitson 2008; Aiken et al. 2008; Youngson 2008; Kirkley et al. 2011)
- Work environment (Van Bogaert et al. 2009; Burston and Stitchler 2010)
- Leadership style (Alimo-Metcalfe et al. 2007; Cummings et al. 2010)
- Complexity of healthcare systems (Kitson 2008; McCormack et al. 2008a, b, Patterson et al. 2010)
- Implementation of evidence into practice (Kitson et al. 1998)

Blamey and Mackenzie (2010) argue that context is crucial in understanding the interplay between a programme and its effects. Furthermore, given that context is multifaceted at a variety of levels (political, social, organisational and individual), they suggest it is important to delineate contextual variation when reporting findings as these are crucial for future recommendations for policy and practice.

## 6.2.1  Study Design

The study used a qualitative, longitudinal research design (Holland et al. 2006) over a 3-year period, with data collection in three phases beginning approximately 6 months after the implementation of the LCC Programme. Ethical approval was sought from the Scotland A Research Ethics Committee (07/MRE00/120) and the university Faculty Ethical Committee. Management approval was obtained from the NHS Research and Development Office (2007/P/UO/03).

## 6.2.2  Sample

Pawson and Tilley (1997 p. 161), identify three stakeholder groups within a realist evaluation. These groups formed the basis of the purposive sampling, with most of the sample being interviewed in each phase of the study:

- *Subjects* (on the receiving end of the LCC Programme)—charge nurses and nurse managers from the Beacon Wards and Development Sites ($n = 14$)
- *Practitioners* (delivering the LCC Programme)—LCC Senior Nurses ($n = 7$)
- *Policymakers* (influencing the direction of the Programme)—senior individuals in the NHS organisation and higher education institution ($n = 5$)

### 6.2.3    Data Collection

A variety of data collection methods were involved (Table 6.2), most of which included direct observations of the context in each of the clinical environments.

Together, these strategies yielded a picture of the context (C) of each ward, the mechanisms (M) utilised by the LCC team and the outcomes (O) for patients, relatives, ward staff and the charge nurses. The longitudinal design led to the prospective examination of the CMO configurations of the LCC Programme and its aim of embedding compassionate care in practice. This process led to the recognition of variation in the 'level of adoption' of the LCC Programme in each ward in relation to the LCC team's analytic framework for compassionate care (Adamson et al. 2011, p. 159–161) presented in Box 6.2. Criteria were developed (Box 6.3) to identify the levels of this summative outcome.

---

**Box 6.3 Criteria for 'Level of Adoption' of the LCC Programme**
1. Engagement with the LCC Programme during the period of facilitation
2. Engagement with the LCC team once the initial period of facilitation had come to an end
3. Self-association with the LCC Programme, including self-identification as a Beacon Ward/Development Site
4. Continued adoption of the appreciative approaches within the setting
5. Continued use of some of the key LCC Programme technique

---

**Table 6.2**  Data collection methods and research outputs (MacArthur et al. 2017)

| Data collection method | Research output |
|---|---|
| Semi-structured interviews ($n = 39$) and focus groups ($n = 3$) with key stakeholders | • Views, experiences and perceptions of LCC Programme<br>• Understanding practice development tools in action<br>• Outcomes for patients, relatives and staff |
| Informal observation of practice in clinical settings | • Outputs from engagement with LCC team—patient stories, photo-elicitation, beliefs and value statements<br>• Developments in practice |
| Attendance at LCC meetings | • Views and experiences of LCC team<br>• Emerging themes on compassionate care from action research |
| Review of research outputs from LCC team | • Emergent understanding of compassionate care in practice<br>• Development of practice development methods that have potential to impact on embedding compassionate care |
| Attendance at three LCC conferences | • Outcomes for individuals and clinical teams following participation in LCC Programme |
| Access to Health Board data systems | • Contextual data on staffing establishment, absence rates, number of beds, percentage bed occupancy and average length of stay |

## 6.2.4    Analysis

Inductive thematic analysis (Boyatzis 1998) was employed, which involved initial immersion in the interview transcripts ($n = 42$) and field notes drawn from the other data sources identified in Table 6.2, followed by coding within QSR NVivo 9. A realist evaluation framework shaped the emergent themes, which highlighted the contextual elements of the CMO configurations within and across the eight wards and how these interacted with the LCC Programme mechanisms to influence final outcomes for different patients, families and staff.

## 6.3    Results

## 6.3.1    Ward Characteristics

Data from Wards A–D were collected over 3 years and from Wards E–H over 2 years. The findings in Table 6.3 are summaries from all forms of data collection and show considerable heterogeneity across the eight wards in terms of specialty, size, bed occupancy, length of stay, team composition, management support and leader experience.

**Table 6.3**  Contextual information and characteristics of the Beacon Ward and Development Sites (MacArthur et al. 2017)

| Ward (level of adoption) | Patient group | Ward profile *Number of beds; % occupancy; average length of stay* (where data is available) | Team characteristics and involvement in LCC Programme | Management support | Experience of leader |
|---|---|---|---|---|---|
| Ward A (high) | Older people Acute medicine | 24 beds 95.1% 19.4 days | Established team Strong involvement multidisciplinary team | Mainly stable but some change Supportive at higher level | New charge nurse |
| Ward B (high) | Older people Mental health | 30 beds Long stay | Established team Minimal multidisciplinary involvement | Stable and supportive at immediate and higher level | Established charge nurse |
| Ward C (low) | Mainly older people Acute medical specialty | 22 beds 90% 8.7 days | Established team Stable multidisciplinary team—no medical staff involvement | Variable and number of changes Supportive at higher level | Acting charge nurse |

(continued)

**Table 6.3** (continued)

| Ward (level of adoption) | Patient group | Ward profile Number of beds; % occupancy; average length of stay (where data is available) | Team characteristics and involvement in LCC Programme | Management support | Experience of leader |
|---|---|---|---|---|---|
| Ward D (low) | Mixed age Acute and long-term medical specialty | 46 beds 122.1% 6.6 days | Established nursing team Minimal multidisciplinary involvement | Variable and number of changes Supportive at higher level | Experienced charge nurse during year 1 Two changes of charge nurse during year 2 and 3 |
| Ward E (high) | Mixed age Mental health rehabilitation | 25 beds Medium stay | Established nursing and multidisciplinary team Strong involvement | Strong at all levels | New charge nurse |
| Ward F (high) | Older people Frail health Continuing / palliative care | 34 beds Long stay | Established nursing team Minimal multidisciplinary involvement | Stable and very supportive at immediate and higher level | Experienced charge nurse |
| Ward G (medium) | Mixed age Acute assessment | 72 beds 70.6% 0.6 days | Very large team High turnover of medical/nursing staff Partial involvement | Mainly stable but some change Supportive at higher level | Three charge nurses, only one directly involved in LCC Programme |
| Ward H (high) | Mixed age Rehabilitation National centre | 19 beds Medium-to-long stay | Small established multidisciplinary team Good involvement | Good local management support | Several changes in leadership New charge nurse |

### 6.3.2 Level of Adoption

The 'level of adoption' of the LCC Programme varied across the wards. According to the criteria outlined in Box 6.3, wards were judged to show 'high' (4–5 criteria), 'medium' (=3 criteria) or 'low' (≤2 criteria) adoption as indicated in Table 6.4.

MacArthur et al. (2017) present the overarching study findings which focus on the views, experiences and impact of the LCC Programme, highlighting the principal outcomes in the high adoption wards in terms of: (1) positive changes in *relationships* (with patients, relatives and between staff); (2) new approaches, attitudes and behaviours in *care delivery* that demonstrated a compassionate person-centred approach to care; and (3) specific action projects that led to *developments in practice* such as methods for seeking patient and staff feedback, approaches to person-centred assessments and proactive engagement with relatives. In addition, the study

**Table 6.4** Level of adoption of Beacon wards and development sites

| Beacon wards | Development sites |
|---|---|
| Ward A→high→(5) | Ward E→high→(5) |
| Ward B→high→(5) | Ward F→high→(4) |
| Ward C→low→(1) | Ward G→medium→(3) |
| Ward D→low→(2) | Ward H→high→(4) |

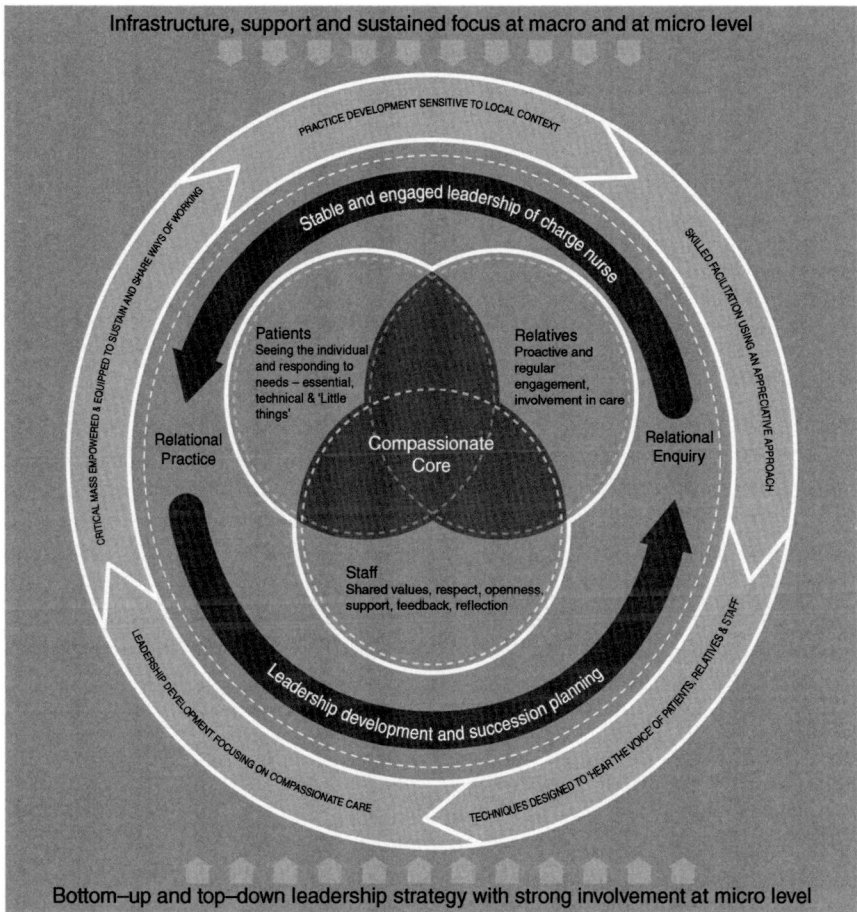

**Fig. 6.2** Conceptual model of enabling factors to enhance organisational capacity to deliver compassionate care (MacArthur et al. 2017)

emphasised the importance of the LCC Programme mechanisms, including the ways of working (such as appreciative inquiry, relationship-centred care, facilitation skills of the senior nurses and pace of implementation) and specific practice development techniques that were influential in leading to sustainable change (in particular emotional touchpoints and beliefs and values clarification).

Figure 6.2 illustrates the conceptual model of factors seen to enhance organisational capacity to develop and sustain a culture of compassionate care (MacArthur et al. 2017). At its centre is a 'compassionate core', reflecting both the distinct and interrelated needs of patients, relatives *and* staff. This core is supported by relationship-centred care involving what Patterson et al. (2010) describe as 'relational practice' (creating and sustaining a culture change to promote compassionate care) and Doane and Varcoe (2007) focus on 'relational inquiry' (recognising the contextual and personal elements that can affect relationships).

The outer layers of this model are very much shaped by the organisational context in which the LCC Programme was delivered, particularly at the meso and micro level. These centre on the leadership of the charge nurse, investment in a practice development infrastructure involving skilled facilitation to support cultural change (such as that proposed by McCormack et al. 2013) and a strategic commitment to prioritising compassionate care alongside other corporate business.

### 6.3.3   Importance of Context

It was possible to delineate promoting (actual and potential), neutral and limiting factors that all had a relationship to work environment and agreed with the original 'folk theories' identified prior to data collection.

#### 6.3.3.1 Promoting Factors

Five contextual factors were identified as having a strong influence on achieving 'high adoption' of the LCC Programme: (1) committed strategic leadership (macro level), (2) an infrastructure of managerial support and expectation (meso level), (3) leadership skills of the senior charge nurse (micro level), (4) stability of leadership (and/or effective succession planning) (meso and micro levels) and (5) experienced facilitation skills (micro level).

Luxford et al. (2011) stress strong committed leadership as a critical factor in changing and sustaining a more patient-centred approach within healthcare organisations. This was evident for the LCC Programme and was exemplified by its delivery being a *corporate objective* for the Board, regular executive visits to the Beacon Wards and Development Sites and showcasing of LCC Programme outcomes in Board meetings and reports. In England, the King's Fund[5] is promoting the concept of 'compassionate leadership', which it argues is a fundamental enabling factor that will create a culture of improvement and radical innovation across healthcare (West et al. 2017). They further propose that in order to nurture a culture of compassion, organisations must require their leaders (which they describe as the 'carriers of culture') to embody compassion in their leadership.

Clinical nurse managers had a crucial role in establishing a *local infrastructure* to support and maintain the profile of the LCC Programme within the directorate: examples included their establishment and leadership of directorate-wide LCC Groups and/or the Programme being a standing agenda item at directorate meetings. Also important was the expectation of regular reporting on processes and outcomes

---

[5] The King's Fund is an English health charity that shapes health and social care policy and practice and provides NHS leadership development (https://www.kingsfund.org.uk/).

of the Programme to the clinical nurse manager and wider peers. In a systematic review of quality improvement models in healthcare, Powell et al. (2009) identified sustained managerial focus and attention as one of the 'necessary but not sufficient' (p. 7) conditions necessary for successful implementation. They concluded that managers need to be actively involved for both symbolic and practical purposes to ensure alignment of activities with strategic objectives and effective organisation of and resources for activities. In addition, managers are instrumental in addressing barriers to change.

In their research study conducted in acute hospitals, Patterson et al. (2010) found that whilst 'support from the top' was important for the overall strategic direction of initiatives, the critical organisational culture element was a positive local team ethos. The *leadership skills* of charge nurses in the high adoption wards were used to engage ward teams, maintain momentum and role model compassionate behaviours towards patients, families and colleagues. The importance of effective leadership style and authority of senior charge nurses has been widely recognised (Cummings et al. 2010; Royal College of Nursing 2010). In recent years the Scottish and Welsh Governments have developed strategies to redirect the charge nurse's role towards a stronger emphasis on patient experience as well as broader organisational objectives (Scottish Government 2008, Welsh Assembly Government 2008). Within the Health Board, charge nurses were simultaneously participating in the 'Leading Better Care' programme (Scottish Government 2008); however, they reported that the LCC Programme was more oriented towards achieving person-centred compassionate care and equipped them with a unique set of skills to enhance their leadership skills.

In addition to leadership style, leadership *stability* at meso (directorate) and micro (ward) level also emerged as an important contextual factor. Complex healthcare systems frequently experience organisational change, natural turnover of staff and unplanned absences, all of which lead to leadership instability. Wards C and D were particularly affected by such factors. However Ward H, which also went through a number of changes, was protected from negative effects on programme implementation through clear succession planning, including the participation of the deputy charge nurse in the 12-month LCC Leadership Programme.

LCC Senior Nurses' *facilitation* skills in practice development emerged as a crucial contextual factor. Referring back to Patterson et al. (2010) assertion that policy promotes aspirational visions without always fully considering the complex processes needed to enact visions, this study supports Manley et al. (2008) assertion that practice development has the potential to translate complex organisation agendas into practice realities. They argue that practice development is rooted in the work of facilitators who have the skills and ability to address culture change. In the interviews, nursing staff articulated the strengths of senior nurses' facilitation approaches: (1) having the ability to 'draw people out and make them think', (2) adopting an open partnership based on inclusivity and approachability, (3) demonstrating leadership and role modelling that allayed staff anxieties and (4) displaying a 'second sense' that allowed staff to focus on the positives in their practice. The LCC Programme involved a unique investment to support practice development opportunities for engagement of multidisciplinary staff in exploratory and reflective techniques to create shared values about compassionate care at a local level.

The contextual factors that *may* have influenced the level of adoption and had some impact on wards outside the high adoption group of wards included: the larger staff teams (e.g. Ward G had 140 staff), which presented challenges for facilitating the key practice development techniques; the pressures of 'patient flow[6]', which created a preoccupation with admissions and discharges; and the 4-hour waiting time targets,[7] which particularly affected Wards D and G, although it also affected Ward A, a high adoption ward.

### 6.3.3.2 Neutral Factors

The contextual factors that *did not* seem to influence the level of adoption of the LCC Programme included: the specialty of the ward in terms of a focus on older people, mental health or uni-specialty; the 'pace' of care in terms of whether the patient group were having high care needs or showed clinical instability, were in rehabilitation or were receiving continuing care; the location (i.e. whether the ward was embedded within a major service or isolated/self-contained); and the experience of the charge nurse.

### 6.3.3.3 Limiting Factors

Four contextual factors were seen to limit the level of adoption and primarily affected Wards C and D. The first two were contrasts to the previously identified promoting factors: firstly *instability* or change of leadership at both local (micro) and middle management (meso) level and secondly a *lack of interest/support at middle management level*, which meant that ward staff and the LCC team had little success in effectively engaging in the Programme activities or sustaining any meaningful change. A third factor was evident where there was *active opposition* to participation in LCC activities by an important leadership figure at the local level, which resulting in a divided staff team. This became a particular issue in Ward D following the departure of the original charge nurse who had been a strong advocate of the Programme and resulted in the development of cliques amongst the staff team, who were either 'for' or 'against' the Programme.

*Coexisting pressures* on the wards were the fourth main contextual factor limiting adoption of the Programme. These included high unplanned absences and budget shortfalls that led to barriers to employing supplementary staffing that would have allowed greater opportunities for participation of the ward team in the LCC practice development activities. In addition, the LCC Programme was implemented concurrently with unexpected clinical pressures in the form of the H1N1 pandemic in 2009, which led to competing training demands, higher patient acuity and greater throughput particularly on Ward D.

---

[6] 'Patient flow' is a term used in the UK to denote the continuous process of discharge or transfer of patients from one in-patient setting to the next to permit admissions from 'front door' services such as the Emergency Department or medical admissions unit.

[7] This is a target imposed by the English and Scottish Governments in 2004 that 95% of patients should wait no longer than 4 h from arrival to admission, discharge or transfer for A&E treatment.

## 6.4    Implication for Practice

The LCC Programme was only one of several initiatives and programmes that regularly emerge in the UK NHS to address perceived deficits in care or to pave the way for organisational change. What is crucial to the success of any planned initiative is that organisational context (at macro, meso and micro levels) be considered when defining each programme's strategic aims, ways of working, resourcing and engaging in more detailed project planning. The findings and resultant conceptual model arising from this study (MacArthur et al. 2017) have informed a template for such planning (Table 6.5), and this has more recently influenced the design and implementation of a programme in NHS Lothian known as Care Assurance Standards (CAS). The CAS Programme is organised around a set of 13 standards of care (pressure area care; falls; promoting bladder and bowel health; deteriorating patient; medicines management; pain management; infection, prevention and control; food, fluid and

**Table 6.5** Application of key concepts of LCC Programme to Care Assurance Standards Programme

| Key concept drawn from LCC Programme | Relevance to Organisational Context | NHS Lothian Care Assurance Standards Programme |
| --- | --- | --- |
| Strategic buy-in (macro) | Corporate priority; resourcing; expectation of outcomes | Executive Nurse Director and Deputy Chief Executive sponsor programme; Nurse Director (Acute) chairs Programme Board and funds core facilitation resource |
| Theoretical underpinning | Establishment of values-based approach; agreement of ways of working | Appreciative approach (Cooperrider et al. 2008) rather than scrutiny; emphasis on developing relationships and trust with clinical areas (Nolan et al. 2006) |
| Leadership at meso level | Support crucial for local resourcing; dealing with barriers to change; expectation of outcomes | Associate Directors of Nursing all members of CAS Programme Board and fully involved in decision-making around pace and delivery of programme; resource site-based facilitation according to own preferred model |
| Facilitation | Recognition of the importance of facilitation to support clinical teams and enable organisational change (McCormack et al. 2013) | Clinical areas only brought into CAS Programme where they can resource site-based facilitator to work with core facilitation team |
| Recognition of complexity of clinical environments | Programme planning around pace and timing of phased approach to implementation | Adaptability of programme working; trusting relationships between CAS facilitators and charge nurses; recognition of winter clinical pressures |
| Leadership of charge nurse (micro level) | Leadership style and support from facilitators; local ownership of programme delivery | Charge nurse determines order of assurance of standards according to local priority; embedding supported system of link practitioners to develop wider leadership |

nutrition; person-centred care; older people in acute care and adult protection; end of life care; effective management of resources and staff governance; and working effectively in the multidisciplinary team). In addition to these standards, it incorporates McCance et al. (2012) key performance indicators for nursing and midwifery care. After an initial pilot of the CAS Programme in four wards in 2015–2016, a phased implementation plan is currently in progress. Since September 2016, it has been extended in three phases to 34 wards across three adult teaching hospitals.

## Conclusion

Whilst the initial assertion in this chapter that embedding compassionate care necessitates placing patients at the centre of organisational structures and function is undoubtedly correct, the research presented here demonstrates the key importance of fostering an organisational culture and context that demonstrates compassion for staff. There are clearly elements of the work environment in the NHS (and other health systems) that have undergone irreversible changes in response to demographic and workforce changes. Nonetheless, it is possible to shape initiatives to embody a more compassionate approach to change. Compassion is linked to situational awareness of an individual's 'suffering' and needs, responsive actions and relational abilities, and these qualities can and should be directed at creating work environments that support and enable staff to deliver high-quality patient care.

## References

Adamson E, Dewar B, Donaldson JH, Gentleman M, Gray M, Horsburgh D, Smith S, Waugh A. Leadership in compassionate care programme: final report. Edinburgh, Scotland: NHS Lothian/ Edinburgh Napier University; 2011. http://www.napier.ac.uk/~/media/worktribe/output-192596/compcarefinreptallapr13pdf.pdf. Accessed 25 April 2017.

Aiken LH, Buchan J, Ball J, Rafferty AM. Transformative impact of Magnet designation: England care study. J Clin Nurs. 2008;17(24):3330–7.

Aiken LH, Sermeus W, Van der Heed K, Sloane DM, Busse R, McKee M, et al. Patient safety, satisfaction, and quality of hospital care: cross sectional surveys of nurses and patients in 12 countries in Europe and the United States. Br Med J. 2012;344:e1717.

Alimo-Metcalfe B, Alban-Metcalfe J, Samele C, Bradley M, Mariathasan J. The impact of leadership factors in implementing change in complex health and social care environments. Department of Health, NHS SDO P22/2002; 2007. http://www.netscc.ac.uk/hsdr/files/project/SDO_FR_08-1201-022_V01.pdf. Accessed 19 May 2017.

Atkins PWB, Parker SK. Understanding individual compassion in organisations: the role of appraisals and psychological flexibility. Acad Man Rev. 2012;37(4):524–46.

Baillie L, Gallagher A. Evaluation of the Royal College of Nursing's 'Dignity at the heart of everything we do' campaign: exploring challenges and enablers. J Nurs Res. 2010;15(1):15–28.

Beach MC, Inui T. Relationship-centred care: a constructive reframing. J Gen Intern Med. 2006;21:3–8.

Blamey A, Mackenzie M. Theories of change and realistic evaluation: peas in a pod or apples and oranges? Evaluation. 2010;13(4):439–55.

Bloomberg K, Griffiths P, Wengström Y, May C. Interventions for compassionate nursing care: a systematic review. Int J Nurs Stud. 2016;62:137–55.

Boorman S. NHS Health and Well-Being Review: Interim Report London: Department of Health; 2009. http://webarchive.nationalarchives.gov.uk/20130107105354/http://www.dh.gov.uk/prod_consum_dh/groups/dh_digitalassets/documents/digitalasset/dh_108910.pdf. Accessed 5 May 2017.

Boyzatis RE. Transforming Qualitative Information: Thematic Analysis and Code Development California: Sage Publications; 1998.

Bradshaw A. Measuring nursing care and compassion: the McDonaldised nurse? J Med Ethics. 2009;35:465–8.

Brown J, Nolan M, Davies S, Nolan J, Keady J. Transforming students' views of gerontological nursing: realising the potential of 'enriched' environments of learning and care: a multi-method longitudinal study. Int J Nurs Stud. 2008;45(8):1214–32.

Burston PL, Stitchler JF. Nursing work environment and nurse caring: relationship among motivational factors. J Adv Nurs. 2010;66(8):1819–31.

Cooperrider DL, Whitney D, Stavros JM. Appreciative inquiry handbook. Bedford, OH: Lakeshore Communications Inc & San Francisco: Berrett-Koehler Publishers Inc.; 2008.

Cornwell J, Goodrich J. Exploring how to enable compassionate care in hospital to improve patient experience. Nurs Times. 2009;105(15):14–6.

Crawford P, Gilbert P, Gilbert J, Gale C, Harvey K. The language of compassion in acute mental health. Qual Health Res. 2013;23:719–27.

Cummings GG, MacGregor T, Davey M, Lee H, Wong C, Lo E, Muise M, Stafford E. Leadership styles and outcome patterns for the nursing workforce and work environment: a systematic review. Int J Nurs Stud. 2010;47(3):363–85.

Dewar B. Using creative methods in practice development to develop and understand compassionate care. Int Pract Dev J. 2012;2(1):1–11.

Dewar B, Mackay R. Appreciating compassionate care in acute care setting caring for older people. Int J Older People Nursing. 2010;5:299–308.

Dewar B, MacKay R, Smith S, Pullin S, Tocher R. Use of emotional touchpoints as a method of tapping into the experience of receiving compassionate care in a hospital setting. J Res Nurs. 2011;15(1):29–41.

Doane GH, Varcoe C, Relational practice and nursing obligations. Adv Nurs Sci. 2007;30(3):192–205.

Firth-Cozens J, Cornwell J. The point of care: enabling compassionate care in acute hospital settings. London: The Kings Fund; 2009.

Frampton S, Goodrich J. Current initiatives for transforming organizational cultures and improving the patient experience. In: Shea S, Wynyard RT, Lionis C, editors. Providing compassionate healthcare; challenges in policy and practice. London: Routledge; 2014.

Francis R. The Mid Staffordshire NHS Foundation Trust Inquiry Independent Inquiry into care provided by Mid Staffordshire NHS Foundation Trust January 2005 – March 2009, vol. I. London: The Stationary Office; 2010.

Francis R. Report of the Mid Staffordshire NHS Foundation Trust Public inquiry executive summary. London: The Stationery Office; 2013.

Holland J, Thomson R, Henderson S. Qualitative longitudinal research: a discussion paper Families & Social Capital ESRC Research Group Working Paper No. 21 London South Bank University; 2006. https://www.lsbu.ac.uk/__data/assets/pdf_file/0019/9370/qualitative-longitudinal-research-families-working-paper.pdf. Accessed 30 May 2017.

Kirkley C, Bamford C, Poole M, Arksey H, Hughes J, Bond J. The impact of organisational culture on the delivery of person-centred care in services providing respite care and short breaks for people with dementia. Health Soc Care Community. 2011;19(4):438–48.

Kitson A. The need for systems change: reflections on knowledge translation and organisational change. J Adv Nurs. 2008;65(1):217–28.

Kitson A, Harvey G, McCormack B. Enabling the implementation of evidence-based practice: a conceptual framework. Qual Health Care. 1998;7(3):149–58.

Lown BA, Dunne H, Mancer SJ, Chadwick R. How important is compassionate healthcare to you? A comparison of the perceptions of people in the US and Ireland. J Res Nurs. 2017;22(1-2): 60–9.

Luxford K, Safran DG, Delbanco T. Promoting patient-centered care: a qualitative study of facilitators and barriers in healthcare organizations with a reputation for improving the patient experience. Int J Qual Health Care. 2011;23(5):510–5.

Maben J. Care, compassion and ideals: patient and healthcare providers experiences. In: Shea S, Wynyard RT, Lionis C, editors. Providing compassionate healthcare; challenges in policy and practice. London: Routledge; 2014. p. 117–38.

Maben J, Latter S, Macleod C. The challenges of maintaining ideals and standards in professional practice: Evidence from a longitudinal qualitative study. Nurs Inq. 2007;14(2):99–113.

Maben J, Adams M, Peccei R, Murrells T, Robert G. Poppets and parcels': the links between staff experience of work and acutely ill older peoples' experience of hospital care. Int J Older People Nursing. 2012a,7(2).03 94.

Maben J, Pecci R, Adams M, Robert G, Richardson A, Murrells T, Morrow E. Patients' experiences of care and the influence of staff motivation, affect and well-being. Final report NIHR Service Delivery and Organisation programme; 2012b. http://www.netscc.ac.uk/hsdr/files/project/SDO_FR_08-1819-213_V01.pdf. Accessed 5 May 2017.

MacArthur J. Embedding compassionate care in local NHS practice: a realistic evaluation of the Leadership in Compassionate Care Programme. (Thesis) Edinburgh Napier University; 2014. http://researchrepository.napier.ac.uk/id/eprint/7248. Accessed 8 May 2017.

MacArthur J, Wilkinson H, Gray M, Matthews-Smith G. Embedding compassionate care in local NHS practice: developing a conceptual model through realistic evaluation. J Res Nurs. 2017;22(1–2):130–47.

Manley K, McCormack B, Wilson V. International practice development in nursing and healthcare. Oxford: Blackwell Publishing Ltd; 2008.

McCaffery G, McConnell S. Compassion: a critical review of peer-reviewed nursing literature. J Clin Nurs. 2015;24:3006–15.

McCance TV, Telford L, Wilson J, MacLeod O, Dowd A. Identifying key performance indicators for nursing and midwifery care using a consensus approach. J Clin Nurs. 2012;21(7&8):1145–54.

McCormack B, McCance TV. Development of a framework for person-centred nursing. J Adv Nurs. 2006;12(3):472–9.

McCormack B, McCance TV. Person-centred nursing: theory and practice. Oxford: Wiley Blackwell; 2010.

McCormack B, Mitchell EA, Reed J, Childs S. Older persons' experiences of whole systems: the impact of health and social care organisational structures. J Nurs Manag. 2008a;16(2):105–14.

McCormack B, Manley K, Walsh K. In: Manley K, McCormack B, Wilson V, editors. International practice development in nursing and healthcare. London: Wiley-Blackwell; 2008b.

McCormack B, Manley K, Titchen A. Practice development in nursing and healthcare. 2nd ed. London: Wiley; 2013.

McMahon A, White M. Compassion in practice: connected, contested, conflicted, conflated and complex. J Res Nurs. 2017;22(1–2):3–6.

Meyer J. Qualitative research in healthcare: using qualitative methods in health related action research. Br Med J. 2000;320(7228):178–81.

NHS England. Five Year Forward View – NHS England; 2014. https://www.england.nhs.uk/wp-content/uploads/2014/10/5yfv-web.pdf. Accessed 21 May 2017.

NHS Lothian. The External Reference Group for Older People's Services. Unpublished Report; 2006.

Nolan, M, Brown J, Davies S, Nolan J, Keady J. The senses framework: Improving care for older people through a relationship-centred approach GRIP: University of Sheffield; 2006. Accessed online from https://shura.shu.ac.uk/280/1/pdf_senses_framework_report.pdf. Accessed 6 June 2017.

Nursing and Midwifery Council (NMC). The code: professional standards of practice and behaviour for nurses and midwives. London: NMC; 2015.

Patterson M, Nolan M, Rick J, Brown J, Adams R, Musson G. From metrics to meaning: culture change and quality of acute hospital care for older people. Report for the National Institute for Health Research Service Delivery and Organisation programme; 2010. http://www.netscc.ac.uk/hsdr/files/project/SDO_FR_08-1501-93_V01.pdf. Accessed 5 May 2017.

Pawson R, Tilley N. Realistic evaluation. London: Sage Publications; 1997.

Powell AE, Rushmer RK, Davies HTO. A systematic narrative review of quality improvement models in healthcare. Social Dimensions of Health Institute of the University of Dundee and St. Andrews: NHS Quality Improvement Scotland; 2009. http://www.healthcareimprovementscotland.org/previous_resources/hta_report/a_systematic_narrative_review.aspx. Accessed 26 May 2017.

Ramunujam R, Abrahamson K, Anderson JG. Influence of workplace demands on nurses' perception of patient safety. Nurs Health Sci. 2008;10(2):144–50.

Royal College of Nursing. Making the business case for ward sisters/team leaders to be supervisory to practice; 2010. https://www2.rcn.org.uk/__data/assets/pdf_file/0005/414536/004188.pdf. Accessed 26 May 2017.

Schantz M. Compassion: a concept analysis. Nurs Forum. 2007;42(2):48–55.

Scottish Government. Leading Better Care: Report of the Senior Charge Nurse Review and Clinical Quality Indicators Project; 2008. http://www.gov.scot/Resource/Doc/225218/0060938.pdf. Accessed 26 May 2017.

Scottish Government. A Route Map to the 2020 Vision for Health and Social Care; 2013. http://www.gov.scot/Resource/0042/00423188.pdf. Accessed 21 May 2017.

Scottish Government. Health and Social Care Standards: My support, my life; 2017. http://www.gov.scot/Resource/0052/00520693.pdf. Accessed 28 May 2017.

Van Bogaert P, Meulmans H, Clarke S, Vermeyen K, Van de Heyning P. Hospital nurse practice environment, burnout, job outcomes and quality of care: test of a structural equation model. J Adv Nurs. 2009;65(10):2175–85.

von Dietze E, Orb A. Compassionate care: a moral dimension of nursing. Nurs Inq. 2000;7:166–74.

Welsh Assembly Government. Free to Lead, Free to Care: Empowering Ward Sisters/Charge Nurses Ministerial Task and Finish Group; 2008 http://www.wales.nhs.uk/documents/Cleanliness-Report.pdf. Accessed 26 May 2017.

West M, Baker R, Dawson J, Dixon Woods M, Lilford R, Martin G, McKee L, Murtagh M, Wilkie P. Quality and Safety in the NHS: Evaluating Progress, Problems and Promise; 2013. http://www.lancaster.ac.uk/media/lancaster-university/content-assets/documents/lums/cphr/quality-safety-nhs-e.pdf. Accessed 5 May 2017.

West M, Eckert R, Collins B, Chowla R. Caring to change: how compassionate leadership can stimulate innovation in health care; 2017. https://www.kingsfund.org.uk/sites/files/kf/field/field_publication_file/Caring_to_change_Kings_Fund_May_2017.pdf. Accessed 26 May 2017.

Youngson R. Futures debate: compassion in healthcare – the missing dimension of healthcare reform? NHS Confederation Futures Debate Series May: Paper 2, p. 3; 2008. http://www.nhsconfed.org/~/media/Confederation/Files/Publications/Documents/compassion_healthcare_future08.pdf. Accessed 19 May 2017.

# Learning and Innovation in Health-Care-Based Teams: The Relationships Between Learning, Innovative Behavior at Work, and Implementation of Innovative Practices in Hospitals

**7**

Olaf Timmermans, Bart Van Rompaey, and Eric Franck

**Abstract**

Non compliance with implementation of innovations is a major problem in health-care-based teams. In the literature, (team-) learning is proposed as a facilitator for the process of implementing innovations. Still, a comprehensive exploration of learning in health-care-based teams and the relation with innovation is scarce. This chapter explores (team-) learning activities in health-care-based teams and the relation between learning processes at individual, team, and organizational levels and implementation of innovations. A review of the literature was conducted. Theoretical aspects of learning on individual, team, and organizational levels are summarized, as well as the concepts of innovative work behavior and implementation of innovations. In addition, we used data and insights from the studies we performed on learning and innovation in health-care-based teams. Insights from separate empirical studies are synthesized to underbuild the relationships between (team) learning, innovative work behavior, and implementation of innovations in health-care-based teams. Learning in health-care-based teams exists on individual, team, and organizational levels. Especially for learning on team level, the relation with innovative behavior at

O. Timmermans (✉)
Nursing and Midwifery Sciences, Centre for Research and Innovation in Care (CRIC),
Faculty of Medicine and Health Sciences, University of Antwerp, Antwerp, Belgium

Professorship Healthy Region HZ University of Applied Sciences, Vlissingen, Netherlands
e-mail: olaf.timmermans@uantwerpen.be

B. Van Rompaey
Nursing and Midwifery Sciences, Centre for Research and Innovation in Care (CRIC),
Faculty of Medicine and Health Sciences, University of Antwerp, Antwerp, Belgium

E. Franck
Nursing and Midwifery Sciences, Centre for Research and Innovation in Care (CRIC),
Faculty of Medicine and Health Sciences, University of Antwerp, Antwerp, Belgium

Karel De Grote University of Applied Sciences, Antwerp, Belgium

© Springer International Publishing AG 2018
P. Van Bogaert, S. Clarke (eds.), *The Organizational Context of Nursing Practice*,
https://doi.org/10.1007/978-3-319-71042-6_7

work and implementation of innovations was demonstrated in different studies. Finally, we show how the theories can be used in practice, by showing how we used the theoretical assumptions on learning in building a master's-level program in nursing science.

**Keywords**

Learning and innovative behavior in health-care-based teams • Process and implementations of novelties in health care

## 7.1    Introduction

This chapter examines the implementation of innovations in health-care settings by looking at the importance of learning at individual, team, and organizational levels. The ability of teams to perform on a day-to-day basis as well as to innovate is a hallmark of their effectiveness in the twenty-first century. In hospitals, nursing and multidisciplinary work teams are the key factors in these processes. Beyond daily delivering of nursing and medical care, teams in hospitals are expected to continuously implement innovations to ensure care meets state-of-the-art standards. Nonetheless, in various health-care settings, a low compliance with widely accepted/ evidence-based clinical guidelines and protocols has been reported, and strong attachments of hospital-based teams to routines and rituals have been documented even when better provided care exists (Timmermans et al. 2012a).

There are many different definitions and ways of describing events related to innovation in hospital settings (Timmermans et al. 2011). In general, innovation in this context is the implementation of new initiatives to bring about minor, as well as major, changes in hospitals whereby health-care professionals learn and modify their knowledge, skills, and behaviors (Grol and Grimshaw 2003; Timmermans et al. 2012a). For example, in the implementation of a new protocol for hand hygiene or early warning scores, learning for the involved employees relates to acquiring or consolidating knowledge of protocols, as well as some combination of psychomotor, communication, and cognitive skills. Truly new or novel approaches representing complex departures from work practices, such as implementation of the bedside handover method, working with Lean, or adoption of clinical pathways, each create different learning tasks at an even higher level of complexity for the individuals on the team (Timmermans et al. 2012b).

To elevate standards of care to the state of the art, successful implementation of innovations is crucial. Yet, many teams in hospitals fail to achieve the expected benefits of innovations. A key reason for this is not necessarily found in the innovation itself, but rather in failures of implementation, especially a lack of attention to the role of learning. Reviewing the implementation process and understanding the reasons of impaired implementation, we detected the importance of learning to enhance successful implementation (Timmermans et al. 2012b). Therefore, the aim of this chapter is to explore (team) learning activities in hospital-based teams and examine the relation between learning processes at individual, team, and organizational levels and implementation of innovations.

The chapter starts with an in-depth overview of learning on individual, team, and organizational levels, as well as the concept of innovative work behavior. The chapter continues with an overview of research on relationships between (team) learning, innovative work behavior, and implementation of innovation. It concludes with an explanation of how practical application of the theories discussed is taught in a master's-level program in clinical leadership.

## 7.2 Levels of Learning in Health-Care Settings

### 7.2.1 Individual Learning

In individual learning, the learner is an individual such as a nurse or physician. Individual learning focuses on the uptake of new knowledge and/or skills. Mostly individual learning is connected with cognitive and emotional efforts where the learner actively builds or expands existing knowledge or thinking schemes. A number of definitions of individual learning exist. According to Dixon (1994), learning involves selecting, recording, processing, integrating, capturing, and using new information. Crossan et al. (1999) linked individual learning to understanding new ideas and fusing in one's own thinking. Simons et al. (2000) characterized individual learning as the creation or setting up of changes in knowledge, attitude, and skills, through a process of selecting, recording, processing, integrating, and using information. Homan (2001) described learning as the giving up of old behavior. Synthesizing these definitions, individual learning involves selection, uptake, and the use of new information that merges with existing knowledge and thinking schemes, resulting in new behavior or skills.

In health-care settings, individual learning is mostly linked to the growth of clinical skills in students during their clinical time in various areas. In other words, individual learning is linked to learning a profession, e.g., nursing or medicine. Not surprisingly, much research on learning and teaching in health-care settings focuses on professional education, typically in clinical practice, where success typically leads to academic credits and ultimately certificates or diplomas. Eraut (2004) defined this as the formal educational process in health-care settings. However, beyond formal learning, also informal learning takes place in hospital settings. Informal learning in the workplace takes places through interactions between individuals and expands learning opportunities. Bjørk et al. (2013) estimate that 80% of the learning in health-care settings is informal in nature and is an experiential, non-routine learning that takes place incidentally and sometimes unconsciously.

In contrast to formal learning, informal learning occurs without specific, predetermined learning goals or outcomes and takes place in a wide variety of settings. Often informal learning is triggered by unexpected situations in clinical work that provoke discussion with colleagues. The connection of informal learning to delivery of state-of-the-art care in hospitals, as well as during implementation of innovations, is obvious. To be sure, working with some innovations requires formal learning to acquire skills, for example, hand hygiene protocols or communication with the standardized Situation, Background, Assessment, and Recommendation or SBAR method. Informal learning, however, provides opportunities to discuss the logistics of executing new tasks.

Illeris (2003) categorized the results of individual learning into four levels (see Table 7.1). It is obvious that the results of learning are stored before they can be retrieved. This storing takes places in one's memory, but different forms of learning lead up to different ways of processing and storing. Illeris (2003) used these differences to distinguish four levels of learning. The levels differ in terms of how the learning occurs, the way it is linked to preexisting structures in memory, and how retrieval of stored learning material takes place.

The first level of learning is called *cumulative* or *mechanical* learning. This level of learning is characterized by learning something completely new and has no existing structure to link with, no meaning or personal importance. This level of learning is most prevalent in the early years of life, when one learns a lot of things or skills unrelated to previously acquired knowledge and skills. Reuse of learned material often occurs automatically and involves retrieval and application in situations similar to the learning situation.

The second, and most common, level of learning is *assimilative* learning. In this level of learning, material is linked to an existing structure or scheme in one's memory. This is what most people consider learning and is dominant in educational

**Table 7.1** Levels of individual learning

| Level of learning | Characteristics | Linking with existing structures | Retrieval |
|---|---|---|---|
| Cumulative or mechanical learning | Most frequent during the first years of life | No existing structure to link with, no meaning or personal importance | Recalled and applied in situations mentally similar to the learning context |
| Assimilative learning | Learning in school | New element is linked as an addition to a scheme or pattern that is already established | Relatively easy to recall and apply toward the field in question |
| Accommodative learning | Relinquishes and reconstructs | One breaks down (parts of) an existing scheme and transforms it so that the new situation can be linked in and can be painful, requiring mental energy | Recalled and applied in many different, relevant contexts |
| Transformative learning | A far-reaching type of learning | Personality changes and is characterized by simultaneous restructuring in the cognitive, the emotional, and the social-societal dimensions | Personality change presented in all next situations, new perspectives of reality |

settings, where new material gradually builds on what has been previously learned. Transfer or translation is relatively easy in the setting in question, but relatively hard in new contexts.

The third level of learning is *accommodative* learning. In this type of learning, one has to (at least partially) break down existing structures or schemes, in order to store new learned materials in one's memory. This happens especially when one encounters situations that cannot directly be understood or linked with earlier learning. This level of learning can be emotionally difficult and painful and requires efforts because one has to go out of their own comfort zone. An example is the adaptation to project-based teaching/learning strategies for students who are used to individual learning. The results of accommodative learning can be retrieved and applied in many different situations, because this type of learning involves acquiring new mental models or cognitive skills.

The fourth and most far-reaching level of learning is *transformative* learning. This level of learning results in personality changes and is characterized by simultaneous restructuring existing cognitive and/or emotional structures. Transformative learning is triggered by a crisis situation or challenges which one only can encounter by change in one's deepest insights, values, thoughts, and feelings. An example of transformative learning is the so-called stimul-experience, an educational setup to enhance dignity in care, wherein professional caregivers adapt and simulate for 48 h a client-like role to experience what it is like to receive care (Timmermans et al. 2013). After being in the "stimul-experience," participants expressed deep personal changes and major changed perspectives toward what is good care. The result of transformative learning is applied in all situations that the learner encounters from that point forward; the personality change and new perspectives on reality are at work in all new situations, personal and professional, a person experiences (Table 7.1).

The four different levels of learning can be used in setting up educational interventions; first, it is important to define the goals of the learning interventions. To extend existing knowledge or skills, mechanical or assimilative learning will do the job. But if the goal of the education intervention is to change existing thinking schemes, accommodative or transformative learning is needed.

## 7.2.2   Learning in Teams

In addition to individual learning, also teams can learn to accomplish different tasks (Timmermans et al. 2012a). Edmondson et al. (2001) defined team learning as a team-level construct that enfolds the learning activities that team members undertake to gather and process information which allows the team to develop and perform: in teams, caregivers can offer and receive feedback, ask others for help to solve problems, or share and apply knowledge on novelties in their field of practice (Timmermans et al. 2011). These team learning activities benefit the cognitive, attitudinal, and behavioral changes of the individuals in the teams when they have to modify their own routines (Edmondson et al. 2001).

Transferring research on ambidexterity, team learning, and innovation to nursing teams, Timmermans et al. (2012b) created the perspective that nursing teams are becoming ambidextrous. Raisch and Birkinshaw (2008) defined ambidexterity as the ability of a team to manage simultaneously production-oriented and development-oriented processes (Raisch and Birkinshaw 2008). To transform into an ambidextrous team, team learning activities are essential. The productive and innovative tasks of a team lead to different learning tasks, possibly at the same time (Van Linge 2006). Timmermans et al. (2012a) reported team learning tasks can be divided in production- and development-oriented learning tasks. Production-oriented learning is a reaction to learning tasks that are triggered from the daily production process and results in adjustments in the way caregivers in hospital-based teams work together to produce nursing care or nursing education. On the other hand, development-oriented learning is triggered from the gap between current practice and new developments in the environment of the teams of caregivers. Development-oriented learning includes active seeking and processing of new knowledge and results in fundamental changes in the provision of care by the team (Timmermans et al. 2013). Overall, Timmermans et al. (2012a) defined five clusters of team learning activities in ambidexter teams: (1) gathering production-oriented information, (2) gathering development- oriented information, (3) processing information, (4) storage/retrieval production-oriented information, and (5) storage/retrieval development-oriented information. Production-oriented and development-oriented learning differ on the type of information processed. Information needed to execute the production process, such as information on patients and planning, creates production-oriented learning tasks in teams. Information used to reflect on the congruence between the current ways of practicing in the production process and developments outside the team, such as information on evidence-based practice or clinical guidelines, brings up development-oriented learning tasks in the nursing team. Because each learning task includes its own type of information, teams are challenged to handle different types of information at the same time (Timmermans et al. 2013).

Team learning activities result in constructing shared mental models and storing these in the memory of the team members. Throughout the team learning activities, teams transfer and apply new insights in their practice to find innovative approaches to problems. Teams become more efficient over time, acquire and apply new skills, and change values, norms, and procedures (Timmermans et al. 2013). Moreover, team learning activities in nursing teams led to improvement of performance on organizational learning and team effectiveness, such as the way nursing teams handle patient safety and the implementation of innovations.

## 7.2.3  Organizational Learning

Although learning is conventionally thought of as an individual process and recently extended to a team-level phenomenon, organizations can also learn. Organizational learning can be thought of as the way organizations adapt to continuous changes in their environments. Hospitals exist in a direct environment, e.g., a city with other hospitals nearby, or in a rural area where they are the only hospital in a wide area. No matter what direct environment hospitals are in, the environment is changing. Examples are the new possibilities for treatment of chemotherapy in home care instead of in hospitals or the possibilities of care on distance with telecare. A striking example of an organizational learning failure outside health care is the story of the decline of Kodak. Kodak is an international company founded in the nineteenth century and failed to successfully sell consumer products in the digital era, despite having itself developed digital technology. No one on Kodak's management team recognized the changes toward digital products, such as digital photography or music. This organizational non-learning directly caused Kodak's decline as trending manufacturer of film materials (see https://hbr.org/2016/07/kodaks-downfall-wasnt-about-technology).

The main asset of a learning organization is its constant scanning on the external environment for important developments. The author on learning at organization level is Peter Senge, who presented his learning organizational model back in 1990. Senge defined a learning organization as "an organization where people continually expand their capacity to create the results they truly desire, where new and expansive patterns of thinking are nurtured, where collective aspiration is set free, and where people are continually learning how to learn together" (Senge 1990). In his model, Senge (1990) presented five disciplines: (1) system thinking, (2) personal mastery, (3) shared mental models, (4) shared vision, and (5) team learning.

Systems thinking is the ability to use holistic viewpoint toward what happens in organizations, instead of being focused on single elements or situations. System thinking underlines that all situations in an organization are related to one another, whereby the relationship presents (not directly viewable) patterns in an organization. Personal mastery reflects the learning process of really mastering his/her tasks in the organization. Personal mastery is reflected in continually improving one's level activates and energizes individuals in the organization. Two factors that are of importance in this discipline are (1) being able to know and define what is really important and (2) having the ability to see the current reality as it is. Mental models are deeply underlying and non-visible values, premises, and generalizations that affect how individuals perceive their reality. Moreover, mental models display the underlying assumptions and values which influence the perception of reality and the actions individuals undertake. In organizational learning, shared mental models are pursued, wherein the individuals in a team have the same underlying premises and generalizations and the same perception of reality. This fits in with the discipline of shared vision, which reflects the collaborative sharing of goals, values, and missions of the organization. This means that if a shared vision is present, all members of a team or an organization know where they want to go to and what the team or organization stands for. Lastly the discipline of team learning is described earlier in this chapter. Each of these five learning disciplines is essential in building a learning organization and is dependent on one another (Senge 1990). In other words, organizations that develop only one of the disciplines cannot become learning organizations.

## 7.3    Innovative Work Behavior and Team Learning

Mesdagh et al. (2016) stated that organizations need members who are flexible and innovative and act proactively, because such people are more likely to redefine and construct their roles broadly and take up new roles and goals as circumstances change. Creative individuals will generate and implement new ideas. Based on West and Farr (1989), innovative work behavior (IWB) comprises individual actions aimed at intentionally introducing new and useful ideas, processes, products, or procedures within the work environment (Janssen 2004). Both the development of new ideas and their implementation are encompassed within IWB (Janssen 2004; De Jong and Den Hartog 2010; Knol and Van Linge 2009).

Innovative work behavior (IWB) is a four-stage process consisting of (1) idea exploration, (2) idea generation, (3) idea promotion, and (4) idea implementation (De Klerk-Jolink et al. 2016). IWB can be observed and studied at the individual level but also at the team level (Messmann 2012) and involves both observable behavior and cognitive processes such as reflection and construction of new knowledge and ideas. IWB components are knowledge of entrepreneurship, adaptability, self-efficacy, creative thinking, networking, and teamwork skills (Van Dam et al. 2010). This means that, although the definition of IWB is based on individual behavior, it is necessary to be aware that the individuals in hospitals mostly operate in a team.

A number of studies present results on the influence of personal factors on the prevalence of IWB. In the studies, personal factors are divided into individual characteristics (age, gender, educational level) and personality traits (proactive attitude, confidence, creativity, personal empowerment, self-efficacy, and a learning goal orientation). De Prins et al. (2012) and Thurlings et al. (2014) reported no clear relation of age and gender with IWB. This is in contrast to Messmann (2012) who classified age as a predictor for IWB. Bouwhuis (2008) reported a relationship between higher education and IWB, hypothesizing that education encourages the continuous improvement clinical practice because highly educated care professionals actively follow latest trends. Regarding personality traits, studies indicate that there is a relationship between IWB and a proactive attitude, personal empowerment, self-efficacy, and a learning goal orientation whereby there is an individual willingness to learn and improve (De Klerk-Jolink et al. 2016).

De Klerk-Jolink et al. (2016) studied the relation between individual characteristics, team learning, and IWB in a study among lectures at universities of applied sciences, and reported team learning was a significant predictor of IWB. More specific, especially the gathering, processing and storage/reuse of development-oriented information significantly related to all four stages of IWB. These findings indicate the importance of team learning for innovative behavior at work and support the outcomes of earlier research, where team learning positively coincided with innovation (Hoogveld et al. 2003; Stalmeijer et al. 2007) and research into the importance of team learning for the effectiveness of education innovations in higher education (Donderwinkel 2010; Timmermans et al. 2012a, b).

## 7.4    Team Learning and Implementation of Innovations

A specific connection between team learning and implementation of an innovation was first demonstrated in a qualitative study by Edmondson et al. (2001) exploring team learning activities during the introduction of minimally invasive cardiac surgery (MICS). Before the introduction of MICS, cardiac surgery was a major operation, but after its implementation, care needs changed dramatically because patients recovered more quickly and were discharged sooner. Not surprisingly, this technological innovation affected team routines. Edmondson et al. (2001) reported that teams that used team learning activities to explore the fit between the effects of MICS and their routines experienced smoother implementation trajectories. Team learning activities, such as gathering information from external sources and forming shared mental models of the effects of MICS on the organization and delivery of patient care, were tied to changes in practices. A higher level of motivation, greater psychological safety, and greater willingness to develop new team behaviors characterized the teams. In contrast, teams with unsuccessful implementation outcomes reported fewer team learning activities (Edmondson et al. 2001).

Timmermans et al. (2013) explored the factors that enhance implementation effectiveness and compliance of nursing teams using a contingency perspective on learning and innovation. More specific, they explored the effect of team learning activities on the knowledge and use of nurses in teams toward an incremental and a radical innovation. Similar to the findings of Edmondson et al. (2001), the results of the study indicated that nurses in teams simultaneously activated different team learning activities to handle information regarding delivery or innovation of nursing care. Nurses shared and applied knowledge on strategies either to produce or to innovate their nursing or care (Timmermans et al. 2013). In this study, the implementation of Nutrition Risk Screening guideline or NRS-2002 was defined as an incremental innovation. During the implementation of the NRS-2002, nurses individually participated in a hospital-wide training day, whereby knowledge was gathered throughout individual learning. In the use of the NRS-2002 in daily practice, however, team learning activities affected the implementation effectiveness of this incremental innovation. In contrast, the implementation process of a radical innovation in this study (adopting the Neuman systems model in a different setting) included longitudinal team-oriented activities. Nurses in the teams studied received collaborative training and education, what made team learning activities most relevant (Van Linge 2006; Holleman et al. 2009). Overall, the study findings suggested a relationship between production-oriented team learning processes and incremental innovations, as well as another between development-oriented team learning processes and implementation of a radical innovation.

Managers can apply this contingency framework in work with hospital-based teams to promote production-oriented as well as innovation-oriented team learning processes and promote team learning by providing adequate time and a suitable infrastructure. Elements that are known to influence team learning such as psychological safety in the team and team learning competencies of individual nurses in the team should be considered. It is also important to remember that individuals in teams undertake individual and team learning activities within a context that includes elements that can either facilitate or hinder team learning, such as underlying values and belief systems of the nurses in the team and team culture (Van Linge 2006; Edmondson et al. 2001; Holleman et al. 2009; Timmermans et al. 2011).

## 7.5 Practical Applications in the University of Antwerp's Master in Nursing and Midwifery Sciences Program

A central assumption of the Master's program in Nursing and Midwifery at the University of Antwerp is that its graduates will work in environments and on monodisciplinary, multidisciplinary, and/or interprofessional teams that must deliver care as well as innovate. Its graduates will work in and set up ambidextrous (efficient and adaptable) teams (Timmermans et al. 2011). Thus, it is vital that students in the program acquire a broad range of competencies in establishing and working with different types of teams. However, team-based learning is a recent development in health care, and teaching monodisciplinary, multidisciplinary, and interprofessional cooperation is, however, not widespread in most current professional education programs in nursing, medicine, and the allied health professions.

Cooperative learning consists of activities whereby students collect, process, and reproduce information with others (Cheng et al. 2014; Timmermans et al. 2012b). The emphasis is on working, learning, and creating together. Cooperative learning is an active, development-oriented learning method. Students ask each other questions; ask and give feedback; discuss unexpected situations, errors, and unwanted results; and reflect on how they dealt with the situation. To build cooperative learning skills in the Master in Nursing and Midwifery at the University of Antwerp, students are introduced to a vision of peer learning where there is a tight connection between learning and working in teams. Cooperative learning is a key theme throughout the courses in the program.

While many academic programs in a variety of disciplines have implemented cooperative learning experiences, to our knowledge, few do it in as comprehensive a manner as the Nursing and Midwifery program. This program uses three levels of cooperative learning: (1) peer studying (learning in a study group), (2) peer feedback (targeted feedback to peers using preestablished evaluation criteria), and (3) peer assessment (assessing a specific competence based on preestablished criteria, which is taken into account in final grades).

Peer studying consists of collecting, interpreting, applying, and saving/re-using information in a study group of peers (fellow students) or in a multidisciplinary study group. Peer feedback requires students to exchange targeted feedback about a number of preestablished characteristics relating to a specific learning objective, e.g., composing a study protocol. Peer assessment follows from peer feedback. Here students work with a preestablished assignment and criteria. However, the students must assess each other based on the criteria, and the final assessment also counts toward the student's final grades.

A first example of the use of cooperative learning is the implementation of the care project in the first year of the program. The care project is about an existing problem in a health-care setting and is built on learning assignments and program components from the learning domain management and innovation. Here cooperative learning is implemented as project-based learning and is based on the jigsaw method (Anderson and Palmer 2001). The jigsaw method involves that students are divided in subgroups that solve parts of the existing problem in a health-care setting and combine and share their learning in the overall project group to solve the overall problem. Project-based learning and the underlying jigsaw method enable the formulation of challenging problems/assignments, based on a practical problem that care institutions are facing. Moreover, project-based learning in combination with the jigsaw method establishes the preliminaries for cooperative learning, such as mutual positive dependence, individual accountability, personal contact, the experience that students gain from certain aspects of cooperating such as helping one another and responding to each other's input, and the potential for learning how to process and understand the complex relation between large quantities of related knowledge and organizing it into conceptual frameworks (Anderson and Palmer 2001; Felder and Brent 2001).

Building blocks for the care project come from the content in courses in the learning domain of "management and innovation," which focuses on knowledge and insight in terms of management and innovation in health care. In the diverse courses on management and innovation, concepts and processes are transposed into specific topics such as leadership, organizational culture, result-oriented management, and quality and result-oriented management and implementation of innovations. For the content aspect of the care project, students themselves develop the scientific substantiation of the care project. Also, students must incorporate guidelines developed by the Registered Nurses' Association of Ontario (Registered Nurses' Association of Ontario 2012), specifically the guidelines on "Developing and Sustaining Nurse Leadership," "Developing and Sustaining Interprofessional Health Care" and "Person- and Family-Centered Care." Furthermore, students are encouraged to integrate RNAO guidelines that fit the specific content of their care project. The cohesion between management and content is a complex matter, requiring knowledge of the separate components and their cohesion and interaction. In other words, the entire care project is a complicated puzzle, but it can be subdivided into separate puzzle pieces, which are easily pieced together. Building blocks also come from the innovation tool kit developed by the Registered Nurses' Association of Ontario (Registered Nurses' Association of Ontario 2012). This toolbox provides a comprehensive overview of theory and research on implementation and is for the students a practical manual toward implementation issues in the care project.

During the care project, the overall emphasis is on working together, on cooperative learning and creation. Eight to ten students work together in a project group throughout the first year on one care project assignment. The students subdivide themselves into pairs/threesomes per project component, working on one piece of the overall problem. At the end of the first year, students put together the puzzle as a whole in the project group and present innovative solutions to the practical problem of the health-care organization. The project-based learning is implemented by a combination of peer teaching and peer feedback. In the first and second semester, peer feedback is given on the specific component that the groups of two to three students develop (feedback on content) and on the cooperation in a project group (feedback on project skills). In the second semester, this is supplemented with peer assessment. The feedback that is given based on criteria counts toward the final exam result.

A second example of a cooperative learning project involves a case study of a fictitious health-care system/network organization, which we call Scheldeboord that is confronted with evolving conditions, opportunities, pitfalls, and problems that are currently widespread in health-care organizations. Students working in study groups pick out four problems in the case and develop a solution, based on integrating clinical and nursing scientific knowledge with knowledge on learning and working in health-care settings. Here, students participate in cooperative learning, as well as develop their competences to set up ambidextrous, learning teams in health-care setting to encounter all kinds of different problems, together with their peers. Students are expected to share and apply specific knowledge and insights from various health-care domains and devise a solution based on cooperation, cooperative learning, and the dynamics of producing and innovating simultaneously. Peer feedback is given within the study group to which the student belongs as well as by the students as a whole when students present their own solution and receive feedback from their fellow students (based on a list of criteria).

Both examples show cooperative learning can be positively influenced by already facilitating this during the student's training. As a result, this becomes a basic attitude for alumni in their daily practice. Ultimately, the aim is to improve care quality through cooperation, as the combination of learning and cooperating contributes to the up-to-date quality of the care provided. Overall, the implementation and expansion of collaborative learning in the Master of Nursing and Midwifery has ensured that the intended end level of training differs from similar programs in Belgium. For prospective and current students, this signature approach distinguishes our program from a number of competitors.

## Conclusion

The aim of this chapter was to explore (team) learning activities in hospital-based teams and to examine relations between learning processes at individual, team, and organizational levels and implementation of innovations. To do so, we used literature on learning and implementation of innovations in health-care-based teams, synthesized data and insights from studies we performed on learning and innovation in health-care-based teams, and (finally) described how theoretical aspects of learning can be used in setting up an educational program. Results in this chapter show learning in health-care-based teams exists on individual, team, and organizational levels. Individual learning can be defined on four different levels, differencing in the level of deepness and whether or not that what is to be learned can be linked to existing thinking schemes or not. The deeper the level of learning and the incongruence with existing thinking schemes, the more learning leads to changes in one perception and personality. Especially for learning on team level, the relation with innovative behavior at work and implementation of innovations was demonstrated in different studies.

In setting up educational strategies, the insights in individual and team learning can be used. In setting up strategies for implementation of innovations in health-care-based teams specifically, the insights on team learning should be used. Throughout team learning, teams in health-care organizations can enhance their implementation effectiveness on innovations. Using the provided insights, effective team learning processes can be developed that enable teams to improve implementation effectiveness of different types of innovations.

## References

Anderson FJ, Palmer J. The jigsaw approach: students motivating students. Education. 2001;109:59–62.

Bjørk IT, Tøien M, Sørensen AL. Exploring informal learning among hospital nurses. J Work Learn. 2013;25:426–40.

Bouwhuis L. Explanation of innovative behavior of teachers: a PhD study on individual variables, self-efficacy and learning-goal-orientation (in Dutch). Enschede: Universiteit Twente; 2008.

Cheng CY, Liou SR, Hsu TS, Chang C. Preparing nursing students to be competent for future professional practice: applying the team-based learning–teaching strategy. J Prof Nurs. 2014;30(4):347–56.

Crossan MM, Lane HW, White RE. An organizational learning framework: from intuition to institution. Acad Manag Rev. 1999;24:522–37.

De Jong J, Den Hartog D. Measuring innovative work behavior. Creat Innovation Manage. 2010;19(1):23–6.

De Klerk-Jolink N, van der Klink M, Timmermans O. Innovative behavior of university of applied sciences lecturers (in Dutch). Tijdschrift voor Hoger Onderwijs. 2016;34(1):37–55.

De Prins P, Segers J, De Vos A, Brouwers S. The influence of new and hard-working career practices on the sustainability of careers (in Dutch). Tijdschrift voor Arbeidsvraagstukken. 2012;28(4):413–33.

Dixon NM, The organizational learning cycle: how we can learn collectively. New York: McGraw-Hill; 1994.

Donderwinkel F. Implementation of "Skills online": the relationship between individual factors of Nursing lecturers, team learning and the implementation effectiveness of the education innovation "Skills Online" (in Dutch). Utrecht: University Utrecht; 2010.

Edmondson AC, Bohmer RM, Pisano GP. Disrupted routines, team learning and new technology implementation in hospitals. Adm Sci Q. 2001;46(4):685–716.

Eraut M. Informal learning in the workplace. Stud Contin Educ. 2004;26(2):247–73.

Felder RM, Brent R. Effective strategies for cooperative learning. J Coop Collab Coll Teach. 2001;10:69–75.

Grol RPTM, Grimshaw J. From best evidence to best practice: effective implementation of change in patients' care. Lancet. 2003;362:225–1230.

Holleman G, Poot E, Mintjes-de Groot J, Van Achterberg T. The relevance of team characteristics and team directed strategies in the implementation of nursing innovations. A literature review. Int J Nurs Stud. 2009;46:1256–64.

Homan T. Team learning: theory and facilitation (in Dutch). Schoonhoven: Academic Service; 2001.

Hoogveld A, Paas F, Jochems W. Application of an instructional systems design approach by teachers in higher education: individual versus team design. Teach Teach Educ. 2003;19:581–90.

Illeris K. Towards a contemporary and comprehensive theory of learning. Int J Lifelong Educ. 2003;22(4):396–406.

Janssen O. How fairness perceptions make innovative. J Organ Behav. 2004;25:201–15.

Knol J, Van Linge R. Innovative behavior: the effect of structural and psychological empowerment on nurses. J Adv Nurs. 2009;65(2):359–70.

Mesdagh E, van Rompaey B, Beekman K, Boogaerts A, Timmermans O. A concept analysis of proactive behaviour in midwifery. J Adv Nurs. 2016;72(6):1236–50.

Messmann MA. Innovative work behavior: investigating the nature and facilitation of vocational teachers contributions to innovation development. Regensburg: Universität Regensburg; 2012.

Raisch S, Birkinshaw J. Organizational ambidexterity: antecedents, outcomes, and moderators. J Manag. 2008;34(3):375–409.

Registered Nurses' Association of Ontario. Toolkit: implementation of best practice guidelines. 2nd ed. Toronto: Registered Nurses' Association of Ontario; 2012.

Senge PM. The fifth discipline – the art & practice of a learning organization New York: Doubleday; 1990.

Simons PRJ, Van der Linden J, Duffy T. New learning: three ways to learn in a new balance. Dordrecht: Kluwer Academic Publishers; 2000.

Stalmeijer R, Gijselaers W, Wolfhagen H, Harendza S, Scherpbier A. How interdisciplinary teams can create multi-disciplinary education: the interplay between team processes and educational quality. Med Educ. 2007;41:1059–66.

Thurlings M, Evers AT, Vermeulen M. Toward a model of explaining teachers innovative behavior: a literature review. Rev Educ Res. 2014;20(10):1–42.

Timmermans O, Van Linge R, Van Petegem P, Elseviers M, Denekens J. Team learning and team composition in nursing. J Work Learn. 2011;23:258–75.

Timmermans O, Van Linge R, Van Petegem P, Denekens J. Team learning and innovation in nursing; results of a comprehensive research project. J Nurs Educ Pract. 2012a;2(4):10–21.

Timmermans O, Van Linge R, Van Petegem P, Denekens J. Team learning and context; assessing the relationship between team-learning activities and contextual factors of team-learning environment and team-configurations. Nurs: Res Rev. 2012b;1:1–8.

Timmermans O, Van Linge R, Van Petegem P, Van Rompaey B, Denekens J. Contingency perspective on team learning and innovation in nursing. J Adv Nurs. 2013;69(2):363–73.

Van Dam K, Schipper M, Runhaar P. Developing a competency-based framework for teachers' entrepreneurial behavior. Teach Teach Educ. 2010;26(4):965–71.

Van Linge R. Innovation in health care: theory, practice and research (in Dutch). Maarssen: Elsevier Gezondheidszorg; 2006.

West MA, Farr JL. Innovation at work: psychological perspectives. Soc Behav. 1989;4:15–30.

# Project Management and PDSA-Based Projects

# 8

Stijn Slootmans

**Abstract**

In this chapter, healthcare today is characterized by innovation and organizational change. The implementation of innovations is mainly directed toward improvement of quality, patient safety, or patient satisfaction, taking the financial and human resources of healthcare organizations into consideration. Healthcare systems have to change their focus from cost-efficiency to a more value-based approach. In this approach, value for patients is calculated by dividing cost by quality. To increase value for patients, we have to implement innovations that improve the quality and reduce the costs of services. This chapter explores how two specific strategies, project management (PM) and plan-do-study-act (PDSA) or plan-do-check-act (PDCA) cycles, can promote the implementation of innovations and thus improve the value of care.

**Keywords**

Quality improvement • Project management • PDSA-cycles • PDCA-cycles • Lean • A3 reporting method • Productive ward • Value of care

## 8.1 Introduction

Healthcare today is characterized by innovation and organizational change (Aubry et al. 2011). The implementation of innovations is mainly directed toward improvement of quality, patient safety, or patient satisfaction, taking the financial and human

S. Slootmans
Chief Medical Officer Department, Antwerp University Hospital, Antwerp, Belgium

Nursing and Midwifery Sciences, Centre for Research and Innovation in Care (CRIC), Faculty of Medicine and Health Sciences, University of Antwerp, Antwerp, Belgium
e-mail: stijn.slootmans@uza.be

© Springer International Publishing AG 2018
P. Van Bogaert, S. Clarke (eds.), *The Organizational Context of Nursing Practice*,
https://doi.org/10.1007/978-3-319-71042-6_8

resources of healthcare organizations into consideration. The Institute for Healthcare Improvement (IHI) stated that healthcare systems have to change their focus from cost-efficiency to a more value-based approach (Institute for Healthcare Improvement 2017). In this approach, value for patients is calculated by dividing cost by quality. To increase value for patients, we have to implement innovations that improve the quality and reduce the costs of services. The previous chapter explained the relationships between (team) learning, innovative work behavior, implementation of innovations, and improved patient outcomes. This chapter will explain how two specific strategies, project management (PM) and plan-do-study (PDSA) or plan-do-check-act (PDCA) cycles, can promote the implementation of innovations and thus improve the value of care.

Project management (PM) methodology is for the most part relatively new in healthcare and tends not to be formally taught in nursing education programs (Aubry et al. 2015; Overgaard 2015). However, nurses have many reference points they can use in learning to think about and manage projects in daily practice. For instance, like project management, the nursing process, familiar to nurses and managers alike, is a systematic approach based on assessment, diagnosis, planning, implementation, and evaluation and offers many parallels.

PM includes the following steps: initiation, planning, monitoring and controlling, and closing. The initiation phase parallels the assessment and diagnosis steps in the nursing process where those working on a unit project need to define the goals and objectives for the improvement by clarifying the desired outcome. Next, the underlying problems/challenges need to be identified and solutions to address them need to be identified in the planning phase. A project plan should identify the human resources, materials, and education needed. Third is the execution phase, where the plan is put into motion (which is the implementation phase in the nursing process). The fourth phase, monitoring or evaluation is found in PM as well as in nursing. Optimal project results are seen when teams constantly evaluate and adapt their approaches until desired results are obtained. The final step is the closing of the project where the results are completed and sustained (Overgaard 2015).

Quality improvement (QI) methods have been introduced in healthcare settings to enhance quality, patient safety, satisfaction, and efficiency. Achieving improvements in healthcare requires its application within complex social systems. Local contexts have great impacts on the success of an intervention. It is also clear that "single-bullet" approaches (involving only one set of actions and communications) do not tend to deliver consistent improvements. Improvement projects need to have complex and multifaceted interventions that are developed iteratively in response to obstacles and unintended effects (Taylor et al. 2014).

The PDSA (PDCA) cycle and the concept of iterative tests are methods central to many QI approaches like Lean, Six Sigma, and Total Quality Management (Reed and Card 2015; Taylor et al. 2014). PDSA represents a practical method for testing changes in complex systems in a manner based on the scientific method (Taylor et al. 2014). The PDSA cycle is focused on making changes that translate ideas into action. Rapid learning cycles allow for quick feedback so that the effectiveness of interventions is clear. Sustainable change is said to have been achieved when results suggest that no further adjustments are needed. Another important benefit of PDSA cycles lies in learning opportunities for healthcare workers and teams (Reed and Card 2015; Taylor et al. 2014). The method gives healthcare workers skills to learn from their experiences and to act to improve patient safety and conditions in their organizations. PDSA forces teams to predict likely outcomes of their interventions and measure the outcome of the improvement to assess their actual impact (Taylor et al. 2014). The chance to make and document meaningful change, connect multiple stakeholders to the intervention, and increase confidence in the intervention are also important benefits of PDSA. In Lean management, the PDSA cycle is operationalized with A3 problem solving.

A systematic review by Taylor et al. (2014) described the application of the PDSA method in healthcare. A theoretical framework to assess the use of PDCA in peer-reviewed publications was developed based on literature that assessed the use of iterative cycles, prediction of the outcome, small-scale testing (mini-experiments), the use of longitudinal data, and documentation. Of the 73 publications included in the review, only 2 demonstrated all 5 principles. However, the lack of standardized reporting in the publications rendered the assessment difficult. This paper found that the use of iterative change cycles and longitudinal data were described in 20% and 14% of the publications, respectively. Among the publications describing iterative change cycles, only 15% ($N = 2$) appeared to use small-scale tests. These data suggest that PDSA cycles are not being used optimally, leaving much room for greater consistency and attention to the use of the method as originally described that would likely yield benefits in terms of improved outcomes.

Reed and Card (2015) examined opportunities, complexities, and challenges in the use of PDSA cycles in healthcare. Many consider PDSA cycles to be an approach easily applied to QI purposes but while a certain simplicity in the methodology is a great strength, users need to be aware that tackling different problems often requires need more extensive knowledge and skills. The exploration and framing of problems is a very important aspect of PDSA and is one where staff often need the support of experts. Unfortunately, the planning and reflection stage of the method is sometimes considered a luxury time instead of a necessity. Following the structure of the cycle also forces healthcare workers to avoid the pitfalls of rushing to interventions prematurely. There are opportunities for inductive and double-loop learning of frontline staff when the application of the scientific principles is rigor in the "do" phase. Methodological expertise and sustained effort is necessary to maximize the benefits of PDSA.

## 8.2 Background of PM, Lean Management, and UZA Journey to Magnet Excellence

In Belgium, acute hospitals exist in a system with an increasing level of competitive pressure. This competition is increasing even more steadily given the movement toward limiting the volume of services provided in hospitals based on quantitative and qualitative criteria. Designating specific hospitals as the providers of care programs was initiated by the government to increase the quality and efficiency of care (Policy Cell Ministry of Social Affairs and Public Health Belgium 2017). Furthermore, there is increasing competition between Belgian hospitals, like healthcare organizations internationally, for highly educated physicians, nurses, and other healthcare workers. All of this evolution in the external environment has had tremendous impacts on internal operations. Increasing quality standards, higher expectations of patients, financial challenges, and multiple impacts of the competitive environment made the need for a transformation of practices at the Antwerp University Hospital (abbreviated UZA in Dutch) obvious.

Over a decade ago, to increase the performance of the hospital at every level and to prepare the hospital for the future, the UZA's board proposed a new strategy built around a vision to provide more value for the patient through the empowerment of frontline staff. To operationalize this new strategy, many different change programs were initiated over a 10-year period. In 2007 a strong need to support the different improvement projects with a project management structure was identified. Under the title PM@UZA, a nurse staff member and a manager of the HR department were assigned to evaluate the state of the science in project management (PM). After a review of different PM methods, the hospital decided to adopt and translate the *Project Management Body of Knowledge* (PMBOK®) for its organizational context.

The organizational PM structure is described in the literature as both a facilitator and as a barrier to harnessing the potential of project management. The impact of the PM structure is determined by its place within the organizational structure. In most organizations, PM is supported by a PM office or PMO that develops organizational PM capacity for achieving strategic goals. Unfortunately, it is challenging, if not impossible, to directly measure return on investment of a PMO. What is clear is that a good fit of the organization's PM structure has very significant effects and can add value to an organization (Aubry et al. 2011). Hurt and Thomas (2009) mentioned that PMOs must continually change and reinvent themselves to keep adding value to their organizations. PMOs generally typically start out addressing specific identified problems in PM within the institution. Later on, effective PMOs set new goals or objectives such as ensuring adherence to processes. New structures and/or processes can be necessary, but as long as a carefully PM vision and focus can be maintained, more value can be added to the organization. Finally, building PM capabilities is not a one-time effort but requires an ongoing, continuous investment that must be managed by qualified, visionary effective leaders (Hurt and Thomas 2009).

Aubry et al. (2011) present a case study where a PMO was assigned to guide a relocation and reorganization of six hospital sites into three in the McGill University Health Centre (MUHC) located in Montreal, Quebec. This case provides insights into the potential power of a PMO as well as into the facilitators of project management in healthcare settings. Because of the massive change the hospitals were undergoing, the PMO was called a Transition Support Office, which nonetheless met the definition of a PMO because this department managed a wide range of projects and offered services to different project managers and other stakeholders (Aubry et al. 2011). The TSO was launched in 2008 and was assigned to help key players coordinate the organization transition, support improvement in care processes, and create a culture of learning and innovation (Biron et al. 2012; Aubry et al. 2011). The TSO included staff members from a variety of backgrounds, such as nursing, management, and engineering, as well as students, and was led by a nurse (Lavoie-Tremblay et al. 2012). The TSO was under supervision of the CEO and a steering committee composed of by senior managers (Aubry et al. 2011).

An important task for the TSO was introducing performance management with not only a focus on productivity but also on measuring the impact of their efforts and various projects on quality and patient safety outcomes. For this purpose, the hospital designed an evaluation framework where structure, process, and patient and provider outcomes elements were specified. The overall goals of the activities were clinical effectiveness, patient centeredness, and patient safety, which were aligned with the hospital's strategic direction. By using performance management, the hospital could select outcomes aligned with the vision, determine opportunities for improvement, and follow up the effectiveness of the action plans. The TSO supported the project teams in optimizing and sustaining clinical and work processes within this framework (Biron et al. 2012).

Beyond the use of performance management, the TSO was also responsible for dissemination and implementation of evidence-based processes. Therefore, the project charter, based on the PMBOK, helped the project manager to coordinate, identify the stakeholders, and determine the aim and objectives of the projects. Important facilitators of change created by the TSO included their credibility as internal coaches for project management within the organization; their expertise in and advocacy for evidence, change management, direction and facilitation of projects; and, last but not least, their support for driving organizational culture change (Aubry et al. 2011; Lavoie-Tremblay et al. 2012).

The innovative role of the TSO as described here lies in its facilitation of organizational change, where mostly PMOs are traditionally oriented to monitoring and controlling narrower areas of operations (Lavoie-Tremblay et al. 2012). In addition, in healthcare, PMOs are often mandated to guide projects around implementation of technology, while the TSO at MUHC was extensively involved in guiding evidence-based improvement projects.

At UZA, our PMO consists of enthusiastic employees from different departments of the hospital, such as medicine, nursing, allied health disciplines, and others, primarily managers and middle managers. In our vision of project management structure, the PMO offers coaching to project managers. Because of the limited time that the PMO members can spend on initiatives outside their daily work, responsibility over the different projects falls to local project managers. Members of the PMO were asked to join a steering committee responsible for project management development, training, and follow-up. It is of note that no specific personnel resources were assigned to the PMO. Nevertheless, our PMO has trained internal project managers, mostly physicians, (nurse) managers, and staff members; to date, more than 300 colleagues have been certified in the local PM methodology.

Research shows that on-the-job training for project management capabilities in healthcare has positive results. Professionals reported high satisfaction and perceive the usefulness of the training, especially in terms of fulfilling otherwise unaddressed needs for skills and knowledge about PM. In pre-post assessment, professionals also reported gains in self-efficacy in carrying out project tasks, teamwork behaviors, goal clarity, and coordination. Together, these study findings suggested that improvement of knowledge and performance of new behaviors targeted by the program was reached (Chiocchio et al. 2015).

At the beginning of the PM@UZA program, various templates were designed using Microsoft Office applications. These templates were based on the PMBOK project management processes (see below). After an internal review, the lack of oversight of the different ongoing projects was identified as an area for improvement in the PMO. At the beginning of 2017, an Enterprise Project Server was installed to gather and analyze data to allow prioritization of resource allocation to different projects based on strategic, financial, and operational criteria. Now, the PMO can also follow the progress of every project and thereby coach project managers confronted with various barriers, issues, and problems.

After expanding the organization's performance to achieve process changes through project management, Lean management was chosen as an organization-wide strategy for operational excellence. The focus of the Lean approach on value creation for clients (patients, units, departments, and/or colleagues) is an excellent fit for the institutional needs to make efficient use of limited resources and continuously improve the quality of care processes to add value for patients.

Our Lean journey began 6 years ago in Birmingham, UK, after we visited two English hospitals that were implementing the Productive Ward: Releasing Time to Care™ program. Productive Ward (PW) is a modular program focusing on improvements at ward level. Nurses are very familiar with the patient care cycle or nursing process, which is comparable with the generic PDSA cycle. In this model, such a scheme is used to structure improvement projects. During the debriefing that followed on the visits, our HR and CNO convinced the CEO that hospital needed Lean thinking to stay on top of future trends and challenges and hold ourselves to the standard of the hospitals we visited.

We realized that adopting PW would be an advantage for UZA: frontline staff could begin incorporating Lean principles in a form already adapted for a healthcare environment. As reported in the literature on Lean, this bottom-up approach was expected to support empowerment and engagement of frontline staff as well as their leadership (Graban 2012). Other elements of the PW program that were appealing include the focus on data-driven, systematic improvements and process stability.

The human resources (HR) saw in Lean methodology a way to boost healthcare workers' engagement in a manner anticipated to support quality and safety of patient care. Lean empowers frontline staff to improve their work and helps every UZA healthcare worker and staff make continuous improvement both a routine and one of the highest priorities in the hospital. At the same time, the nursing department was seeking to achieve Magnet status or designation for the hospital. The Magnet journey has a strong focus on patient outcomes, continuous improvement of patient care, and nurse's work environment improvement with an untimely goal to attract and retain professional nurses. PW was seen as one way to operationalize the Magnet philosophy. The lean transformation of Antwerp University Hospital started in 2011.

At the end of each project that has been translated into the hospital's PM methodology (called PM@UZA), normally implementation of PW considerations follows. PW is a program and thus cannot be compared with a project, but programs are tackled as a series of projects. The project team decided to divide the implementation of PW in two phases. Firstly, the implementation of PW on two nursing wards was launched on a pilot basis. Later, with the experiences and knowledge of this pilot, the project team planned a hospital-wide implementation plan.

## 8.3    Introduction to Project Management Methods

We will now briefly explain the PMBOK® methodology as described in the PMBOK® guide (Project Management Institute 2004). A project is a temporary endeavor to create a unique product, service, or result. The descriptor "temporary" is temporary because each project has a defined start- and endpoint. A project has reached its end when predefined objectives have been (or cannot be) achieved. This does not mean that every project is a short-term operation or that the delivered service, result, or product is impermanent, but it is always important to clarify project run time when considering the use of resources. Most projects begin with an intention to create a unique result that can be sustainably implemented in the operations of the organization (Project Management Institute 2004) (Box 8.1).

---

**Box 8.1 Project Criteria**
1. Temporary endeavor
2. Unique result
3. Realizing predefine objectives
4. Interaction between the triple constraint
    (a) Time
    (b) Scope
    (c) Resources

---

Projects have existed since the beginning of time. In the 1950s, most of the modern project manager's concepts and tools were initially described by military organizations. In the mid-1970s, the Project Management Institute began exploring project management as a profession. In 1987, the first *Project Management Book of Knowledge (PMBOK)* was formally published with eight knowledge areas (scope, time, cost, quality, human resources, communication, risk, and contracts/procurement). In 1996 a revision of PMBOK changed the manual to *A Guide to the Project Management Book of Knowledge* and added integration as a knowledge area. In the

1990s, different industries and organizations have adopted project management tools and techniques. Project management theories use knowledge, skills, methods, and techniques to realize project requirements. In the late 1990s and early 2000s, other organizations established other project management methods such as the Japanese Project Management Book of Knowledge, Agile software management, and PRINCE2. The latter became very influential particularly in the United Kingdom (Morris 2013). Project activities can be divided in the following project management processes: initiating, planning, executing, monitoring and controlling, and closing (Project Management Institute 2004).

The so-called triple constraint must be borne in mind across the entire life cycle of a project. The triple constraint is the concept of intrinsic connections between time, scope, and resources. This triangle is fundamental in the initiation and planning phase but is also crucial when changes in execution are necessary. When one aspect of the triangle has to be adjusted, it has an impact on the other two. For example, when the original plan for a project cannot be carried out, time, scope, or resource use have to be reevaluated in order to achieve the project goals. Project managers must constantly balance three components to achieve project objectives within a predefined budget (Project Management Institute 2004).

### 8.3.1  Initiation Phase

The initiation phase of the process includes every process that leads to formal authorization of the new project. This phase will in most cases be performed outside of project scope. According to the PMBOK guide, this phase consists of a product description, project mandate, and initial scope document. The initiator or sponsor, who can be a person, team, or department and can be an internal or an external partner, must clearly describe the project. The description has to be adapted to the environmental factors and hospital organizational policies and procedures. A feasibility study may be necessary to explore the different solutions to achieve the initial request as described. In this way, alternative options are explored, and the project team can determine the most ideal solution.

After choosing the best solution to address the request in the description, the approach for the project and the project objectives are defined. A summary of the approach consists of a defined scope and product or services to be delivered, throughput time, and an estimation of necessary resources. Another point of interest in the initiation phase is ensuring that there is a link between the project and the strategic plan of the organization. A number of other structural elements of the project are decided upon: management responsibilities within the project can be clarified and large and complex projects can be divided in different phases.

The initial project scope document describes the tentative, global definition of the project and includes product or service requirements for delivery, boundaries, acceptation method, and the way the scope will be managed. In situations where projects need to be divided into separate projects, it is important to repeat the initiation phase to clarify the goals, necessary resources, and the new starting point for each subproject.

The aim of the initiation phase is received authorizing for the objectives of the project and developing a clear understanding of the link between the product or service to be developed and the operations of the organization. Authorization should be made by the management of the department or if necessary (because of the project scope) by the hospital board (Box 8.2 See further).

---

**Box 8.2 Project Charter Components**
- Business case
  - Background
  - Objectives
- Possible solutions and the one being advocated
- Project structure
  - Steering committee
  - Project team
- Classification project size
- Risks
- Acceptance criteria
- One-minute summary

---

First, in our hospital, when a suggestion is made for a project or a need emerges that needs to be addressed, the request has to be approved by the nurse manager and/or nurse leader. When the proposal matches with the hospital or department objectives, the initiation phase can begin. The initiation phase is then established, guided by a project charter and a structure cost–benefit analysis derived from the PMBOK guide.

The project manager (PM) is normally the manager of the department where the project is being conducted or another individual designated by the head of the department. The project manager drafts the program charter in consultation with all relevant stakeholders. The project charter consists of a business case for the project, possible solutions/approaches, and a presentation of the project structure. The business case contains the background for the project (the need that it would address) in addition to the project's SMART goals (an acronym for goals written in a way that clarifies that they are specific, measurable, achievable, realistic, and time-related). The project objectives need to link clearly with the overall goals and objectives of the organization (Overgaard 2010). The project manager must describe different possible solutions that could meet the project requirements and has to specify which one they believe is the optimal solution that should be funded. A project structure includes a steering committee, and a project team is also defined at this time. In the case of large projects, a liaison within the board of directors is often appointed.

Every project will also be categorized according to complexity and size of the project. Large projects and their necessary resources have to be confirmed by the board of directors (Box 8.2).

---

**Box 8.3 PW Implementation Characteristics**
- Project teams internal to nursing units
- Human resources and project management coaching
- Objectives linked to the nursing department and hospital strategic plans
- Selection criteria pilot wards
  - Strong leadership
  - High nurse satisfaction
  No restructuring
  Development of internal knowledge with respect to PW without consultancy support
  Project rollout schedule based on experiences in the pilot phase
  Module-based program
  Sustainable result by follow-up coaching

---

For small rather straightforward specific projects with limited stakeholders and a lead time of 3–6 months, the PMO suggests the use of the A3 method based on PDSA or PDCA cycles (see below) (Jimmerson 2007). This is a method for tackling specific, well-defined problems. Large projects can subsume multiple A3 projects.

Projects involving optimization of a complex process or a range of different linked processes and/or different bottlenecks are preferably tackled using multiple PDSA improvement projects. However, recently reports have appeared of failures of the PDSA method when tackling complex and multicomponent problems (Reed and Card 2015). Reed and Card argue that the four stages of PDSA are nonetheless useful for bigger projects because of the scientific, iterative, and experimental principles they incorporate. Thus when using PDSA in the context of larger projects, the method needs to be applied in a sophisticated and thoughtful way, in concert with a broader methodological approach like Lean management (such as the PW program), and with appropriate organizational support.

Finally, the risks, influencing factors and criteria required for stakeholder acceptance of this project results are identified in the initiation phase and allow project managers to discover barriers to or facilitators of execution. A one-minute summary is also prepared that is discussed at a board of directors meeting to secure official authorization to go ahead when necessary.

After the decision was made to implement the PW program, a project team was assigned, with a base of a nurse manager and a clinical nurse selected internally for the entire project. This project team received coaching and support from a HR coordinator and internal PM expert. The business case for PW was explained in terms of the significant improvement in quality of patient care and benefits for clinical nurses and the nurse's work environment anticipated, without commitments of additional resources on an ongoing basis. The program also operationalizes a business strategy that aims to achieve nursing excellence and progress in the journey to Magnet recognition (Box 8.3).

The PW program provides selection criteria for selecting appropriate pilot wards, such as evidence of stable and transformational leadership, high nurse satisfaction, and a lack of recent restructuring (NHS Institute for Innovation and Improvement 2008). After extensive discussion within the nursing department, these criteria were used to select the wards most ready pilot to adopt the first PW program modules. The implementation of the three foundation modules and two process modules on the pilot wards over a 9-month period was decided upon, alongside the development of a communication plan for the entire hospital, a plan for data gathering needed for hospital-wide implementation and considerations around sustainability of the program. The further rollout of the program at the ward level and follow-up by the project team was deemed beyond the scope of this initial project.

Choices were narrowed down to two approaches to guide implementation. To achieve and maintain the full capacity of the program, the steering committee decided to develop internal knowledge and not to rely on external consultant expertise. To develop internal knowledge, a steering committee of key stakeholders led by the CEO was established at the hospital board level, and a working group of nurse managers led by the CNO was formed. Criteria for acceptability of the project to the staff were identified, based on an analysis of project scope and risks such as difficulties engaging nurses to devote special efforts needed for the first phase of the project and a possible return to top-down approaches to treat and solve problems.

## 8.3.2  Planning Phase

After a project receives authorization based on the product description, project mandate, and initial scope document, the project team can start to successfully plan and manage the project. The planning phase begins with the collection of complete and valid information required to block out the necessary work. The initial scope document is the starting point for the project plan, but when the scope, costs, or timeline are not very detailed, the project team has to make appropriate clarifications in line with the triple constraint. The project team must identify and resolve roadblocks, requirements, risks, opportunities, and prerequisite conditions that may emerge from any new information obtained. At this stage of the project, the triple constraint is a major area of concern. The predetermined scope and budget will affect the timeline and thus the project plan.

The project plan consists of work breakdown structure or WBS. A WBS is a hierarchical separation of the types or phases work that needs to be formalized to make the project objectives succeed (Project Management Institute 2004). The WBS organizes and defines the work packages in smaller and manageable parts with necessary milestones. These milestones are important deadlines for which parts of the project have to be completed next to decide make "go" or "no-go" decision on forward movement. Most of the time, project teams need to adjust project plans when new information emerges. Detailing the plan in advance is called rolling wave planning. Involving every stakeholder group in the project leads to all relevant knowledge and skills being brought to bear to the development of the project plan and facilitates and accelerates the work to be done.

In our hospital, the planning phase was translated to a specific Microsoft® Excel template. The PMO designed a tool for developing a project plan. Important design aspects of the project plan include the scope, costs, manpower, quality, communication, and a plan for possible risks. The first step in the template is creating the work breakdown structure. The project is divided in work packages with an owner and the estimated workload. The predefined milestones are the initiation for the project, project charter, project plan, execution, and closing of the project. Within the project plan, a Gantt chart is used to specify project scheduling elements and resources needed. Beyond the WBS, an organizational breakdown structure or OBS is also constructed, consisting of a steering committee and at least one working committee. Other stakeholders will be identified and a communication plan for the life of the project will be designed. The entire project plan is validated and approved by the steering committee before execution begins.

Support for project plans was optimized with the installation of the Enterprise Project Server in 2017. Within this web-based application, WBSs and OBSs can easily be set up and adjusted based on the initial template. In addition, with the Enterprise Project Server and with frequent updates from various project teams on actual timing and budget variances, the PMO can evaluate the progress of different projects and follow up with coaching as needed in situations of non-compliance with the project plan.

In the case of the PW program, the steering committee made a positive evaluation after implementation on the pilot wards, and a "go" was given for the further implementation relying on internal expertise. The project team expanded its original scope to the other nursing wards. Based on the experiences with the implementation of PW on the pilot wards, the initial scope was maintained and the roll-out pace was increased to 6 months per nursing ward (time to shortened from 9 months).

The PW program suggests several different types of rollout. One possibility is to start on a limited basis on two pilot wards and expand spread in cohorts with a growing number of wards in order to focus on development of the project team and (nurse) managers. This approach has the advantage that knowledge builds with experience of the initiative's implementation, but the quality of the implementation and self-management of the project on different wards can pose threats to the project goals. A linear rollout with the same cohort size is another approach with the advantage of starting with more pilot wards, but more resources will be needed to lead this approach. The follow-up tends to be more manageable, but the project still spreads quickly within the hospital ((NHS Institute for Innovation and Improvement 2008). The steering committee decided to combine these two approaches so a limited pilot phase can create knowledge and experience and a manageable rollout in cohorts of 4–5 nursing wards to expand the program in the hospital within 2.5 years

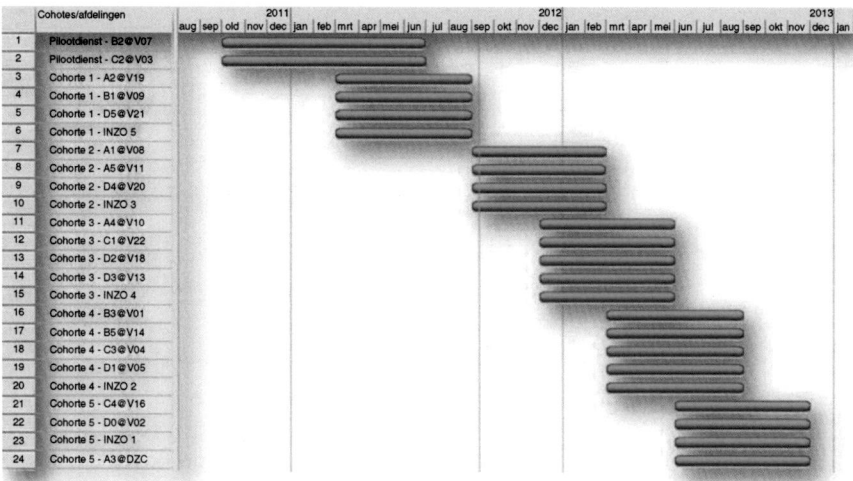

**Fig. 8.1**   Project rollout schedule

(see Fig. 8.1). The chosen approach made it possible to start a hospital-wide program in a short period with a limited effort of nursing department resources.

### 8.3.3   Execution, Monitoring and Controlling, and Closing Phases

The project team must steer the processes necessary for executing the project including the coordination of manpower and resources and the integration and execution of activities described in the project plan. If a project team was not already assigned, the project coordinator now has to set up and develop the team before proceeding. Ensuring the quality of the service, product or result of the project is the most important aspect of managing the project and requires close follow-up of all communication from both technical and organizational sides. Throughout the execution phase, the project team needs to gather information in the form of progress reports about the work packages that in turn can be used to provide feedback to management and stakeholders regarding achievement of the different milestones and completion of the project.

The scope and the project objectives specified in the original scope document will drive monitoring and control to identify potential bottlenecks or deviations from the plan so that corrective adjustments can be made in a timely manner. Deviations from the original project plan will lead to necessary rescheduling and can affect throughput time, productivity, and availability of resources and will uncover unrecognized risks. These deviations may or may not affect the project plan; an analysis is required to find out. PDSA cycles using relevant data or results may help here. This analysis may signal conditions that can result in a change of

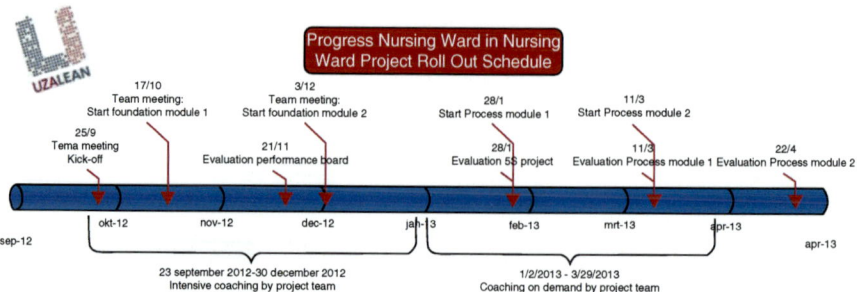

**Fig. 8.2** Project rollout schedule at ward level

project plan after approval by project manager or steering committee. When the project is finished, the project team can formally close down all project processes.

In PM@UZA methodology, the first step in the execution phase is a kickoff meeting. The objective of the formal kickoff of the project is to provide a general overview of the project and the planned approach for the stakeholders. The attendees of this official launch will primarily be the steering committee, working group, and important stakeholders. Next, the project team executes the work packages defined in the project plan, follows timing of activities, and provides status updates to all the stakeholders. Feedbacks about progress, scope changes, use of resources, and potential risk are provided to the steering committee. This committee is in place to make strategic decisions; otherwise, the working group provides operational input to the project team. At the end of the project, a final report and presentation of project deliverables is provided to the management of the hospital (or the relevant department, depending on the scope of the project). The project ends when results have met acceptability criteria. Reviewing the lessons learned from the project can be a meaningful exercise for both the project team and stakeholders.

In the execution of the implementation of PW at UZA involving rollout of the three foundation modules and two process modules, the project team educated and coached the nurse managers in briefing meetings. The introduction of the structure and tools of PW to the nursing teams was provided in a stepwise manner in relation to the introduction of modules. Within 6 and 9 months, nurses and nurse managers of the pilot wards were sufficiently prepared to continue the program as a team. The project team provided structured coaching sessions and feedback for the steering committee to facilitate monitoring and controlling. The working group of nurse managers provided operational and practical support (Fig. 8.2).

## 8.4 Introduction of PDSA Thinking and A3 Method

A problem-solving methodology that is receiving a lot of attention and has been adopted by many healthcare organizations is "A3" (Graban 2012; Graban and Swartz 2012). A3 problem solving has links to both the nursing process and PDSA cycles (Jimmerson 2007).

## 8.4.1  A3 Reporting Method

The A3 reporting method is a systematic approach to address bottlenecks or problems based on teamwork. The method is heavily based on Deming's improvement cycle or PDSA cycles. The improvement steps are displayed in an A3 report, originally designed by the Toyota company—the founders of Lean thinking (Graban 2012; Jimmerson 2007). The name of the method comes from the size of the paper that was originally chosen because it is "faxable"—Toyota employees could share their work with colleagues around the world by printing their reports on A3 paper and sending them along with a facsimile machine.

The outstanding features of the Toyota Production System, as it was originally developed by Toyota, or the Lean management system as those who followed it came to call their method, are reflected in the successes of Toyota as a company. Toyota achieved a level of quality, safety, satisfaction, and financial results whereby the company is now a world-class organization. Other companies followed the Toyota example of problem solving, and they also accelerated and sustain exemplary quality (Jimmerson 2007). The need for Lean in the healthcare sector is very clear, where issues with quality, patient safety, costs, waiting times, and staff morale are widespread (Graban 2012).

The A3 reporting method embodies the concept and strategy of Lean thinking through a transformation from a command and control culture to one where thinking organizations are created, and bottom-up initiatives are supported from the top. The method is focused on adaptive change. An A3 report is characterized by a brief presentation of the analysis of the problem, the improvement process, and has a visual aspect to keep all team members informed about the problem-solving process. In addition, A3 reports are always data-driven (Jimmerson 2007).

More important than the size of paper is the structured manner of problem analysis and PDSA thinking that is the foundation of the methodology (Graban 2012). The A3 method is a step-by-step plan to uncover root causes of a well-identified problem. The aim is to avoid both delayed and/or repeated inadequate responses to relevant issues and problems and jumping to conclusions based on incorrect assumptions without involving staff and stakeholders. The solutions for underlying causes are presented visually and are expected to be guided by data and facts rather than assumptions. The left side of the document describes current practices and focuses on the planning. The right side however contains the improvement. Thus, the do, study, and adjust phases of a PDSA cycle are addressed (Graban 2012; Jimmerson 2007). The report is a living document that can be used as a report of the group's thought process during a meeting and can be used as a communication medium (Jimmerson 2007). While this method may slow down the process of taking actions to solve a problem, if consensus regarding root causes and solutions can be achieved, the resulting plan has much more support and commitment from the group; this improves the likelihood of successful implementation and sustainable outcomes of a project.

An A3 report contains a very brief presentation of the improvement cycle through text and especially through visual tools such as graphs, figures, fishbone diagrams, and process maps. Different templates are used around the world, but the PDSA cycle is the basis for all of them. In our hospital, a 7-step template is used (Box 8.4).

**Box 8.4 7-step A3 Improvement Project**
1. Background
2. Current situation and problem statement
3. Ideal situation and objectives
4. Root cause analysis
5. Identified countermeasures and action plan
6. Evaluation of the improvement results
7. Consideration of sustainability, expansion of scope, and communication plan

1. The team describes the background of the improvement idea. The first step in improving current practice is the clear understanding of the problem, risks, or bottlenecks (Jimmerson 2007). The problem needs to be specific with a clear defined scope and a sense of urgency or link to organizational goals and priorities. When other stakeholders are involved, the team needs to contact them and discuss the problem. The patient is the most important "customer" or stakeholder in healthcare, so improvement projects are preferably patient-centric and/or person-centered. Stating the central objective to improve the outcomes for the patient enables all healthcare workers to be involved in problem solving (Jimmerson 2007).

2. Current practices are analyzed, preferably using graphics, tables, or some other visual presentation. The results of this phase serve provide baseline measurements for evaluating the improvement. Moreover, an observation of daily practice processes and circumstances can improve understanding of the real context so the team can "grasp the situation" (Graban 2012). Establishing baseline data is essential to check the results of the improvement in the study phase, but it also avoids healthcare workers engaging in speculation, jumping to conclusions, or blaming coworkers. The feedback and validation of frontline staff is essential. Group consensus ensures accuracy and clarity of the formulation of the problem and buy-in for the improvement (Jimmerson 2007). Within our hospital, we focus on patient outcomes such as falls, infection prevention and control, patient safety, as well as patient experiences and satisfaction, but compliance or process indicators can also be used. The description and insights of current practices need to be validated within the team and with other stakeholders. Beside current practices, the A3 report asks for a description of desirable practices and tangible goals. Therefore, the gap between current and desirable or ideal practices as well as the aims of the project becomes clear (Jimmerson 2007). Goals are described using the SMART method (see the Initiation phase above).

4. The fourth and most essential and important step is a root cause analysis or RCA. Solving a problem should start with the question *why*? The focus must be on

eliminating barriers to preventing problems or risks, so these barriers need to be uncovered (Graban 2012). It is preferable to use "real" data in an RCA, but a team can also gather relevant data by brainstorming. These (root) causes identify gaps between current and ideal practices. Links between problems and causes need to be clear by a detailed and in-depth investigation of bottlenecks. It is hoped that after a successful implementation of a proper intervention, root causes will all be addressed, and the problems will no longer occur.

In the fourth step, different tools can be used. There are a number of these, the most common of which are fishbone or Ishikawa diagrams, 5-Why analysis and the problem analysis tree. The 5-Why analysis is a framework: sometimes only three questions can reveal the root cause but sometimes the list is longer and more complex. The intention of all of these tools is to drill into the problem and understand its root causes (Graban and Swartz 2012; Jimmerson 2007). These tools steer the team to investigate the nature of errors systematically rather than blame the healthcare worker at the point of care (Graban and Swartz 2012). Because it is rare that a problem is caused by a single cause, a fishbone diagram or problem analysis tree can visualize the connection between the (root) causes and the problem or risk (Graban 2012; Graban and Swartz 2012).

5. After the RCA is completed, the team can start to find and implement countermeasures. The term "countermeasure" is used to underline that these actions are made within the journey of continuous improvement (Graban 2012). The countermeasures need to have a clear link with the RCA and every root cause needs an identified countermeasure (Jimmerson 2007). In situations where there are many different causes, the contributors may need to be prioritized (Graban and Swartz 2012). The team only needs to address only the most relevant causes, identified and selected based on a principle—for example, the Pareto principle. This principle states that 80% of the problems can be tracked to 20% of the possible root causes. Finally, a sufficiently detailed action plan that also describes in addition accountabilities and deadlines is developed and can be supported by a time and resource schedule such as a Gantt chart. This plan sets accountability for the tasks that need to occur for countermeasures to be implemented. Short pilot tests with a limited scope can be performed to evaluate feasibility of countermeasures (Jimmerson 2007). The ideal practices, the countermeasures, and the action plan comprises the "do" phase of the PDSA cycle (Graban 2012; Jimmerson 2007).

6. After implementation of the countermeasures, the study or check phase is performed by collecting results to verify whether the project aims have been achieved. The effectiveness of the action plan will be evaluated with the same method as those used to describe deviations from best practices (Graban 2012; Jimmerson 2007). Improvements need to be established and be sustainable to consider a program a success. In our hospital, the sustainability of the improvements is tracked with measures at three points post-intervention in our hospital. Benefits of successfully implemented changes in practice based on active participation and involvement of team members are of special value; such successes can motivate staff and provide sustainable solutions for key problems on units. Performing a

check on the effectiveness of the action plan by a post-measurement and acting by redoing the RCA or taking more countermeasures ensures that the study and act phase are performed (Graban 2012). In cases where the project aims have not been met (in part or in whole) and additional measures are necessary, a continuous process of improvement can be set up.

7. Once project aims are met, new practices can be standardized and systematized. A follow-up or recurring review of the action plan or results may be needed and must occur (Jimmerson 2007).

An A3 problem-solving project is a team learning exercise rather than a solitary pursuit. Writing the A3 report needs to be an iterative process; continuously refining and adjusting can improve the outcome of the PDSA cycle. The feedback of frontline staff will provide in-depth understanding of the actual current practices (Graban 2012). The role of leaders within A3 problem solving is crucial. Shifting from top-down decision delegation to coaching and approving changes is essential. Leaders can have oversight of the A3 report so that appropriate verification around the improvements and outcomes can be conducted (Jimmerson 2007). When coaching is provided, the expert can ask challenging questions and provide constructive feedback. The outcome of the improvement will also be based on consensus and agreement of the entire team so sustainability can be maximized (Graban 2012).

### 8.4.2 Implementing A3 Problem Solving in Nursing Practice

In our hospital, the management of the nursing department created a strategic plan that is updated every 2 years. This strategic plan is aligned with the hospital mission, vision, and strategy—which is illustrated in a model named K2 (see Fig. 8.3). K2 stands for quality and knowledge (both words *Kennis en Kwaliteit* begin with a K in Dutch): the central organizational aims of a university hospital. In this model, short-term objectives grouped by the categories quality and patient safety, employees, and knowledge are presented alongside the mission, vision, and core values. The foundations for implementing this strategy are evidence-based practice, Lean mindset, leadership, and research.

The organizational objectives are translated into specific goals for nurses and nursing services. Every nursing ward needs to pursue six goals annually based on the nurse strategic plan.

Four further hospital-wide goals are mandatory for all units and involve reduction of hospital-acquired pressure ulcers, falls with injury, catheter-associated urinary tract infection rates, and central line-associated bloodstream infection rates. These goals are measured by outcome indicators. These indicators are nurse sensitive so nurses have a great impact on the results but other healthcare workers like physicians have also responsibilities in achieving great patient outcomes. The results are benchmarked against the National Database of Nursing Quality Indicators or NDNQI. More than 2000 US hospitals and 95% of Magnet®-recognized facilities

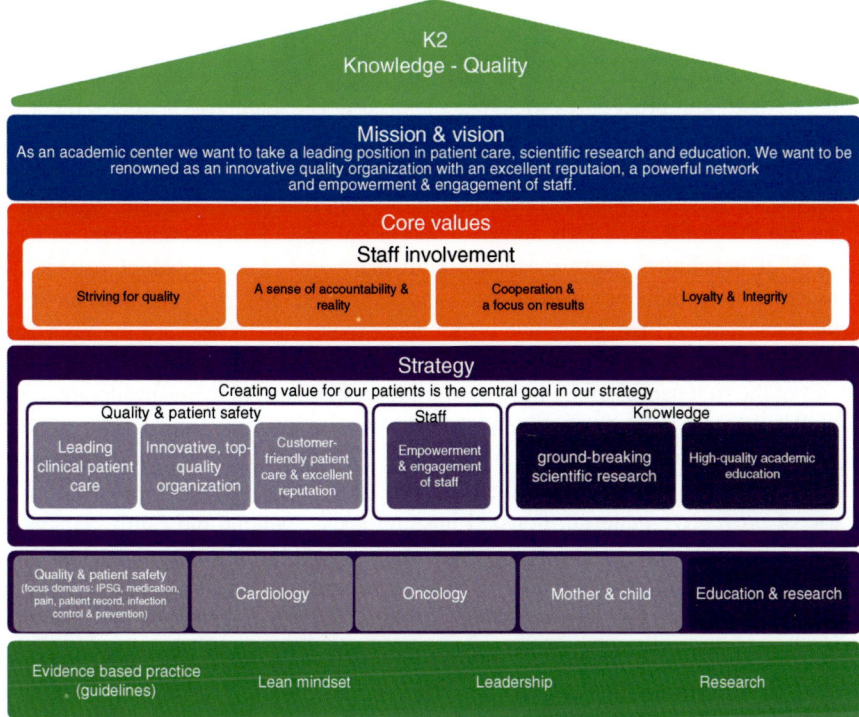

**Fig. 8.3** K2 Strategic plan

participate (Press Ganey Associates, Inc 2017). With these benchmarks, our hospital can compare its performance on the nurse-sensitive indicators with hospitals having the same characteristics.

Each unit chooses further two goals from a departmental picklist. The picklist contains goals within four categories: patient care, quality and patient safety, nurse's work environment, and cost-efficiency.

To reach the objectives, nursing teams employ A3 problem-solving methodology. Some principles were determined to achieve an excellent and sustainable outcome. The frontline nurses are the most important driver of these improvement projects so structural empowerment is a basic. The nurse manager serves as the coach for the project, equipped with transformational leadership skills and support and coaching by the Lean program project leaders. Baseline and post-intervention measurements need to involve patient outcomes that bookend an intervention period where the RCA and evidence-based action plan is implemented. The team also must describe how they plan to share improvements and their evaluation with other departments or externally. These improvement projects are the operationalization of our "journey to nursing excellence."

### 8.4.3 Practical Examples of PDSA Improvements

In our hospital, an expert team has been given responsibility for setting and improving policies and procedures to address fall risks. The team also analyzes reports of fall incidents. After a hospital-wide analysis of trends, a decision was made to do an aggregated root cause analysis of all the fall incidents occurring on two nursing wards where there were significantly more reported falls. First the background around the problem of falls and data on current and ideal practices related to the NDNQI benchmark were discussed with the teams. The causes of patient falls reported in the incidents were merged and categorized in a problem analysis tree by the nurses, nurse manager, nurse leader, and expert team. Afterward the team could include additional causes, and using the 5-Why method, root causes were identified. Out of the root causes at the nursing ward level discovered, the team identified care of disorientated patients, the use of preventive materials, influential medication, and inappropriate footwear as the most important. Next, countermeasures were identified and an action plan was drafted. The most important countermeasures were the use of preventive material, nonskid hospital socks, patient and family education, and communication of the risk within the nursing team. After the intervention, decrease of fall rates was noted. Next steps were decided upon at a team meeting, and the results are now followed up at weekly quality and patient safety huddles.

Central line-associated bloodstream infections or CLABSI increase the cost of hospitalization, in part by increasing length of stay. In intensive care units, the incidence of this complication has been estimated at around 80,000 infections per year worldwide. A decrease in incidence can greatly improve patient outcomes and reduce healthcare costs. CLABSI is the most common nosocomial infection at the intensive care unit (ICU) and thus has a tremendous impact on mortality and morbidity for this patient population (O'Grady et al. 2011). The physician head of the department, the nurse leader, and nurse managers of the various ICUs noticed that the results for the critical care units were worse than the NDNQI benchmark (respectively, 2.38 vs. 1.26 CLABSIs per 1000 catheter days) and decided to start an A3 problem solving (see Fig. 8.4). The team performed an RCA based on literature and observations of practices. Three main causes of infection occur within the care process, namely, (1) the insertion of the catheter, (2) daily care of the catheter, and (3) the catheter remaining in place longer than clinically necessary. These aspects of care were drilled down to identify root causes (see problem analysis tree). The procedures for the insertion, daily care of central line catheters and daily evaluation of necessity for central lines were changed and new procedures adopted. The ICU nurses began using chlorhexidine wash gloves because of the evidence that this technique can reduce the incidence of CLABSI at the ICU by 28% (Climo et al. 2013). The results for the 4th quarter of 2014, 1st quarter of 2014, and 2nd quarter of 2015 improved to 1.94, 0.98, and 1.99 CLABSIs per 1000 catheter days, respectively. The team continues to follow the results on the quality and patient safety dashboard and at team huddles. The improvement in rates has been sustained and even appears to still be decreasing (Fig. 8.5).

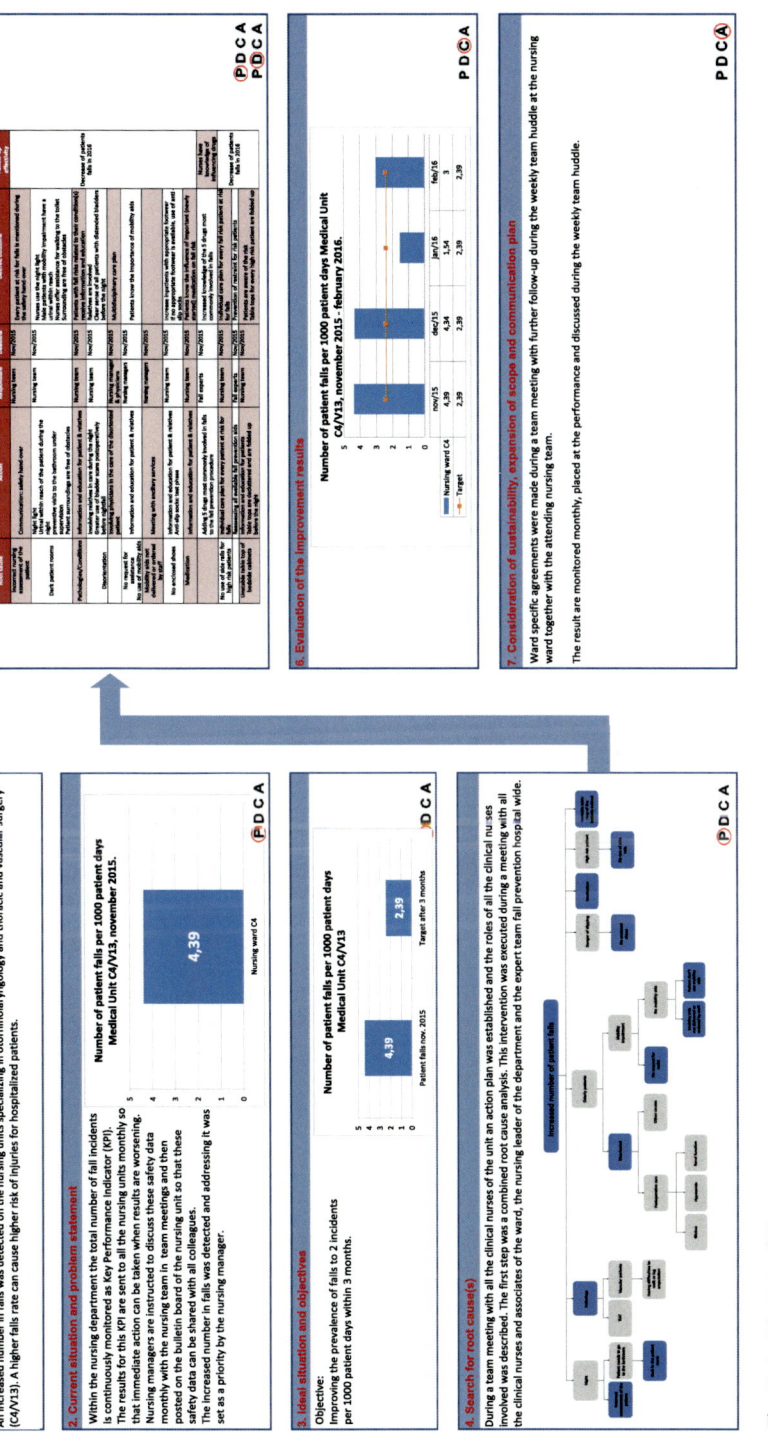

**Fig. 8.4** A3 report falls

## A3-report: CLABSI at Intensice Care

| Owner: | Prof. Dr. Jorens, Brigitte Claes & Infection Prevention and Control | Department | Intensive cae unit |
| Participants: | All caregivers at ICU | Start Date: | Q1 t014 |
| | | End date: | Q2 t015 |

### 1. Background

Central Line Associated Bloodstream infections increase the cost of hospitalization and length of stay. On Intensive Care, the incidence of this hospital-acquired infections is estimated to be around 80,000 infections per year worldwide. A decrease in incidence can significantly improve patient outcomes and reduce healthcare costs (CDC, 2011)

### 2. Current situation and problem statement

As stated in the background, CLABSI is one of the most common nosocomial infection on ICU. CLABSI has a large impact on morbidity and mortality for this patient population. This nurse sensitive clinical indicator is a key performance indicator for the nursing wards hospital-wide. The management team of ICU noted that the result of this indicator is noticeably worse than the benchmark of the National Database of Nursing Quality indicators or NDNQI compared with similar teaching hospitals.

CLABSI rate per 1000 central line days, ICU, Q1 2014

2,38

CLABSI at ICU

P D C A

### 3. Ideal situation and objectives

Objective: To reduce the incidence CLABSI below NDNQI benchmark in a period of 1 year.

CLABSI rate per 1000 central line days, ICU

2,38 → 1,26

CLABSI at ICU    Target

P D C A

### 4. Search for root cause(s)

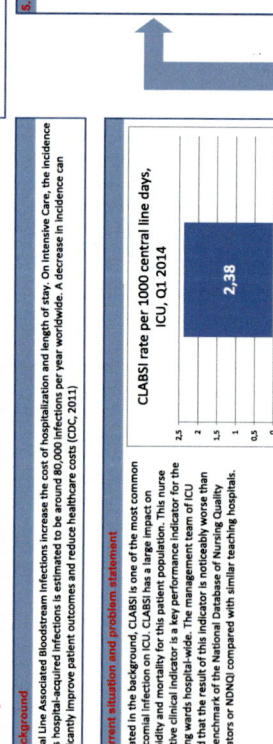

Causes of CLABSI at ICU

P D C A

In the root cause analysis, the head of department, the nurse leader, the nurse managers and infection prevention and control department were involved. Improvements are determined on evidence bases practice and observations by clinical nurses of the infection prevention and control department

### 5. Identified countermeasures and action plan

| Root cause | Action | Responsible | Deadline | Most important action |
|---|---|---|---|---|
| Patient and caregiver are maximally covered at the time of line insertion (surgical mask, cap, apron and hand gloves) | Changing central venous catheter kit | Infection prevention & control department | June 2014 | |
| | Adjusting procedure | Nurse managers | Q2 2015 | |
| Surgical disinfection | Training | Nurse managers | Q2 2015 | |
| | Making available of surgical hand disinfection | Infection prevention & control department | Q2 2014 | |
| Daily multidisciplinary evaluation of the necessity of the central line | Determine criteria of necessity of the central line | Nurse managers and physicians | Q2 2014 | x |
| Incorrect execution of nursing care procedures | Refreshing departmental procedure | Nurse managers | Q2 2014 | |
| Incorrect use of the replacement procedure of IV administration site | Refreshing departmental procedure | Nurse managers | Q3 2014 | |
| Missing caps/failure of disinfect caps | Refreshing departmental procedure | Nurse managers | Q3 2014 | |
| | Application of principles for hand hygiene as the basis of the hospital wide procedure, fincers, compliance with the WHO-designated five moments for hand hygiene, use of cues, monitor, addressing attitudes towards hand hygiene | Infection prevention & control department | Continuous | |
| Migration of bacteria from other locations of the body | Use of chlorhexidine impregnated single-use washcloths | Infection prevention & control department | Q2 2014 | x |
| Recording/hosting of CLABSI | Tracing of CLABSI with feedback mechanism of the nursing wards | Infection prevention & control department | Q2 2014 | x |

P D C A
P D C A

### 6. Evaluation of the improvement results

Follow-up based on the results of the nurse sensitive clinical indicator CLABSI available at the hospital business intelligence center database. Action plan effectiveness is monitored.

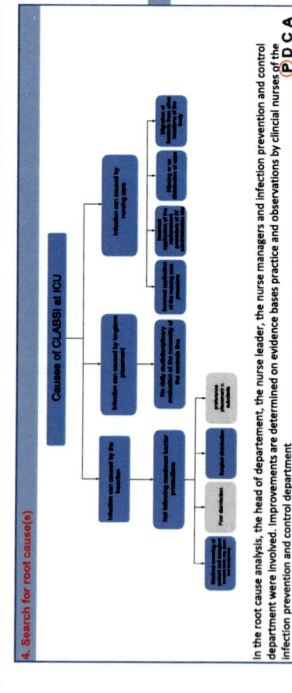

P D C A

### 7. Consideration of sustainability, expansion of scope and communication plan

Monitored results at the weekly team performance huddle involving the infection prevention and control nurses on a monthly base to evaluate the hospital acquired conditions: catheter associated urinary tract infections, central line associated bloodstream infections and ventilator associated pneumonia.

P D C A

**Fig. 8.5** A3 report CLABSI

## Conclusion

This chapter reviewed project management structures and approaches, as well as PDSA cycles as tools for improving the quality and safety of nursing care as well as patient outcomes. These descriptions were amplified with details of the steps involved in the use of these frameworks in practice and many examples of how these principles have been implemented at Antwerp University Hospital. These strategies are intended to be used again and again, and many believe that their successful use changes work environments for the better at the level of clinical teams as well as institution-wide. Given that change and adaptation have been and will always be critical to the survival of healthcare organizations, familiarity with team-based quality improvement initiatives is an essential part of leaders' toolkits for optimizing the delivery of care.

## References

Aubry M, Richer M-C, Lavoie-Tremblay M, Cyr G. Pluralism in PMO performance: the case of a PMO dedicated to a major organizational transformation. Proj Manag J. 2011;42(6): 60–77.

Biron A, Vézina M, St-Hilaire C, Lavoie-Tremblay M, Richer M-C. Role of performance measurement in a major redevelopment project: the case of the McGill University Health Centre Transition Support Office. Healthc Q. 2012;15(1):34–40.

Chiocchio F, Rabbat F, Lebel P. Multi-level efficacy evidence of a combined interprofessional collaboration and project management training program for healthcare project teams. Proj Manag J. 2015;46(4):20–34.

Climo NW, et al. Effect of daily chlorhexidine bathing on hospital-acquired infection. N Engl J Med. 2013;368(6):533–42.

Graban M. Lean hospitals: improving quality, patient safety, and employee engagement. Boca Raton: CRC Press; 2012.

Graban M, Swartz JE. Healthcare kaizen Engaging front-line staff in sustainable continuous improvements. Boca Raton: CRC Press; 2012.

Hurt M, Thomas JL. Building value through sustainable project management offices. Proj Manag J. 2009;40(1):55–72.

Institute for Healthcare Improvement. Quality, Cost, and Value, Overview. 2017. Retrieved from http://www.ihi.org/Topics/QualityCostValue/Pages/Overview.aspx.

Jimmerson C. A3 problem solving for healthcare: a practical method for eliminating waste. New York: CRC Press; 2007.

Lavoie-Tremblay M, Richer M-C, Marchionni C, Cyr G, Biron AD, Aubry M, Bonneville-Roussy A, Vézina M. Implementation of evidence-based practices in the context of a redevelopment project in a Canadian Healthcare Organization. J Nurs Scholarsh. 2012;44(4):418–27.

Morris P. Reconstructing project management reprised: a knowledge perspective. Proj Manag J. 2013;44(5):6–23.

NHS Institute for Innovation and Improvement. Releasing time to care productive ward: executive leader's guide. Coventry: NHS Institute for Innovation and Improvement; 2008.

O'Grady, N.P. et al. Guidelines for the prevention of intravascular catheter-related infections. 2011. Retrieved from https://www.cdc.gov/hai/pdfs/bsi-guidelines-2011.pdf.

Overgaard PM. Get the keys to successful project management. Nurs Manag. 2015;41(6):53–4.

Policy Cell Ministry of Social Affairs and Public Health Belgium. Hervorming van het ziekenhuislandschap en de ziekenhuisfinanciering. 2017. Retrieved from http://www.inami.fgov.be/nl/professionals/verzorgingsinstellingen/ziekenhuizen/financiering/Paginas/default.aspx#.WTBcPLcrJD8.

Press Ganey Associates, Inc. Improve care quality, prevent adverse events with deep nursing quality insights. 2017. Retrieved from http://www.pressganey.com/solutions/clinical-quality/nursing-quality.

Project Management Institute. A guide to the project management body of knowledge (PMBOK® guide). 3rd ed. Amsterdam: Project Management Institute (PMI); 2004.

Reed JE, Card AJ. The problem with plan-do-study-act cycles. Q Saf. 2015;25(3):147–52.

Taylor MJ, McNicholas C, Nicolay C, Darzi A, Bell D, Reed JE. Systematic review of the application of the plan–do–study–act method to improve quality in healthcare. Q Saf. 2014;23(4):290–8.

# Reporting and Learning Systems for Patient Safety

**9**

Danny Van heusden and Peter Van Bogaert

**Abstract**

Safety in healthcare is arguably a constantly moving target. The field of patient safety has expanded and as a result, more types of harm are now preventable. Healthcare providers need to be able to achieve ever-evolving targets dealing with a seemingly infinite variability of safety issues. Therefore, they need to analyze situations and take appropriate actions that fit specific contexts and settings. Two systems related to learning systems for patient safety are highlighted in this chapter. Firstly, we examine registration, reporting, and learning systems for patient safety incidents and examine insights from the literature and practice regarding how reporting systems should be constructed. The various requirements of a learning system are discussed, including shifting from a centralized approach, where experts serve as intermediaries, to a decentralized unit-based approach, as well as a shift from recording/data gathering to learning. Subsequently, we discuss our experiences in organizing an incident learning system—including examples of successes and barriers we encountered in implementing a system based on findings from the literature translated to the context of the Antwerp University Hospital. Secondly, we discuss an approach for developing a learning culture using an internationally recognized nurse-sensitive patient outcomes benchmarking dataset embedded in a professional practice model to align quality and patient safety improvement efforts across all levels of

D. Van heusden (✉)
Nursing Department, Antwerp University Hospital, Edegem, Belgium

Nursing and Midwifery Sciences, Centre for Research and Innovation in Care (CRIC), Faculty of Medicine and Health Sciences, University of Antwerp, Antwerp, Belgium
e-mail: danny.van.heusden@uza.be

P. Van Bogaert
Nursing and Midwifery Sciences, Centre for Research and Innovation in Care (CRIC), Faculty of Medicine and Health Sciences, University of Antwerp, Antwerp, Belgium

© Springer International Publishing AG 2018
P. Van Bogaert, S. Clarke (eds.), *The Organizational Context of Nursing Practice*, https://doi.org/10.1007/978-3-319-71042-6_9

our hospital. The second strategy was part of our journey to nursing excellence as we worked toward Magnet hospital designation.

**Keywords**

Patient safety reporting system • Comprehensive unit-based safety program Learning organization • Unit-based improvements • Nurse-sensitive patient outcomes

## 9.1    Introduction

The well-known report from the Institute of Medicine (IOM) *To Err is Human* drew worldwide attention and created a sense of urgency around improving patient safety. Many recommendations and initiatives followed, along with a sharp increase in the number of safety-related research studies and publications (Mitchell et al. 2016; Stelfox et al. 2006). All these publications and initiatives had one common goal—reducing patient harm in healthcare. To date, there is still no agreement about proven methods for improving patient safety; furthermore, evidence that healthcare has been truly improved is scant (Mitchell et al. 2016). However, it is clear that there will never be exact solutions to the problems of patient safety. Vincent and Amalberti described safety in healthcare as *a constant moving target*. The perimeter of patient safety has expanded—it appears that more types of harm are now preventable (Vincent and Amalberti 2015). Healthcare providers need to be able to reach *moving targets* by addressing a seemingly infinite variety of safety issues. Therefore, we need to learn to analyze situations and adopt solutions appropriate to specific contexts and settings (Leistikow et al. 2017).

The World Alliance for Patient Safety of the World Health Organization (WHO) emphasized the importance of a valid reporting system to identify patient safety problems and provide data for organizational and system learning (Organization 2006). Also, the European Commission has suggested the use and implementation of reporting and learning systems in the European Union's member states. Although many European countries have used the WHO report as the basis for designing their systems, there are still important variations across the reporting systems in the different member states (European Commission 2014). Two learning systems for patient safety are highlighted in this chapter. Firstly, we lay the focus on registration, reporting, and learning systems for incidents. Secondly, we discuss the follow-up for outcomes in the context of patient safety.

In terms of systems for learning from incidents, we examine insights from the literature and experiences in application in practice how such reporting systems should be constructed. The various requirements for such learning system are discussed. We discuss shifting from a centralized approach, mediated by experts, to a decentralized unit-based approach and shifting from an emphasis on registration to emphasizing learning. Subsequently, we will focus more on the organization of an incident learning system and potential barriers, examples, and recommendations.

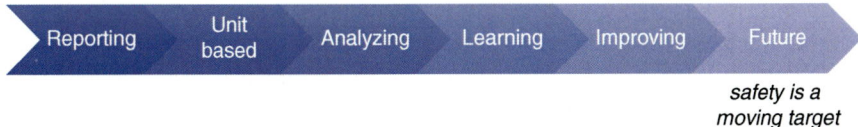

Reporting | Unit based | Analyzing | Learning | Improving | Future

*safety is a moving target*

**Fig. 9.1** Model from pure registration system toward a future learning system

These findings are based on scientific literature translated for the contexts and the experiences of Antwerp University Hospital (UZA) (Fig. 9.1).

## 9.2 Building a Patient Safety Reporting and Learning System: Experiences and Lessons Learned

### 9.2.1 Preliminary Phase: Paper-Based Patient Safety Reporting System

For more than 20 years, the patient care department in Antwerp University Hospital (UZA) has tracked written incident reports. Responses to these reports have been on an ad hoc basis most of the time, and a structured follow-up and feedback had never been developed. In 2005, as a result of an increasing number of reports (2004 = 101, 2005 = 216), a strategy was developed to structure the incident reporting system with the following objectives: (a) encouraging incident reporting to learn about the type of incidents, the circumstances, and the influencing factors; (b) organizing feedback to nursing units and services; and (c) taking intentional steps to prevent incidents.

Following the rewriting of procedures around incident reports, an awareness campaign was initiated among the nurse managers and clinical nurses with the slogan, *"From incident reports to safety reports."* The shift involved a change from recording incidents to a culture of safe patient care. This initiative was part of a broader strategy for safe patient care in the hospital. Reporting on a blame-free basis was encouraged at all levels within the patient care department.

Blame-free reporting is the cornerstone of a systems approach to incidents. Not punishing employees for reporting incidents is an essential component of an organizational culture for effective incident reporting. However, in one study, 78% of nursing students were concerned that they would face disciplinary action if they made a serious error; numerous other studies have illustrated that nurses see fear of punishment as a barrier for reporting incidents (Institute 2017; Polisena et al. 2015; Rabøl et al. 2017; Usher et al. 2017; Vrbnjak et al. 2016). It is known that physicians generally do not use voluntary incident reporting systems. In an auditing study of a Scottish adult intensive care unit, the medical staff submitted only ten percent of the almost 700 reported incidents (Network 2017; Evans et al. 2006; Johnson 2003). International patient safety experts have concluded that there is a lack of medical engagement in these processes that often leads to reporting bias and skewed data (Mitchell et al. 2016). Therefore, in our hospital, nurse leaders, nurse managers, and clinical nurses were urged to involve the medical staff of their units in reporting.

We decided not to make major changes to the structure of the original paper reporting form, which was comprised of several different parts. After identifiers, the core of the report asks for a description of the incident and its consequences. All items in these safety incident reports were entered into a central database and coded for analysis. In addition, space was provided for comments and a coding as to how the form is filled in. Each incident report received a unique identifier in the database and on the form so that the information was easily available. Analyses were based on classification codes. Five nurse leaders each performed the coding of the incidents from their units and services. Classification systems need to be practical and flexible (Macrae 2016). Based on the literature, a coding system called the UZA-Taxonomy was developed that classified the incident (1), the cause (2), the extent of harm (3), and the influencing factors (4).

### 9.2.2   UZA Reports and Learns: An Electronic Patient Safety Reporting and Learning System

A new *UZA Reports and Learns* reporting system for incidents and near-misses was initiated in October 2013, supported by software from The Patient Safety Company (TPSC). When reports are received, it is important that each incident or near-miss be evaluated in terms of (a) circumstances, (b) harm or potential harm, and (c) likelihood of recurrence. After this assessment, a decision can be made to carry out a thorough analysis to better determine the causes and to develop a corrective plan. We consider that unawareness of weaknesses and latent shortcomings in care— which occur relatively frequently along with limited patient harm—increase the risk of preventable adverse events (Box 9.1).

---

**Box 9.1 Pillars of UZA Reports and Learns**
- Systematic reports can be made by any healthcare provider and/or other employees of the hospital, regardless of function in the organization or position within the hierarchy, and on a blame-free basis.
- Reporting of near-misses as well as errors and incidents, meaning reporting of all situations that may potentially or practically endanger quality and safety of patient care.
- Learning is supported by thorough analyses conducted by a multidisciplinary team of experts (at the hospital level or unit level), intended to generate well-thought-out improvement plans that have a real effective impact on structures and processes of care.

---

*UZA Reports and Learns* is aimed at learning from incidents and near-misses— in other words, learning from both serious incidents and latent weaknesses and shortcomings in care. To achieve this goal, it was decided that ownership of *UZA Reports and Learns* should be at the unit level (nursing departments, medical-technical services, etc.) rather than at higher organizational levels. Our experiences with the neonatology and hematology unit, where there have been established traditions of evaluating each reported incident and generating action plans by members of multiple disciplines, support us in this vision. The neonatology unit manages a very vulnerable group of patients where care-related harm is rarely trivial. In hematology, learning from reports addresses the quality monitoring criteria required by organizations such as Joint Accreditation Committee of the ISCT and the EBMT (JACIE) for special accreditations of bone marrow transplant services (Samson et al. 2007). It has been reported that some units and specialties in the same organization are more involved and focused on reporting and learning from incident reports and patient safety than others, suggesting a need for a unit-based approach and an organizational-wide model (Yoo and Kim 2017).

### 9.2.2.1 Learning

The first shift we made was from emphasizing reporting alone to emphasize learning from incidents, which is challenging because the available information is often incomplete. Furthermore, is it not always clear which incidents are preventable or which solutions will optimally address their causes (Anderson and Kodate 2015). Many organizations struggle to reduce incident numbers, which could be partially attributable to a failure to learn from incidents. By detecting and reflecting on adverse event, by treating them as opportunities for growth, and by putting these lessons into practice, future incidents can be avoided (Drupsteen et al. 2013; Drupsteen and Guldenmund 2014). Drupsteen et al. (2013) developed a model of the process of learning from incidents that can be used to guide actions. The main stages of this model are (a) investigating and analyzing incidents, (b) planning interventions, (c) intervening, and (d) evaluating interventions (Drupsteen et al. 2013).

*UZA Reports and Learns* consists of three steps: reporting, analyzing, and learning. The final step, learning, is a part of a bigger framework integrated in our hospital—the Lean approach, where we strive in a continuous culture of improving. Based on the analysis of an incident, evaluation of causes leads to a classification into one of five categories. These categories provide direction to any interventions likely to be helpful and prevent recurrent. They are:

(a) Technical issues
(b) Training and education (human and/or organizational if knowledge is not systematically present)
(c) Inconsistence processes
(d) Patient characteristics that have rendered the patient vulnerable in ways that may or may not have been
(e) External causes beyond the control of the organization

Identifying multiple causes is common, and in such cases an approach that considers multiple causes is then necessary. Regarding the action plans, it is also important to determine what can be dealt with within the service and if when involvement of others (organization-wide departments or services, management etc.) is necessary. It is important to avoid draconian and/or unrealistic measures. Careful thought about the feasibility and the expected impact of measures is necessary.

### 9.2.2.2 Unit-Level

This learning process that must occur at the unit level is very important. Learning at the unit level and involving clinical nurses can reduce resistance. Furthermore, it can improve top-down and bottom-up information flow. Finally, it can also promote a more prompt response to errors (Drach-Zahavy et al. 2014). Clinicians working together at the unit level in peer communities are able to harness peer learning strategies and professional motivation (Pronovost et al. 2016). It has been demonstrated that positive attitudes toward incident reporting can increase when there is active communication and greater participation of direct care nurses in decision-making (Yoo and Kim 2017).

The Comprehensive Unit-Based Safety Program (CUSP) toolkit was developed by teams at the Johns Hopkins Quality and Safety Research Group with funding by the US Agency for Healthcare Research and Quality (AHRQ). The advantage of the CUSP approach is that it supports and can be used in conjunction with a range of quality and safety improvement models (AHRQ 2017) (Box 9.2). This approach has been successfully used to reduce CLABSI rates (Miller et al. 2016; Pronovost et al. 2016).

---

**Box 9.2 The CUSP Toolkit's Modules Include**
- Learn About CUSP
- Assemble the Team
- Engage the Senior Executive
- Understand the Science of Safety
- Identify Defects Through Sense-making
- Implement Teamwork and Communication
- Apply CUSP

---

CUSP (AHRQ 2017) was specifically designed to improve hospital culture. It is perhaps the only strategy that has been demonstrated empirically to improve teamwork and safety culture on a large scale (Wick et al. 2012). Miller et al. (2016) found that CUSP can also be used as a strategy to improve culture and learn from mistakes. It is flexible enough that units can focus on risks they perceive as important, taking unit context into account (Miller et al. 2016). Thus, we were successful in using CUSP as a foundation for *UZA Reports and Learns*. Unlike earlier, the focus is now on unit-based examination and resolutions instead of a centralized approach mediated by experts.

The follow-up of incidents/events and near-misses is the responsibility of the nurse manager and the unit's "nurse champion" for patient safety and infection

**Table 9.1** Modes of feedback

| Mode | Type |
| --- | --- |
| Bounce back | Information to the reporter |
| Rapid response | Action within local work systems |
| Raise risk awareness | Information to all frontline personnel |
| Inform staff of actions taken | Information to the reporter and wider community of reporters |
| Improve work systems safety | Action within local work systems |

Benn et al. (2009)

prevention and control, as well as the physician in charge of a service or physician team(s) practicing on the unit. Positioning responsibility at the unit level is based on the view that healthcare providers know local processes best; unit-level staff are provided with support to continuously improve their care processes. Thus, teams at the unit level are responsible for generating feedback about the handling of the incidents. Incident reports are handled at unit level and the resulting data are verified for completeness. Effective feedback from incident reports is essential if organizations want to learn from failures in delivering care. Research regarding the forms in which feedback is best delivered is limited. Much of the knowledge has come from high reliability organizations within high-risk industries. Benn et al. (2009) presented five modes of feedback that can be used for incident reporting (Table 9.1).

Unit-level teams are aware of and entrusted to respect a *no blame culture* throughout the process. Another task of the team is conducting analyses of serious incidents and retrospective analyses of frequently recurring incidents or recurring incidents of particular importance. Involving the frontline staff in analysis and learning from incidents provides an opportunity to engage team members in a dialogue with patient safety representatives (Moeller et al. 2016). The analysis of incidents launches improvement processes.

### 9.2.2.3 Multidisciplinary Expert Team

A multidisciplinary expert team (or MET) was established under the guidance of the hospital's medical director. This team is composed of physicians, nurses, pharmacist, clinical laboratory worker, and quality employee. Everyone with sufficient clinical experience is potentially allowed to oversee *UZA Reports and Learns* in the form of the monthly follow-up of the number and type of reports and the support and monitoring of the reporting and learning process. Therefore, the MET can always provide advice and suggest various reporting, analysis, and improvement services. Serious incidents with injury to the patient (those that lead to serious complications or death) are always emotional experiences for all concerned, including physicians, nurses, other caregivers and of course, not least of all patients and their families. *UZA Reports and Learns* offers the ability to analyze such incidents (often referred to as sentinel events) thoroughly and to draw appropriate lessons from them. The MET can provide significant support for the analysis process in order to block emotions and an instinct to assign blame that can interfere with learning real lessons. Learning from latent defects is also important in estimating and reducing potentially avoidable risks in care processes. Here, the MET can also provide advice and support. The main tasks of the MET are monitoring and supporting the reporting process for anonymous follow-up at the hospital level. This support is meant for further analyses, evaluations, improvement processes, and prospective analyses of care processes (HFMEA). Lastly, the MET monitors the overall incident reporting system and makes recommendations for change to different stakeholders to enhance the value of the system (Pham et al. 2013).

### 9.2.2.4 Training

Training about the incident reporting system and how to use it must be tailored for the different healthcare disciplines and functions (Ontario 2017). Since October 2013, *UZA Reports and Learns* has been introduced to the yearly nursing department educational training program called 8H4every1 and in workshops. Nurse managers and nurse champions attended workshops to become acquainted with the software package and the process. This was organized through five training sessions and five return days during the first semester of 2014. Physicians were invited to one of five training sessions during the first semester 2014.

### 9.2.3   Barriers for Incident Reporting Systems

*To report or not to report?—That is the question.*

Sometimes incident report systems are frustrating to use, and as a result, often users decide not to report or to report only those incidents they deem most important (Drupsteen and Hasle 2014; Hewitt and Chreim 2015; Macrae 2016; Shojania 2008). Furthermore, there are also biases in reporting. This is unavoidable, because an incident report is an individual's view of a complex clinical situation. For research purposes and/or as measurements, the heavy influence of personal interpretation can be a weakness, but it can also be a strength for actual safety management (Macrae 2016). That clinical nurses and other healthcare workers do not report some incidents does not mean that they do not care about safety, because we know that they systematically fix imperfections, near-incidents, and individual patient safety problems. Hewitt and Chreim (2015) have described the choice healthcare workers make: "fix and forget" vs. "fix and report." It is vital to ensure that fixing and forgetting do not become the norm (Hewitt and Chreim 2015). Other reasons for low reporting by staff include perceptions (or realities) of a blame culture, fear of disciplinary action, status differences (hierarchy and power distance), lack of feedback mechanisms, bureaucratic and nonuser-friendly reporting systems, heavy work pressure and lack of time, overlap with other systems, and a lack of intrinsic motivation on the part of clinical staff (Polisena et al. 2015; Veiligheidsprogramma 2009; Vrbnjak et al. 2016).

Failure to see actions as a result of one's reports can have strong negative influences on subsequent reporting. A vicious circle can be set up where eventually frontline staff do not take the time to report any incidents at all and much useful data

**Table 9.2** Reports of incidents and near-misses, Antwerp University Hospital, by year

| Year | 2014 | 2015 | 2016 | 2017[a] |
|---|---|---|---|---|
| Near-misses | 468 | 296 | 279 | *248* |
| Incident | 1038 | 1063 | 1036 | *1102* |
| % near-misses | 31% | 21% | 21% | *17%* |

[a]Data from 2017 is based reports up to September 2017 and prorated to a yearly rate

is missed by the learning system (Shojania 2008). It is obvious that reporting incidents alone is insufficient to improve safety; through analysis, improvement and learnings must occur, with everyone keeping in mind the end goal of preventing incidents in the future. In *UZA Reports and Learns*, we have found that the ratio of near-misses to incidents decreased from 31% in 2014 to 18% in 2017 (see Table 9.2). In learning organizations, there is a strong focus on proactive culture regarding incident reporting. This manifests itself by higher ratios of reports of near-incidents versus incidents. Higher ratio for toward incidents versus near-incidents may indicate a more reactive culture of incident reporting. These results show that our process to improve patient safety through UZA Reports and Learns is vulnerable and needs to be understood and improved as a learning process.

High rates of incident reporting are an attribute of high reliability organizations (HRO) or organizations that have a constant focus on safety culture (Macrae 2016). Typically, a shift is seen in HROs over time from focusing on incidents to attention to hazards and conditions that create safety problems. A common problem with incident reporting systems is that there is the absence of a clear denominator. For instance, we may know how many patients are falling and experiencing an injury but we do not know how many patients are at risk for falls (Shojania 2008). An incident reporting system can promote to a learning system when it can focus on learning. The incident reports have a goal as incident classification a triage. The focus for learning is the inquiry, a trigger for further investigation. Trying to put all the effort in improving the incident data misses this purpose. To improve and to learn from incidents lies in investigating them and not in the reports themselves. But only by analyzing incidents we can't learn (Macrae 2016). The use of incident reporting systems for measuring patient safety or the performance of safety systems should be avoided, as should attempts to use reporting systems to identify unsafe hospitals or healthcare professionals or the incidence of harm in a health system (Macrae 2016; Howell et al. 2017a; Pham et al. 2013).

### 9.2.4 Characteristics of Learning Systems for Incidents

These conditions are based approach of the Dutch "Safety Management System—Safety program," a project supported by the national Ministry of Health, Wellbeing and Sports. The conditions of a learning system for incidents are (1) a safe environment for reporting incidents, (2) training, (3) resources (time and budget), and (4) safety culture (Veiligheidsprogramma 2009). When these conditions are not present, they may act as barriers.

Those who report incidents need a certain degree of protection, and systems should not be used in a punitive way (Safety 2016; Ontario 2017; Rabøl et al. 2017). The incident reporting system and the systems or procedures for disciplining individual employees should be separated. Information from the reporting system should never be provided to third parties, unless law or court order requires it of the institution. Training is necessary in order to analyze the reports in a manner that accurately identifies root causes of an incident. Sufficient resources in terms of time and budget are necessary for a learning system, especially in terms of the teams at the unit level who need time for training and time to investigate and analyze information and formulate action plans for improvement. Experience teaches us that the number of incident reports tends to increase at least initially upon the implementation of a learning system (Kaplan and Fastman 2003). Our report rate increased exponentially from 101 reports in 2004 to 1350 reports in 2017. On the other hand, it is essential that a budget be provided to finance the necessary staff and training costs. The possibility that a budget could be required for the improvement measures that emerge from analyses of incidents should be considered (Pham et al. 2013).

Within the hospital and nursing department, certain standards and values govern patient safety.

Patient safety culture (norms, values, perceptions, and patient safety behaviors taken together) plays an important role in reporting incidents, dealing with causes, and working stakeholders. In a blame-free culture, incidents can be reported freely, without fear of being unfairly penalized, to maximize potential learning from incidents (Kaplan and Fastman 2003).

### 9.2.5    Recommendations for Incident Reporting Systems

Based on our empirical evidence and the scientific literature, we offer a number of

> **Box 9.3 Three Pillars of UZA Reports and Learns**
> - Reporting: easy, with low effort, reflecting safety culture, unit-based
> - Analyzing: use of a simple coding system, trained staff; preferably at the unit level
> - Learning: sufficient feedback; dissemination of lessons learned

key recommendations. We have classified them using the three pillars of *UZA Reports and Learns* (Box 9.3).

Data input for clinical staff should be easy and demand minimal effort from staff (preferably keeping reporting time to 2 min) by avoiding asking too many questions (Institute 2017; Ontario 2017; Pham et al. 2013; Rabøl et al. 2017). Reporting systems may not be used in a punitive way. It must be safe for staff to report voluntary and feel supported. Furthermore, other potential organizational barriers to reporting should be reduced. When all of these elements are in place, an improvement in patient safety culture results (Institute 2017; Safety 2016; Ontario 2017; Pham et al. 2013). Unit-based reporting system provides healthcare workers with specific information for their own practice and therefore makes it easier to design and prioritize improvement action plans (Wagner et al. 2016).

A simple safety classification system that can be coded by clinicians and helps quickly identify relevant improvements in clinical practice is recommended (Williams et al. 2016). Well-trained people should conduct incident analyses in a timely manner using standardized techniques (Ontario 2017; Howell et al. 2017a). Involving frontline staff at the unit level in analysis provides an opportunity to engage them and to stimulate learning from incidents (Moeller et al. 2016). Healthcare workers can lose a sense of ownership of incidents, if report analyses are not presented and applied at the local level (Safety 2016). However, handling of sentinel (severe and rare) events should be done at the organization level or even at the national level (Howell et al. 2017b). Meaningful feedback for those reporting and to those who are disseminating and implementing recommendations is an imperative. This can be accomplished through communication strategies such as empathy, communication on multiple channels, timely feedback to reporters and managers, and sharing reports on incidents with staff. It is critically important for staff to understand the value of incident reporting system (Institute 2017; Ontario 2017; Howell et al. 2017a; Macrae 2016; Pham et al. 2013; Rabøl et al. 2017). The dissemination of lessons learned is crucial, not only to clinical staff but sometimes also with patient and families, communities, and the public. Communication must be tailored to the needs of the specific audience (Institute 2017; Ontario 2017). Sharing of information can happen across units or across organizations (Pham et al. 2013; Rabøl et al. 2017). The end goal is empowering staff to take responsibility for improving safety in their local workplaces. It is important to avoid draconian and/or unrealistic measures (Benn et al. 2009).

### 9.2.6 UZA Reports and Learns: What It Is and What Is Not

To conclude we would like to summarize what UZA Reports and Learns is and is not (see Table 9.3).

**Table 9.3** UZA Reports and Learns: what it is and what is not

| UZA Reports and Learns is not | UZA Reports and Learns is |
| --- | --- |
| A witch-hunt to discover clinician's/workers mistakes | A process for monitoring and improving quality and safety of patient care |
| A system for deciding upon guilty parties during handling and analysis of incidents | Learning from incidents and near-misses, looking beyond the involvement and responsibility of healthcare providers |
| A system to resolve conflicts between healthcare providers | Initiating targeted and meaningful improvement actions |

### 9.2.7 Lessons Learned

#### 9.2.7.1 Top-Down Versus Bottom-Up Approaches

From the outset, it was our strategy to work with outcomes, improvement projects, and learning systems at the unit level. This "bottom-up" approach ensured involvement of clinical nurses. As reported in the literature, involvement at the unit level is crucial (Van Bogaert et al. 2014). Due to conflicting goals, a separate implementation of an international accreditation process used a "top-down" approach by necessity. Nurses were confused and did not see the coherence between the two approaches across concurrent initiatives such as Productive Ward, JCI accreditation, and Magnet Recognition. Experts have noted that effective approaches for reducing preventable harm are to align and synergize policy efforts around common goals and measures (Pronovost et al. 2016). Likewise, it has been noted that accreditation programs can distract healthcare team from their primary clinical goals (Brubakk et al. 2015), especially when these programs are not aligned with unit-level strategy and do not engage frontline staff.

#### 9.2.7.2 From Incidents to Improve Outcomes

Incident reporting systems may perform poorly in identifying patient safety incidents, especially when patient harm occurs (Sari et al. 2007). It is therefore unlikely that incident reporting alone will meet the expectations of identifying the causes of human error (Johnson 2003) and thus it is imperative to expand strategies and look to other sources of data to capture data about incidents. These can include, as examples, mortality and morbidity rounds, analysis of administrative data, chart reviews, electronic medical record, malpractice claim analysis, observation of patient care, executive walk-arounds, and clinical surveillance (Shojania 2008; Thomas and Petersen 2003). Another way to reinforce quality improvement projects is the policy to evaluate and learn as a common and good practice at the patient level.

*It is not possible to learn without measuring, but it is possible—and very wasteful—to measure without learning (Donald Berwick).*

## 9.3 Focus on Nursing Excellence

For decades, the American Nurses Association (ANA) has promoted quality in nursing care and nurse work environments as a means of increasing patient safety (Lewis 2014). The Magnet Recognition Program of the American Nurses Credentialing Center (ANCC) is considered as the highest recognition for nursing excellence in the world. Only 8% of all American hospitals have achieved Magnet designation (Gonzalez et al. 2015). The principles used in the Magnet model are supported by research and provide guidance and suggest strategies for nurse leaders creating work environments conducive to nurse satisfaction and quality patient care (Van Bogaert et al. 2014).

Nurse-sensitive measures are defined as *processes and outcomes that are affected, provided, and/or influenced by nursing personnel, but for which nursing is not exclusively responsible* (Clarke and Donaldson 2008). Since 2012, four specific nurse-sensitive patient outcomes are systematically followed on every unit in out hospital: hospital-acquired pressure ulcers grade 2 or higher (HAPU2+), injury falls, catheter-associated urinary tract infections (CAUTI), and catheter-associated bloodstream infections (CLABSI). Unit-based international benchmarks are available for these measures and are used to inform learning systems as evidence of use of one of the Magnet principles.

## 9.3.1 Use of Benchmarking

Comparing outcomes with peer organizations drives staff to create better conditions and achieve better results for their patients (Luquire and Strong 2011). In the context of meeting data requirements for the Magnet Recognition Program®, we adopted the National Database of Nursing Quality Indicators® (NDNQI®) at our hospital. This database collects nurse-sensitive outcome data on a quarterly basis from more than 2000 hospitals and health systems worldwide, mainly in the USA. The NDNQI also generates reports of these outcomes on a quarterly base that are available at both the organizational and unit levels. We load this information into our hospital business intelligence center for action planning and interventions at the unit level. Reports are also provided to nursing leaders and units for their units and in aggregated form to support nurses in their pursuit of exemplary professional practice.

## 9.3.2 Development of a Professional Practice Model to Achieve Goal Alignment

The professional practice model describes how nurses and their colleagues (patient care assistants, unit clerks, etc.) at the Antwerp University Hospital carry out their work: how they communicate and work together and develop and improve professionalism and quality. It highlights the deeper (what might be called cultural) values that are at the heart of our mission and vision and how we implement them in practice. Our professional practice model is an identity of UZA nurses and UZA staff in-patient care. Two elements are crucial: (a) excellent teams as a basic condition for obtaining good outcomes for the patient and (b) putting patients at the center, where key values for the patient are also preconditions for high team functioning. Clinical nurses developed the professional practice model in workshops and the model was discussed and agreed to in open

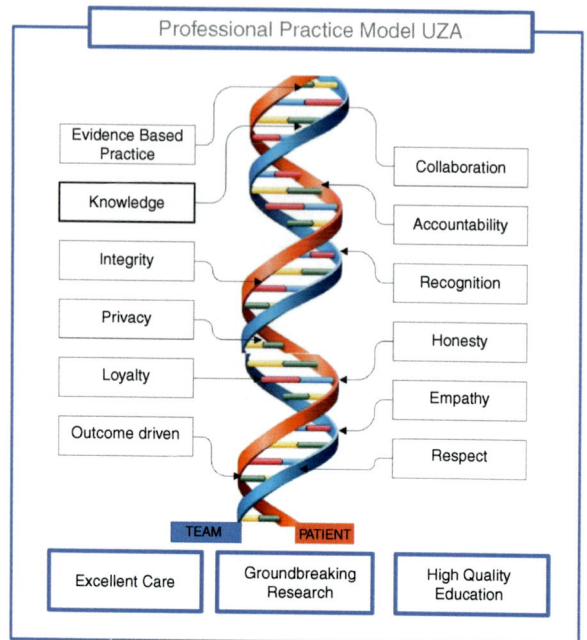

**Fig. 9.2** Professional practice model UZA

sessions. In this model, pictorially depicted as a strand of DNA, 12 competencies are represented (Fig. 9.2).

The rationale for pursuing the main components of the Magnet® hospital model was on the one hand to attract and retain nurses and, on the other hand, to improve results (value) for the patient, including the demonstration of patient outcomes through benchmarking. Because these elements were key to the hospital's strategy, the nursing department's and the hospital's goals were well-aligned.

### 9.3.3    An Example of Improving Outcomes

Staff on units participating in the Productive Ward (Lean) program are instructed to follow outcomes and take improvement actions at the unit level. In addition, the professional practice model at Antwerp University Hospital is based on clinical evidence and adoption of best practices with a continuous focus on quality and awareness of patient safety. Falls with injury (per 1000 patient days) are one of the main nurse-sensitive clinical indicators monitored continuously at Antwerp University Hospital. All healthcare workers and employees involved with patients are informed about the reporting program and have the opportunity to report falls with injury to *UZA Reports and Learns*. A team of experts evaluates the reports and set goals for preventing falls with injury across the hospital and supports units in their efforts to improve practice in this area. The team of experts consists of a

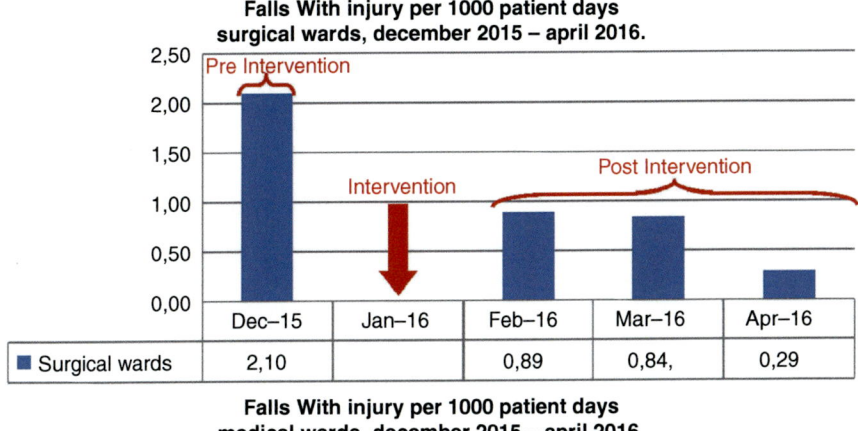

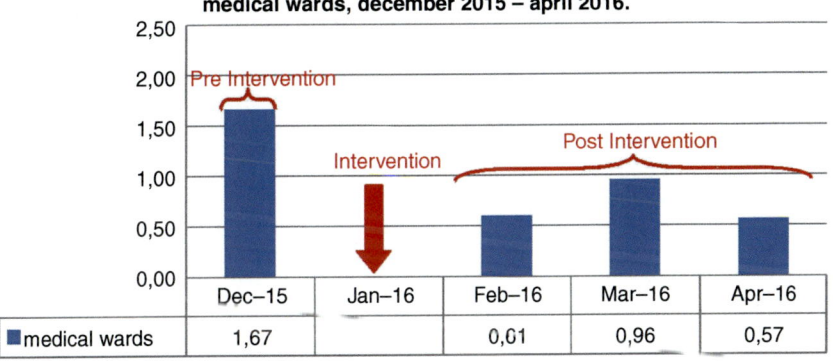

**Fig. 9.3** Falls with injury in surgical and medical wards

clinical nurse and a nurse leader whose main goal has been to reduce fall rates on surgical and medical wards. On surgical wards, monthly falls with injury in February to April 2016 decreased to 0.89, 0.84, and 0.29 per 1000 patient days, respectively, in comparison with 1.67 per 1000 patient days in December 2015. On medical wards, monthly falls with injury in February to April 2016 decreased to 0.61, 0.96, and 0.57 per 1000 patient days in comparison with 1.67 per 1000 patient days in December 2015 (Fig. 9.3).

**Conclusion**

Creating a learning culture across all organizational levels in the hospital is an essential cornerstone in the organizational context of nursing practice and improves practices and patient outcomes. Patient safety reporting systems need to be part of learning systems embedded and supported in hospital governance and policy, but since actions must occur at the unit level and efforts must be interprofessional, the focus of supportive efforts must be both unit level and interprofessional. Tracking incidents as well as monitoring and evaluating relevant outcomes is key to making improvement of care routine and continuous.

# References

AHRQ. CUSP toolkit. 2017.

Anderson JE, Kodate N. Learning from patient safety incidents in incident review meetings: organisational factors and indicators of analytic process effectiveness. Saf Sci. 2015;80:105–14.

Benn J, et al. Feedback from incident reporting: information and action to improve patient safety. Qual Saf Health Care. 2009;18:11–21.

Brubakk K, et al. A systematic review of hospital accreditation; the challenges of measuring complex intervention effects. BMC Health Serv Res. 2015;15:280.

Canadian Patient Safety Institute. Reporting and learning systems. 2017. http://www.patientsafetyinstitute.ca/en/toolsResources/PatientSafetyIncidentManagementToolkit/PatientSafetyManagement/pages/reporting-and-learning-systems.aspx#

Clarke SP, Donaldson NE. Nurse staffing and patient care quality and safety. In: Hughes RG, editor. Patient safety and quality: an evidence-based handbook for nurses. Rockville: Agency for Healthcare Research and Quality; 2008.

Danish Society for Patient Safety. Optimisation of the Danish incident reporting system. 2016. https://patientsikkerhed.dk/content/uploads/2016/09/optimisationofthedanishincidentreportingsystem.pdf

Drach-Zahavy A, et al. How do we learn from errors? A prospective study of the link between the ward's learning practices and medication administration errors. Int J Nurs Stud. 2014;51:448–57.

Drupsteen L, Guldenmund FW. What is learning? A review of the safety literature to define learning from incidents, accidents and disasters: a review about learning from incidents, accidents and disasters. J Contingencies Crisis Man. 2014;22:81–96.

Drupsteen L, Hasle P. Why do organizations not learn from incidents? Bottlenecks, causes and conditions for a failure to effectively learn. Accid Anal Prev. 2014;72:351–8.

Drupsteen L, Groeneweg J, Zwetsloot GI. Critical steps in learning from incidents: using learning potential in the process from reporting an incident to accident prevention. Int J Occup Saf Ergon. 2013;19:63–77.

European Commission. Key findings and recommendations on reporting and learning systems for patient safety incidents across Europe. Brussels: European Commission, Patient Safety and Quality of Care Working Group; 2014.

Evans SM, et al. Attitudes and barriers to incident reporting: a collaborative hospital study. Qual Saf Health Care. 2006;15:39–43.

Forward Programme. World alliance for patient safety. 2006–2007.

Gonzalez JF, et al. Impact of magnet culture in maintaining quality outcomes during periods of organizational transition. J Nurs Care Qual. 2015;30:323–30.

Hewitt TA, Chreim S. Fix and forget or fix and report: a qualitative study of tensions at the front line of incident reporting. BMJ Qual Saf. 2015;24:303–10.

Howell AM, et al. International recommendations for national patient safety incident reporting systems: an expert Delphi consensus-building process. BMJ Qual Saf. 2017a;26:150–63.

Howell AM, et al. Incident reporting: rare incidents may benefit from national problem solving. BMJ Qual Saf. 2017b;26:517.

Johnson CW. How will we get the data and what will we do with it then? Issues in the reporting of adverse healthcare events. Qual Saf Health Care. 2003;12(Suppl 2):ii64–7.

Kaplan HS, Fastman BR. Organization of event reporting data for sense making and system improvement. Qual Saf Health Care. 2003;12(Suppl 2):ii68–72.

Key findings and recommendations on Reporting and learning systems for patient safety incidents across Europe. 2014.

Leistikow I, et al. Learning from incidents in healthcare: the journey, not the arrival, matters. BMJ Qual Saf. 2017;26:252–6.

Lewis L. Magnet supporting patient safety. J Nurs Adm. 2014;44:S1–2.

Luquire R, Strong M. Empirical outcomes. In: Drenkard K, Wolf GA, Morgan SH, editors. Magnet : the next generation : nurses making the difference. Silver Spring: American Nurses Credentialing Center; 2011. p. 194.

Macrae C. The problem with incident reporting. BMJ Qual Saf. 2016;25:71–5.

Miller K, et al. Using the comprehensive unit-based safety program model for sustained reduction in hospital infections. Am J Infect Control. 2016;44:969–76.

Mitchell I, et al. Patient safety incident reporting: a qualitative study of thoughts and perceptions of experts 15 years after 'To Err is Human'. BMJ Qual Saf. 2016;25:92–9.

Moeller AD, Rasmussen K, Nielsen KJ. Learning and feedback from the Danish patient safety incident reporting system can be improved. Dan Med J. 2016;63:A5242.

Ontario HQ. Patient safety learning systems: a systematic review and qualitative synthesis. Ont Health Technol Assess Ser. 2017;17(3):1–23.

Optimisation of the Danish incident reporting system. 2016.

Pham JC, Girard T, Pronovost PJ. What to do with healthcare incident reporting systems. J Publ Health Res. 2013;2:e27.

Polisena J, et al. Factors that influence the recognition, reporting and resolution of incidents related to medical devices and other healthcare technologies: a systematic review. Syst Rev. 2015;4:37.

Pronovost PJ, et al. Fifteen years after To Err is Human: a success story to learn from. BMJ Qual Saf. 2016;25:396–9.

Rabøl LI, Gaardboe O, Hellebek A. Incident reporting must result in local action. BMJ Qual Saf. 2017;26:515–6.

Reporting Patient Safety Events. 2017.

Samson D, et al. Current status of JACIE accreditation in Europe: a special report from the Joint Accreditation Committee of the ISCT and the EBMT (JACIE). Bone Marrow Transplant. 2007;39:133–41.

Sari AB, et al. Sensitivity of routine system for reporting patient safety incidents in an NHS hospital: retrospective patient case note review. BMJ. 2007;334:79.

Shojania KG. The frustrating case of incident-reporting systems. Qual Saf Health Care. 2008;17:400–2.

Stelfox HT, et al. The "To Err is Human" report and the patient safety literature. Qual Saf Health Care. 2006;15:174–8.

Thomas EJ, Petersen LA. Measuring errors and adverse events in health care. J Gen Intern Med. 2003;18:61–7.

Usher K, et al. Self-reported confidence in patient safety knowledge among Australian undergraduate nursing students: a multi-site cross-sectional survey study. Int J Nurs Stud. 2017;71:89–96.

Van Bogaert P, et al. Nursing unit teams matter: Impact of unit-level nurse practice environment, nurse work characteristics, and burnout on nurse reported job outcomes, and quality of care, and patient adverse events–a cross-sectional survey. Int J Nurs Stud. 2014;51:1123–34.

Veiligheidsprogramma VMS. Praktijkgids Veilig Incidenten Melden. 2009.

Vincent C, Amalberti R. Safety in healthcare is a moving target. BMJ Qual Saf. 2015;24:539–40.

Vrbnjak D, et al. Barriers to reporting medication errors and near misses among nurses: a systematic review. Int J Nurs Stud. 2016;63:162–78.

Wagner C, et al. Unit-based incident reporting and root cause analysis: variation at three hospital unit types. BMJ Open. 2016;6:e011277.

Wick EC, et al. Implementation of a surgical comprehensive unit-based safety program to reduce surgical site infections. J Am Coll Surg. 2012;215:193–200.

Williams H, Cooper A, Carson-Stevens A. Opportunities for incident reporting. Response to: 'the problem with incident reporting' by Macrae et al. BMJ Qual Saf. 2016;25:133–4.

World Health Organization. Forward programme 2006–2007. Washington, DC: World Alliance for Patient Safety; 2006.

Yoo MS, Kim KJ. Exploring the influence of nurse work environment and patient safety culture on attitudes toward incident reporting. J Nurs Adm. 2017;47:434–40.

# Team Resource Management and Quality of Care

# 10

Erik Franck, Leen Roes, Sarah De Schepper,
and Olaf Timmermans

**Abstract**

In spite of being characterized by more highly educated professionals and more cutting-edge training facilities, equipment, and more research than ever, healthcare systems are still confronted with serious safety problems. In more than 70% of cases, serious and avoidable medical errors originate in so-called human factors or deficits in "nontechnical" skills—including communication, leadership, teamwork, situational awareness, and decision-making. A major reason behind slow improvement is the cumbersome, hierarchical organizational structure in many healthcare organizations that stand in the way of a safety culture, encourage a "blame culture," and foster communication errors. Resolving these issues requires a fundamental cultural shift from an individual to a group focus where safety is the shared responsibility of all individual healthcare workers and the entire management team working in a hospital (or other healthcare organization). Because safe care relies on the collective individual expertise of team members as well as teamwork, the interdisciplinary performance of care teams goes hand in hand with the

E. Franck (✉)
Nursing and Midwifery Sciences, Centre for Research and Innovation in Care (CRIC), Faculty of Medicine and Health Sciences, University of Antwerp, Antwerp, Belgium
Karel De Grote University College, Antwerp, Belgium
e-mail: erik.franck@uantwerpen.be

L. Roes • S. De Schepper
Centre of Expertise Psychological Wellbeing in Patient Care, Karel De Grote University College, Antwerp, Belgium

O. Timmermans
Nursing and Midwifery Sciences, Centre for Research and Innovation in Care (CRIC), Faculty of Medicine and Health Sciences, University of Antwerp, Antwerp, Belgium

HZ University College of Applied Sciences, Vlissingen, Netherlands

© Springer International Publishing AG 2018
P. Van Bogaert, S. Clarke (eds.), *The Organizational Context of Nursing Practice*,
https://doi.org/10.1007/978-3-319-71042-6_10

217

safety culture of the healthcare organization as a whole. Consequently, investments in multidisciplinary teams in teamwork training (i.e., Team Resource Management training) to build nontechnical skills are essential.

**Keywords**

Patient safety • Nontechnical skills • Culture • Human factors • Teamwork

## 10.1  Introduction

"Happy people deliver happy products" is an often used motto in workforce management. Whereas workforce management was traditionally aimed at staff scheduling to improve time management and efficiency, in the last decades, it has become more and more an institutional process that aims at maximizing performance levels and competency for an organization. This process includes *all* the activities needed to maintain a productive workforce—as measured in terms of the provision of excellent quality of patient care by that workforce. In 1999, the Institute of Medicine's seminal "To Err is Human" report (Kohn et al. 2000) about patient safety offered shocking content. Routine avoidable harm in American healthcare was quantified: between 44,000 and 98,000 hospitalized patients die each year as a result of preventable incidents and deemed very costly. Approximately 2.9–16.6% of all hospital admissions involve unintentional harm to patients and the financial costs of avoidable adverse events have been estimated at 1% of a hospital's total budget. Likewise healthcare was found not always to be effective or of particularly high technical quality (Chassin 2013).

Van Bogaert and colleagues demonstrated that organizational management has an impact on the healthcare workers' practice environment which in turn influences the quality of healthcare delivery (Van Bogaert et al. 2009). In their study, higher ratings by clinical nurses of nursing management at the unit level and of hospital management-organizational support were associated with more favorable outcomes in terms of nurse-assessed quality of care variables. But beyond sound supervision and leadership, multidisciplinary teamwork has also been identified as a defining factor for patient safety and quality of care across different areas of healthcare (Manser 2009). Yet, managing the multidisciplinary healthcare team is challenging.

Aviation is another high-risk industry where there has long been recognition of the importance of effective teamwork. Team mental models have been identified as a prerequisite for successful teamwork (Salas et al. 2005). Although sparse, research demonstrates that programs that build shared mental models to enhance teamwork and communication in multidisciplinary healthcare teams improve patient safety and employee satisfaction and enhance healthcare workers' perception of team-based awareness and safety awareness (McComb and Simpson 2014). In this chapter, we will elaborate on the concept and principles of this shared mental model based on scientific research supplemented with our experiences in training multidisciplinary teams in different healthcare settings using a Crew Resource Management training program.

## 10.2   Background

In the late 1970s, Cockpit Resource Management was developed by NASA (the US National Aeronautics and Space Administration), stimulated by the observation that although airplanes were technically optimized by engineering standards, too many plane crashes were due to failures of flight crews to make use of available strategies and resources. Research indicated that these types of occurrences shared many common features. Most often, the problems that flight crews encountered were associated with ineffective communication, inadequate leadership, poor group decision-making, and poor management. Until the 1970s, training programs for pilots were focused exclusively on acquisition of technical skills. This led to the development of a Cockpit Resource management training program in order to train cockpit crew members to effectively use all available resources, i.e., equipment, procedures, and people, in order to achieve safe and efficient flight operations. Originally aimed only at cockpit crew members, several commercial airline accidents due to serious failures in teamwork and communication between cabin crew members outside the cockpit and pilots led to extension of these principles to the entire flight crew and renaming the approach Crew Resource Management (CRM) training. Today, several airlines have gone as far as renaming the training yet again—calling it Company Resource Management training and thereby highlighting the importance of the entire company staff operating under the same principles.

CRM training emphasizes optimizing nontechnical skills in a complex and stressful high-risk environment to reduce avoidable errors (Flin and Maran 2015). Over the last 30 years, it has been implemented more and more widely. Due to its demonstrated benefits, it is now required in the training and ongoing education of pilots in Europe and the USA (Haerkens et al. 2012). Partly due to the introduction of CRM training, air travel—after elevators (in buildings)—has become the safest means of transportation on the planet and is now truly "high-reliability" sector.

## 10.3   Aviation Industry and Healthcare

Healthcare invites comparison with other high-risk industries. Although the nature of the services they provide is clearly different, aviation and healthcare share many common features. Both are dynamic, highly complex, high technological, intrinsically dangerous undertakings that employ highly educated professionals hired for complementary purposes that are expected to behave appropriately toward each other (Vandijck et al. 2015). The circumstances in which aviation crew members' works are largely comparable to those of medical teams. They are characterized by collaboration in small interdisciplinary teams, time pressure, variable workload and working hours, irreversibility of decisions, frequent intrusions of fatigue and stress, responsibility for people's lives, and the potential for intense media coverage of adverse events (Gaba 2010). In addition, both industries are equally susceptible to human error. This explains the focus of many leaders and researchers on translating aviation safety principles into healthcare to reduce avoidable errors (Haerkens et al. 2012). It might be argued that similarities with aviation are even more striking in intrinsically dynamic and risk-prone healthcare settings such as critical care units, labor and delivery suites, operating rooms, and emergency departments, which might explain the greater popularity of CRM approaches in those specialty areas. However CRM has also been applied to community, outpatient, and long-term settings.

Nearly 20 years ago, the US Institute of Medicine urged the healthcare industry to adopt structurally embedded strategies based on organizational learning perspectives and improvement techniques from aviation to deal with human error and anticipate problems (e.g., checklists, simulation training, notification systems, and standard operating procedures) because of the stakes involved (Vandijck et al. 2015). Portable (or transferrable) CRM skills from aviation can be translated from the cockpit to the multidisciplinary healthcare team (Powell and Hill 2006). By portable CRM skills, we mean skill sets observed in individuals who exhibit excellent performance in such a way that allows their team members to perform better.

## 10.4 Team Mental Models and Organizational Culture

High reliability organizations use a combination of people and systems to maintain an exceptionally safe workplace (Powell and Hill 2006). In healthcare organizations, professionals and workers usually function as a multidisciplinary team. However, in the traditional healthcare team, the nurses and physicians primarily mainly work independently guided by conventional role demarcations. Practitioners have little control over the complex environment of a healthcare setting, and care delivery is often fragmented (Cronin and Wright 2005).

In order to form high-reliability teams, an organization must train their individual members to perform in a well-coordinated manner across situations. High-reliability team members consistently show specific performance behaviors in complex situations under high stress (Wilson et al. 2005). One of the prerequisites of high-reliability teams is that members share the same mental sense or model of how the overall work is performed (Mohammed et al. 2000). Indeed, DeChurch and Mesmer-Magnus (2010) meta-analysis of research covering a wide range of types of teams revealed a significant effect of team mental models (shared across members) on team processes and team performance. Crew Resource Management as a (shared) mental model is about nonhierarchical teamwork, focusing on certain favorable behavioral markers related to communication, leadership, situational awareness, and decision-making (Flin et al. 2008). In healthcare, this means a shift toward a "group" rather than an "individual" culture.

In an individually oriented organizational safety culture, errors are sought out, and the individual or individuals responsible for them are identified and punished on an individual basis. However, in the long run, finger-pointing does not solve the problem, but rather cultivates a culture of "covering up." Improving patient safety requires organizational learning at the system level, meaning that changes in organizational routines must cut across departments, professions, and disciplines (Rivard et al. 2006). After all, an organization's culture is the key to professional practice within the systems designed by an organization (Boysen 2013). Leaders of all departments (medical and allied health) are expected to assume responsibility for creating a group culture of trust and empowerment among all employees in their organizations.

Punishing people without focus on the system rather than solving it only perpetuates the problem. From the perspective of a "what" (versus a "who") model of patient safety, investigations into incidents are analyzed, and where warranted, findings are acted upon. This is only possible in an organization where a shared mental model is adapted and every team member remains vigilant and mindful and maintains continuous surveillance.

A group culture where members feel obligated to report errors and learn from them is a "just culture" (Boysen 2013). Each team member has to take responsibility to do *what* is right, as opposed to a model where people spend effort in finding out *who* is to blame for safety problems after the fact. However, it is recognized that healthcare organization cannot afford to adopt a completely blame-free culture: some errors do warrant disciplinary actions. Finding the balance between blame-oriented and a blame-free culture is the goal of developing a just culture (Dekker 2008). In a just culture, an open and honest reporting climate is constantly complemented by a quality learning environment and culture. The organization has a responsibility toward its employees in the creation of systems and structures, whereas employees are responsible for the quality of their individual choices (Boysen 2013). The focus must be toward system design and individuals' behavioral choices rather than outcomes alone. Just culture means being transparent about responsibility, where checking "testable" assumptions and identifying "vulnerable" points in processes are key principles.

Shifting from an individual-hierarchical organizational culture to a more group-oriented, "bottom-up" culture is challenging but is a key component in improving patient safety and the quality of care in healthcare organizations. Transforming organizational culture is a slow and demanding process of changing the organization's values through changes in managers' leadership style (Mash et al. 2016). In order to successfully implement a just culture in a healthcare organization, the entire management team from medicine, allied health professions and support services must share common values. At the team level, nurse managers and physicians must be aware of the value of teamwork and role model positive team behaviors for others—or in other words, they must lead by example.

## 10.5  Human Factors in Healthcare

In aviation, error management and teamwork skills training programs, often called Crew Resource Management training, have become mandatory for flight crews worldwide since the late 1980s. They are focused on training nontechnical or human factors skills or the cognitive, social, and self-management skills that contribute to safe and efficient task performance (Flin et al. 2008, p. 1). Cognitive skills include situational awareness and decision-making; the social skills are communication, leadership, and teamwork supplemented with skills in relation to self-management of stress and fatigue, error management, and task management (Manser 2009; Nagpal et al. 2010). In healthcare, technical skills form the basis for quality of care, although they alone are insufficient to ensure safe patient care (Yule et al. 2006). Suboptimal nontechnical skills lead to (avoidable) errors, poorer patient outcomes, and exposures to medicolegal liability (Yule et al. 2008). While protocols and guidelines are available for many technical skills and processes (e.g., advanced cardiac life support), those relating to nontechnical skills are sparse. Interestingly, deficits in nontechnical skills, such as suboptimal interprofessional communication and decision-making or unclear leadership and task coordination, often appear to underlie deviations from technical guidelines (De Meester et al. 2013). Ultimately, breakdowns in interpersonal, cognitive, and personal resource skills remain key root causes of medical errors worldwide (Hull et al. 2012).

Most research on nontechnical skills in healthcare has been conducted in operating room settings. The highest rates of documented adverse events are related to surgery, with surgical patients involved in almost 60% of hospital-based adverse events and intensive care, emergency, and labor and delivery departments accounting for the second, third, and fourth most common sources of adverse events, respectively (Yule et al. 2008; de Vries et al. 2009). Patients in high-acuity settings often suffer from severe and complex conditions that require urgent decisions and interventions by multiple disciplines. Especially in these very dynamic healthcare settings, teams are confronted with frequently changing conditions, are sometimes assembled on an ad hoc basis, have dynamically changing team members, tend to draw on specialized professionals and workers who often work together for short periods of time, and frequently involve members contending with different and sometimes conflicting professional cultures (Manser 2009). In the literature, these are called "action teams." Clearly, it is crucial to identify nontechnical skills in these contexts to lower the risk of adverse events.

Weak teamwork makes all healthcare processes more susceptible to errors. This is due to a number of very specific features of healthcare. First, work pressure can be controlled only to a very limited extent in these departments, which often struggle with both staff shortages and surges in demand for services that can overwhelm staff (Hakimzada et al. 2008). Furthermore, care providers in these services treat multiple patients simultaneously, whereby they must constantly change their cognitive mindset and communication approach (Eisenberg et al. 2005). This produces potentially dangerous situations in which, for example, information can be lost. A third factor is the high degree of uncertainty about the accuracy of decisions and treatment. Often in these settings, the patient's medical history is not known, and so caregivers must make difficult decisions concerning treatment with incomplete information (Hakimzada et al. 2008; Richardson et al. 2003). In addition, the care in these settings is often performed under high time pressures, where workers have high workloads, which can place extreme demands on staff attention. Finally, even in high-acuity settings, most of the tasks that caregivers perform are routine, and the riskiest and most challenging scenarios arise only sporadically (Eisenberg et al. 2005).

For all of these reasons, effective teamwork is crucial, and we and others feel that *Team Resource Management* is a preferable term over Crew Resource Management in highlighting the shared responsibility of every team member in a multidisciplinary healthcare team for collaborating and acting from a shared mental model to ensure optimal deployment of all expertise and resources.

## 10.6   Team Resource Management

Team Resource Management (TRM) can be simplified into five core competencies of nontechnical skills that require specific and focused training: communication, leadership, situational awareness, decision-making, and teamwork. We review each briefly.

### 10.6.1 Communication

Poor communication can lead to serious adverse events, especially in critical care settings. One can imagine that in an intensive care unit, emergency department, or operating room, breakdowns in communication can lead to catastrophic harm to patients and even result in patient deaths. Examining data from mandatory root cause analyses of adverse events in the facilities they accredit, The Joint Commission (formerly the Joint Commission on Accreditation of Healthcare Organizations) revealed that in over 60% of sentinel events, communication failure was the primary root cause identified (Joint Commission International 2014). Because communication failures are one of the primary causes of adverse events in healthcare, it is safe to assume that clear, complete communication is the basis for all other nontechnical skills. Effective professional communication conveys information, clarifies responsibilities, and is the most effective way to achieve crucial goals in moments of crisis. In the absence of sound communication, the risk of error increases tenfold due to incomplete shared mental models and/or the emergence of conditions where not all team members feel "safe" raising safety concerns (Leonard et al. 2004). In high-risk environments, high-quality exchanges of information are imperative but are constantly challenged by seemingly endless distractors (such as nonverbal behaviors, verbal cues lost under surgical masks, noise, features of tools and technology, high workloads, cell phones and pagers, and large and constantly changing members of team). The end result is possible miscommunication that can impact performance of individual team members and might result in adverse consequences for both the team and the patient.

Communication failures can also be traced back to historical and contextual factors. First, there are fundamental disparities in the way that nurses and doctors are trained in interprofessional communication (Leonard et al. 2004). Nurses are educated to communicate using very broad narratives to describe clinical situations.

Conversely, physicians learn to be very concise to rapidly arrive at the most critical or immediately relevant aspects of a situation. A different breed of communication barrier is often observed in operating rooms where different styles of communication can lead to difficulties surgeons and other staff in interpreting what is really meant by each other (Powell and Hill 2006) leading to errors and impeding the development team cohesion (Gillespie et al. 2012). Second, hospitals are by tradition rather hierarchical in their management. Hierarchy, or power distance, can create an unsafe environment for team members which inhibits them from speaking up (Leonard et al. 2004), and especially large authority gradients create unnecessarily high risks. The Silent Treatment Study (Maxfield et al. 2011), based on findings from research conducted in 2005, identified nurses' failure to speak up and share their concerns fully. The researchers describe very severe consequences: colleagues see each other make mistakes repeatedly over longer periods of time, demonstrate dangerous levels of incompetence, or violate rules but are unwilling or unable to speak up. Third, a large and persistent cultural barrier in healthcare takes the form of a belief that training for technical competence and emphasizing hard work and effort will result in error-free clinical performance and high quality of care (Leonard et al. 2004). Finally, in addition to the professional culture, organizational, and team factors, interpersonal communication is also influenced by factors intrinsic to individual workers such as speaking and listening skills, conflict resolution techniques, and the use of appropriate assertion and advocacy. All these intrinsic, internal, external, and contextual factors impede shared understandings among team members about their respective roles, tasks, and goals and lead to reduced situational awareness, weaker shared mental models and elevated risks for errors (Westli et al. 2010).

Teaching people how to speak up so that they will be appropriately assertive in expressing their concerns contributes to safer patient care. Also, checklists can facilitate team members speaking up. For example, since the introduction of the Safe Surgery Checklist (a pre-task briefing) in operating rooms, awareness regarding strengthening communication between care providers in order to optimize patient safety has grown (Haynes et al. 2009), and a significant drop in mortality and morbidity by means of optimized team communication has been observed in a number of contexts (Nagpal et al. 2010). Because the lack of a shared mental model and differential places in hierarchies contributes to miscommunication, language and scripting for critical situations is another important tool. Using a clearly agreed upon shared (mental) communication model avoids the natural tendency of less powerful members to speak indirectly and deferentially (and less clearly) (Leonard et al. 2004). SBAR (situation, background, assessment, and recommendation) can be a tool for implementing formal communication flows between care providers in both urgent and nonurgent situations (De Meester et al. 2013). Research has shown that the use of the SBAR technique produces a heightened perception of effective communication, greater collaboration among nurses, and improved quality of nurses' communications in, for instance, telephone communications with physicians. Finally, "read back" and "closed-loop" communication skills, ways of exchanging information accurately and acknowledging receipt of information, are skills often observed in high-reliability team members.

## 10.6.2 Leadership

After communication, leadership is one of the social skills that appear to be the most essential factor for the successful functioning of teams (Parker et al. 2012). Multiple studies have identified associations between good leadership and the effectiveness of cardiopulmonary resuscitation, the duration of surgical procedures, and the incidence of errors (Hull et al. 2012). Especially in crisis decision-making, team performance is associated with effective team leadership (Flin et al. 2006). Team leadership includes directing and coordinating the actions of team members; managing workload and resources; encouraging collaboration; developing team knowledge, skills, and abilities; and overseeing implementation of protocols or plans (and responding to non-compliance) (Flin et al. 2006).

However, the distinction between authority and leadership is not always clear, nor are authority and leadership evenly distributed across team members (Flin and Maran 2015). In clinical practice, different team members of a multidisciplinary team may in principle have equal status, and it can become unclear who is "in charge." In the YouTube video, "Just a routine operation" tells the story of Martin Bromiley, an airline pilot and human factors expert, whose wife died following complications of routine sinus surgery. Among other problems, a lack of clear leadership resulted in a breakdown related to human factors, and poor teamwork was noted in this situation.

In aviation, for example, there are clear agreements on who is flying the airplane. Before takeoff, the question is asked "Who is flying the aircraft?". After a brief summary on current aircraft status, the relinquishing pilot states: "You have the controls," which the second pilot acknowledges by saying: "I have the controls" (Powell and Hill 2006). Following this procedure, it is clear who is in charge especially in the event of a mishap. The pilot flying the aircraft (who had the controls) is the one who flies the airplane manually in case of a failure. The pilot monitoring the aircraft monitors the pilot flying, the system, and the routes and analyzes and attempts to resolve problems in the case of a failure or emergency. In essence, this standard operating procedure is simply a task sharing division, so each person in the cockpit knows at all times what his or her role is, avoiding possible overlap and confusion especially in high workload circumstances. Why not adopt a similar strategy in healthcare where oftentimes leadership roles are unclear?

Good leadership can be considered as a set of skills with behavioral indicators such as use of authority and assertiveness, providing and maintaining standards, and planning and prioritizing and managing workload and resources (Flin et al. 2008). This suggests that formal or intentional training in leadership techniques is necessary (Manser 2009). In environments with increased stress and workload, dividing and delegating tasks reduces the risk of errors. In fact, numerous studies demonstrated that extreme workload is a contributing factor for diagnostic errors both in the emergency department as well as in the operating room (Hull et al. 2012; Kachalia et al. 2007). Of course, leadership styles must be adapted according to specifics of the team's situation, autonomy, and experience (Parker et al. 2012). In high workload situations such as the management of medical emergencies, a *clear directive style* of leadership is appropriate, whereas in routine or non-emergency situations, a more *consultative* leadership style is indicated, especially when experienced well-trained teams are using standard operating procedures. It is important to note that the leader is not necessarily always the most highly educated or experienced (e.g., a physician in a multidisciplinary team) and leadership role may be assumed by different individuals over time as situations evolve. However, a clear leadership role must be communicated at all times in order to maintain situational awareness and efficient teamwork (Deering et al. 2011).

### 10.6.3 Situational Awareness

Situational awareness and decision-making comprise the two key cognitive skills in TRM. The concept refers to "knowing what is going on around you," implying the possession of knowledge and understanding to achieve a certain goal (Flin et al. 2008), and occurs when team members share the same perception of the elements in the internal and external environment, comprehend the meaning of these elements, and can forecast the status of these elements in the near future (Endsley 1995, p. 36; French and Hutchinson 2002; Mitchell et al. 2012). Accurate situational awareness is the basis for optimal decision-making. In fact, a specific assessment of the current situation must be made in order to determine whether or not action should be taken. Optimal situational awareness has a positive impact on performance and thus on the quality of care (Schulz et al. 2013).

Research shows that distractions and interruptions that occur frequently in operating and emergency rooms can cause a loss of situational awareness (Flin et al. 2009). A systematic review by Hull et al. (2012) showed a negative correlation between the nontechnical skills of the entire surgical team (surgeon, anesthesiologist, nurse) and errors in surgeon technical performance. The most relevant nontechnical skill in surgeons proved to be situational awareness—the better the situational awareness, the fewer technical errors (Hull et al. 2012). In addition, Way et al. (2003) found misperceptions (particularly low situational awareness), rather than deficits in technical skills, cause many surgical errors.

Although we consider ourselves to be very observant individuals, practice teaches us the opposite. On YouTube, there is an awareness test called "Whodunnit?". In this video, the viewer is confronted with a small segment of video recording where multiple visual elements are being changed. Most of the time, viewers only observe a fraction of what has been modified. This is a manifestation of the psychological concept called selective attention and is the consequence of the way our brain processes information. Because there is too much information available in the environment at any one time for our brain to process, our attention will shift to some things over others. Past experiences and environmental changes will guide the selection (Flin et al. 2008).

The imperative to develop and foster situational awareness is the consequence of selective attention. Factors that influence a breakdown in situational awareness include incomplete information, knowledge and experience, goals and expectations, individual capacity to absorb information, fatigue, degree of stress, distraction, interruption, stimulus overload, and the complexity of the situation (Schulz et al. 2013).

Interventions that improve situational awareness in multidisciplinary healthcare teams include good briefing communications; well-developed information and communication systems; minimization of external distractors and interruptions such as cellular phones and redundant alarms especially, but not only, during critical tasks (e.g., portable phones, redundant alarms); ensuring fitness for work (dealing with physical and mental health); regular preplanned updates (e.g., time-out mechanisms); monitoring and cross-check; speaking-up; and efficient time management (Flin et al. 2008). In addition, in aviation the rule "sterile cockpit" was introduced to clearly define where and when crew must set aside nonessential activities and tend strictly to the task at hand—the safe operation of the aircraft. After all, it is unrealistic to expect a crew to work together over many hours without ever discussing personal matters, and team members need to talk to get to know each other in order to be most effective.

### 10.6.4  Decision-Making

Various situations in healthcare are characterized by the risk of unforeseen circumstances that require on-the-spot decisions and/or modifications to prearranged plans. In particular in emergency situations, time pressure, rapidly changing or unclear conditions, and a high degree of uncertainty are factors that affect decision-making (Pauley et al. 2011). In a simulation activity, Endacott et al. (2010) found that in responding to cues reflecting patient deterioration, student nurses made decisions partly based on gut feelings. Research indicates that people, including duly credentialed nurses and physicians, make decisions that do not follow normative models, especially under natural conditions characterized by time pressure, vague and competing goals, complex information processing demands, and uncertainty (Resnick 2012). Decision-making is a multifaceted process that includes a team gathering information, detecting the problem, identifying alternatives, considering consequences for each alternative, and selecting the best one (Lipshitz et al. 2001). Deliberating and identifying optimal solutions can be very time-consuming and can challenge the limits of human information processing capabilities. When time is at stake, selecting a satisfactory solution that is not necessarily the optimal one can be the best approach (Lee et al. 2009). However, research has demonstrated that when decision-makers achieve expertise, they move to using an unconscious pattern matching recognition-primed decision-making (RPD) process (Resnick 2012). Because skilled healthcare workers have matched situations against a large number of templates stored in their memories, their responses are both skilled and efficient because of automatic processing that is further speeded up through priming with expectations (Green 2004). In a typical healthcare environment, emotions are all around originating from both external and internal sources. Research has shown that emotions have an often unconscious though powerful impact on decision-making.

Emotions due to sleep deprivation, usability factors of IT systems and medical devices, and a plethora of device alarms negatively impact decision-making (Resnick 2012). Finally, the hierarchical nature of titles and cultures of top-down decision-making in hospitals not only leads nurses to be very careful about asking questions or offering interpretations but also makes attending physicians to be careful when questioning the decisions of other physicians (Powell and Hill 2006). As we all know, holding a title of authority does not always mean that that a person always has the right answer.

Research indicates that team decisions—that is, collectively made decisions—tend to be better ones, especially in conditions where workloads are high (Powell and Hill 2006). Furthermore, some research findings suggest that training in decision-making skills through simulations and classroom-based instruction (often involving case studies) improves the outcomes of emergency care and anesthesia (Riley et al. 2011; Cohn and Dolich 2014). Training appears to create a greater awareness of one's personal decision-making strategies (meta-cognition), which can improve one's clinical effectiveness and can reduce the risk to patients of suboptimal decisions. Finally, the influence of emotion on information processing and decision-making can be neutralized by basic awareness training (Resnick 2012).

## 10.6.5 Teamwork

Interestingly, the perception of teamwork differs among healthcare professionals (nurses tend to perceive quality of teamwork less favorably than physicians), within disciplines (physicians in training report a lower quality of teamwork than senior physicians), and among specialists (Hull et al. 2012). Surgeons and anesthesiologists report higher satisfaction scores than nurses about the collaboration between physicians and nurses. Nurses were found to be less satisfied than physicians about their ability to raise questions ("speaking up"), support, collaboration between disciplines, conflict resolution, and consideration of nurses' input. The cause of this might be sought in fundamental differences between the professions, including social status, authority, historical gender balances in these professions, training, and responsibilities. Nurses tend to feel that good collaboration respects their input, whereas physicians describe good collaboration as nurses anticipating physician needs and following instructions. This may explain why teamwork has been assessed differently by different disciplines (Hull et al. 2012).

A team of experts is not automatically an expert team (Sevdalis 2013). Effective teamwork is only possible with collective efforts of the part of all team members regardless of training or background to manage the team's resources. Complexity in patient care, along with human factors, makes standardized communication and an environment of equality and respect among team members indispensable (O'Daniel and Rosenstein 2008). Weak coordination between care providers at different levels in the organization erodes the quality and safety of care. Moreover, the perception of caregivers concerning good teamwork is also associated with emotional exhaustion, burnout, job satisfaction, and commitment to the organization. Therefore, efforts to improve professional communication that breaks down hierarchies are crucial.

## 10.7  Multidisciplinary Team Training

Improving safety is not just about enhancing knowledge and skills, but also developing nontechnical skills and mitigating human factors that can lead to medical errors (Gordon et al. 2012). Currently, there is a wide variety of team training programs in healthcare with regard to content, method, duration, and focus (Buljac-Samardzic et al. 2010).

Most of the literature divides team training programs into two categories: courses using simulations and classroom-based learning (Lisha 2011). Simulation is a training and feedback method where tasks and processes are practiced under realistic conditions. Based on aviation's CRM training, Gaba et al. (1992) developed the first Anesthesia Crisis Resource Management (ACRM) program—a simulation-based program. In addition, multidisciplinary obstetric simulated emergency scenarios (MOSES) is a simulation course for obstetric teams (Freeth et al. 2006). These training programs use "high-fidelity" simulations as the primary instructional strategy developing nontechnical skills. Examples of classroom-based training, some of which incorporate case study approaches, include Team Strategies and Tools to Enhance Performance and Patient Safety (TeamSTEPPS) (Clancy 2007) and Medical Team Management (MTM) (Clapper and Kong 2012). Pratt and Sachs (2006) suggest that a combination of both classroom training and simulation-based learning is most suitable for team training. Indeed a recent study by Chan et al. (2016) investigated whether a Crew Resource Management classroom-based training had an effect on safety attitudes of doctors and nurses. The results indicated that nurses valued the experience highly and significant safety attitude shifts were observed on nearly all dimensions, suggesting that even classroom-based training programs may have positive impacts.

In our own group, we developed a generic simulation-based team training program for multidisciplinary teams in healthcare settings that frequently deal with emergency situations (Roes et al. 2017). The training program has three phases.

The first phase is a didactic presentation of all five key principles of Team Resource Management, starting with historical background. Although blended learning using e-learning may be preferred by some due to cost-effectiveness, theoretical background can also be provided classroom based. The evidence shows that both are equally effective (Roes et al. 2017).

The second phase involves simulation-based multidisciplinary team training. The training takes place in small groups of four to six team members. It is important that these small teams have a multidisciplinary composition and include at least one physician. Situations where nurses act out the roles of physicians are to be discouraged, because in our experience this renders simulation scenarios less realistic. Furthermore, use of real practice settings is recommended to make simulations as realistic as possible, particularly having team members work in their own environments using their own equipment (which has the side benefit of permitting a critical look at the ergonomics of particular work settings). Each scenario starts with a briefing (about 10 min). The team then goes to the room where the scenario takes place. The facilitator gives instructions. The entire session is video recorded and takes about 20 min. The scenarios used vary according to the department where the participants work: cases for the emergency department staff will be different from those from labor and delivery suite or the intensive care unit. Carefully designing, pretesting, and editing the scenarios is crucial in order to prevent resistance from participants.

The third phase is a detailed debriefing session. This phase is the most important for team learning and takes about 45 min. A facilitator invites participants to share and discuss their experiences during the simulation, leading to clarifications and reflection. In a safe exercise and learning environment, emphasis is placed on positive feedback and improvement points with regard to mutual cooperation and communication. Together Phases 2 and 3 take about 3 h.

Roes et al. (2017) evaluated the effectiveness of this training protocol with 307 participants across 14 units. The mean age of the study participants was 39 years, and the breakdown of backgrounds was 20% physicians, 69% nurses, and 1.5% medical trainees. Participants came from five labor and delivery units, eight emergency departments, and one intensive care unit. The results indicated that participants were highly to very highly satisfied with TRM training. A strong majority of the study participants (81%) were convinced that this type of training would be beneficial for patient safety, and 79% reported that the training led to a change in their behavior in real life emergency situations. In addition, the study also evaluated behavioral changes using the Clinical Teamwork Scale (CTS; Guise et al. 2008), an observational scale for nontechnical skills. Before and after the TRM intervention, nontechnical skills were evaluated in unannounced simulations: a significant improvement in overall teamwork scores after the training was observed ($p < 0.003$). These results are in line with other studies investigating the impact of team training on nontechnical skills of teams and/or subjective outcome indicators (perception of team effectiveness, safety culture, employee satisfaction) (Weaver et al. 2014; Buljac-Samardzic et al. 2010; Lisha 2011). Almost with exception, these studies demonstrate positive impacts between training interventions and team nontechnical skills.

In addition, there is also growing evidence that team training programs may have a positive impact on patient outcomes, including increased safety of care (Neily et al. 2010). For example, a recent intervention study of multidisciplinary simulation training for delivery room staff showed a (lasting) significant improvement of 37% in perinatal morbidity after implementation (Riley et al. 2011). Consequently, both the American College of Obstetricians and Gynecologists and the Institute of Medicine have recommended team training programs and interventions to improve communication as cornerstones of patient safety work (American College of OB/GYN 2009).

## 10.8   Measurement Tools

To assess the nontechnical skills of caregivers, researchers in healthcare have drawn primarily on the NOTECHS tool from aviation. This instrument evaluates four skills assessed during flight simulator training: collaboration, leadership, situational awareness, and decision-making (Chalwin and Flabouris 2013). There are currently a number of tools available both for individual caregivers and for teams and for different settings and contexts. Such systems offer an objective observation of the ability to apply nontechnical skills, which can be used to give feedback to caregivers and/or teams in simulated or real-life scenarios. Examples are (1) nontechnical skills (NOTECHS) for operations teams and trauma nontechnical skills (T-NOTECHS) for trauma teams (Flin et al. 2003), (2) anesthesiologists' nontechnical skills (ANTS) (Flin et al. 2010), (3) nontechnical skills for surgeons (NOTSS) (Yule et al. 2008), (4) scrub practitioners' list of intraoperative nontechnical skills (SPLINTS) (Mitchell et al. 2012), (5) observational teamwork assessment for surgery (OTAS) (Hull et al. 2012), and (6) team emergency assessment measure (TEAM) (Cooper et al. 2010).

## 10.9   Implementation of TRM Principles in an Acute Hospital Setting

### 10.9.1   Implementation in the Organization

Although change is vital to progress, numerous complexities arise when plans need to be translated into actions (Mitchell 2013). Change efforts often fail when change agents take an unstructured approach to implementation (Wright 1998). In order to implement change, however, managers or change agents need a framework for implementing, managing, and evaluating change (Pearson et al. 2005). A number of theories and assumptions about the nature of change can be found in the literature (Kritsonis 2004). Ronald Lippitt and colleagues created a change theory with seven phases focusing on the roles and responsibilities of change agents rather than the unfolding of change itself. After all, change agents or champions are important key components for moving new innovations through the phases of initiation, development, and implementation (Shaw et al. 2012). The seven phases are as follows: (1) diagnose the problem; (2) assess the motivation/capacity for change; (3) assess the change agent(s) resources and motivation; (4) choose progressive change objective(s); (5) the role of the change agents should be selected and clearly understood by all parties so that expectations are clear; (6) maintain the change; and (7) gradually terminate the helping relationship. Lippitt and colleagues argue that changes are likely to be more stable when they are more firmly rooted. The more widespread imitation becomes, the more the behavior is regarded as normal. Although there are many change theories, each with specific assumptions, Lippitt's work is one of the more detailed (Mitchell 2013), and we recommend it to healthcare managers because it incorporates a plan of how to generate change and mirrors the four phases of the nursing process: assessment, planning, implementation, and evaluation (Mitchell 2013; Pearson et al. 2005).

Also, leadership, effective communication, and teamwork are important key components of planned change (Mitchell 2013). To provide inspiration, vision, and support to everyone involved, it is crucial to have passionate team champions in place throughout the change process. Finally, Lippitt's change theory in combination with a democratic leadership style has proven to be a popular and effective combination (Mitchell 2013).

## 10.9.2 Implementation in a Healthcare Team

TRM training may also be challenging to implement in and of itself, depending on team climate. Some general considerations bear mentioning. First, the training only is useful when the whole multidisciplinary team is trained. In our experience, no matter how obvious this seems, we sometimes arrive on clinical units to train a team of healthcare workers and when it comes time to begin training, no physicians are available. Put bluntly, principles of TRM only are useful, and patient safety will be strengthened when all disciplines are trained. Second, the real challenge of the implementation of TRM is changing climate in such a way that healthcare workers of all experience levels and disciplines are engaged to train and adopt the same mental models regarding team collaboration. Individual attitudes toward TRM principles and unit safety climate tend to be interrelated. Consequently, it might be a good start to initiate change by introducing the principles of TRM and start training with a few multidisciplinary teams on a pilot basis. In Rogers' diffusion of innovation theory, these first participants are called innovators or early adopters. Rogers' model provides powerful explanations why some people and settings are more willing to accept change than others. In addition, it is recommended to work with team champions who are responsible in every team to integrate and develop the TRM principles of teamwork. In order to create a shared mental model, it is preferable to make the TRM principles part of the daily routine and culture. Initiatives include developing checklists and standard operating procedures (SOP), using checklists (such as the ISBARR reporting technique), making TRM offerings a standard item at interdisciplinary meetings, ensuring that all (new) personnel receive full TRM training each year, and producing regular information bulletins, posters, and other dissemination tools. Third, power imbalances across different categories and staff and steep hierarchical gradients need to be challenged (Green et al. 2017). The regular use of simple expressions like "there is no I in a team"; models like the assertiveness triangle that distinguishes between passive, aggressive, and assertive behavior; the PACE mnemonic for communication channels (primary, alternate, contingency, and emergency); and the CUS acronym for language to use when escalating communications regarding risk (concerned, uncomfortable, safety is at risk) can be used to focus attention on good teamwork and the shared responsibility of each individual team member in their own roles. The behavior of "toxic individuals" needs to be managed by taking remedial steps in training. If the situation hereafter does not improve, actions need to be taken by the hospital management. If senior colleagues do not realize there is a problem, the team should act as a whole to address the problem. In sum, a "just culture" needs to be in place; healthcare organizations cannot afford a blame-free environment: Some behavior, violations, or errors warrant disciplinary action. Finally, scenario-based simulation is also to be encouraged as refresher or "booster" follow-up training. Additional factors favoring success include guarantees of confidentiality throughout the training/learning process, mandatory participation, TRM training largely delivered by clinicians experienced in high-reliability methods, and leadership by example.

## 10.10   Barriers and Threats

During the years of training experience, we observed a number of barriers that may pose threats to successful implementation of TRM principles. First, healthcare is a sector under pressure due to rapid technological change, the aging of the population, and economic-financial constraints in offering affordable healthcare. It can be difficult to justify human resource development (especially training in nontechnical skills) in light of practical and financial demands on the healthcare system. Second, although there is considerable evidence connecting TRM approaches to improved safety attitudes, evidence regarding impacts on patient outcomes such as mortality and patient safety is still sparse. Finally, the managerial challenges of integrating the TRM principles into a departmental or organizational culture (or colloquially, making TRM part of a unit's DNA) are not to be underestimated. The existing organization or departmental culture may produce counter pressures to changing ways of working. Cultural shifts in medical and nursing staff are necessary if the TRM approach is truly to take root. The entire hospital management needs to operate from a shared mental model that shifts emphasis in the culture from individual performance to teamwork in order to provide safer healthcare.

---

**Conclusion**

Efforts to improve patient safety are a shared responsibility of all healthcare workers and of the entire hospital management team. In spite of being characterized by more highly educated professionals and cutting-edge training facilities, equipment, and research than ever, healthcare systems are still confronted with serious safety problems. In more than 70% of cases, serious and avoidable medical errors originate in so-called human factors or deficits in "nontechnical" skills—including communication, leadership, teamwork, situational awareness, and decision-making. A major reason behind slow improvement is the cumbersome, hierarchical organizational structure in many healthcare organizations that stand in the way of a safety culture, encourage a "blame culture" and foster communication errors. Resolving these issues requires a fundamental cultural shift from an individual to a group focus where safety is the shared responsibility of all individual healthcare workers and the entire management team working in a hospital (or other healthcare organization). Because safe care relies on the collective individual expertise of team members as well as teamwork, the interdisciplinary performance of care teams goes hand in hand with the safety culture of the healthcare organization as a whole. Consequently, investments in multidisciplinary teams in teamwork training such as Team Resource Management training to build nontechnical skills are essential.

# References

American College of OB/GYN. Patient safety in obstetrics and gynecology: committee opinion. Obstet Gynecol. 2009;114:1424–7.

Boysen PG. Just culture: a foundation for balanced accountability and patient safety. Ochsner J. 2013;13(3):400–6.

Buljac-Samardzic M, Dekker-van Doorn CM, van Wijngaarden JD, van Wijk KP. Intervention to improve team effectiveness: a systematic review. Health Policy. 2010;94(3):183–95.

Chalwin RP, Flabouris A. Utility and assessment of non-technical skills for rapid response systems and medical emergency teams. Intern Med J. 2013;43(9):962–9.

Chan CK, So HK, Ng WY, Chan PK, Ma WL, Chan KL, Leung SH, Ho LY. Does classroom-based crew resource management training have an effect on attitudes between doctors and nurses? Int J Med Educ. 2016;9(7):109–14.

Chassin MR. Improving the quality of health care: what's taking so long? Health Aff. 2013;32(10):1761–5.

Clancy CM. TeamSTEPPS: optimizing teamwork in the perioperative setting. AORN J. 2007;86(1):18–22.

Clapper TC, Kong M. TeamSTEPPS: the patient safety tool that needs to be implemented. Clin Simul Nurs. 2012;8(8):367–73.

Cohn SM, Dolich MO. Complications in surgery and trauma. 2nd ed. Boca Raton: CRC Press; 2014.

Cooper S, Cant R, Porter J, Sellick K, Somers G, Kinsman L, et al. Rating medical emergency teamwork performance: development of the Team Emergency Assessment Measure (TEAM). Resuscitation. 2010;81(4):446–52.

Cronin JG, Wright J. Rapid assessment and initial patient treatment team–a way forward for emergency care. Accid Emerg Nurs. 2005;13(2):87–92.

De Meester K, Verspuy M, Monsieurs KG, Van Bogaert P. SBAR improves nurse-physician communication and reduces unexpected death: a pre and post intervention study. Resuscitation. 2013;84(9):1192–6.

de Vries EN, Ramrattan MA, Smorenburg SM, Gouma DJ, Boermeester MA. The incidence and nature of in-hospital adverse events: a systematic review. Qual Saf Health Care. 2009;17(3):216–23.

DeChurch LA, Mesmer-Magnus JR. The cognitive underpinnings of effective teamwork: a meta-analysis. J Appl Psychol. 2010;95(1):32–53.

Deering S, Johnston LC, Caollachio K. Multidisciplinary teamwork and communication training. Semin Perinatol. 2011;35(2):89–96.

Dekker S. Just culture: balancing safety and accountability. Burlington: Ashgate Publishing; 2008.

Eisenberg EM, Murphy AG, Sutcliffe K, Wears R, Schenkel S, Perry S, et al. Communication in emergency medicine: implications for patient safety. Commun Monogr. 2005;72(4):390–413.

Endacott R, Scholes J, Buyckx P, Cooper S, Kinsman L, McConnell-Henry T. Final-year students' ability to assess, detect and act on clinical cues of deterioration in a simulated environment. J Adv Nurs. 2010;66(12):2722–31.

Endsley MR. Toward a theory of situation awareness in dynamic systems. Hum Factors J. 1995;37(1):32–64.

Flin R, Maran N. Basic concepts for crew resource management and non-technical skills. Best Pract Res Clin Anaesthesiol. 2015;29(1):27–39.

Flin R, Martin L, Goeters K-M, Hörmann H-J, Amalberti R, Valot C, et al. Development of the NOTECHS (non-technical skills) system for assessing pilots' CRM skills. Hum Factors and Aerosp Saf. 2003;3(2):95–117.

Flin R, O'Connor P, Crichton M. Safety at the sharp end: a guide to non-technical skills. Surry: Ashgate Publishing Limited; 2008.

Flin R, Winter J, Sarac C, Raduma M. Human factors in patient safety: review of topics and tools. Geneva: World Health Organization; 2009.

Flin R, Yule S, McKenzie L, Paterson-Brown S, Maran N. Attitudes to teamwork and safety in the operating theatre. Surgeon. 2006;4(3):145–51.

Flin R, Patey R, Glavin R, Maran N. Anaesthetists' non-technical skills. Br J Anaesth. 2010;105(1): 38–44.

Freeth D, Ayida G, Berridge EK, Sadler C, Strachan A. Multidisciplinary obstetric simulated emergency scenarios. J Interprof Care. 2006;20(5):552–4.

French HT, Hutchinson A. Measurement of situation awareness in a C4ISR experiment. In: Proceedings of the 7th international command and control research and technology symposium. Quebec City: CCRP; 2002.

Gaba DM. Crisis resource management and teamwork training in anaesthesia. Br J Anaesth. 2010;105(1):3–6.

Gaba DM, Howard SK, Fish KJ, Smith BE, Sowb YA. Simulation-based training in anesthesia crisis resource management (ACRM): a decade of experience. Simulation and Gaming-Symposium on medical and healthcare simulation. 2001;32:175–93.

Gillespie BM, Chaboyer W, Fairweather N. Interruptions and miscommunications in surgery: an observational study. AORN J. 2012;95(5):576–90.

Gordon M, Darbyshire D, Baker P. Non-technical skills training to enhance patient safety: a systematic review. Med Educ. 2012;46(11):1042–54.

Green B, Oeppen RS, Smith DW, Brennan P. Challenging hierarchy in healthcare teams – ways to flatten gradients to improve teamwork and patient care. Br J Oral Maxillofac Surg 2017;55(5):449–53.

Green M. Nursing error and human nature. J Nurs Law. 2004;9(4):37–44.

Guise JM, Deering SH, Kanki BG, Osterweil P, Li H, Mri M, Lowe NK. Validation of a tool to measure and promote clinical teamwork. Simul Healthc. 2008;3(4):217–23.

Haerkens MH, Jenkins DH, van der Hoeven JG. Crew resource management in the ICU: the need for culture change. Ann Intensive Care. 2012;2(1):39.

Hakimzada AF, Green RA, Sayan OR, Zhang J, Patel V. The Nature and occurrence of registration errors in the emergency department. Int J Med Inform. 2008;77(3):169–75.

Haynes AB, Weiser TG, Berry WR, Lipsitz SR, Breizat A-HS, Dellinger EP, et al. A surgical safety checklist to reduce morbidity and mortality in a global population. N Engl J Med. 2009;360(5):491–9.

Hull L, Arora S, Aggarwal R, Darzi A, Vincent C, Sevdalis N. The impact of non-technical skills on technical performance in surgery: a systematic review. J Am Coll Surg. 2012;214(2):214–30.

Joint Commission International. Joint Commission International Accreditation Standards voor Hospitals. 2014.

Kachalia A, Gandhi TK, Puopolo AL, Yoon C, Thomas EJ, Griffey R, Brennan TA, Studdert DM. Missed and delayed diagnoses in the emergency department: a study of closed malpractice claims from 4 liability insurers. Ann Emerg Med. 2007;49(2):196–205.

Kohn L, Corrigan J, Donaldson M. To err is human: building a safer health system. Washington, DC: N.A. Press; 2000.

Kritsonis A. Comparison of change theories. Int J Sch Acad Intellect Div. 2004;8(1):1–7.

Lee L, Amir O, Ariely D. In search of homo economicus: cognitive noise and the role of emotion in preference consistency. J Constr Res. 2009;36(2):173–87.

Leonard M, Graham S, Bonacum D. The human factor: the critical importance of effective teamwork and communication in providing safe care. Qual Saf Health Care. 2004;13(suppl 1):85–90.

Lipshitz R, Klein G, Orasanu J, Salas E. Taking stock of naturalistic decision making. J Behav Decis Making. 2001;14(5):331–52.

Lisha L, Teamwork and communication in healthcare. A literature review. Edmonton, AB, Canada: The Canadian Patient Safety Institute. 2011. http://www.patientsafetyinstitute.ca/en/toolsResources/teamworkCommunication/Documents/Canadian%20Framework%20for%20Teamwork%20and%20Communications%20Lit%20Review.pdf

Manser T. Teamwork and patient safety in dynamic domains of healthcare: a review of the literature. Acta Anaesthesiol Scand. 2009;53(2):143–51.

Mash R, De Sa A, Christodoulou M. How to change organizational culture: action research in a South African public sector primary care facility. Afr J Prim Health Care Fam Med. 2016;8(1):1–9.

Maxfield D, Grenny J, Lavandero R, Groah L. The silent treatment: why safety tools and checklists aren't enough to save lives. 2011. http://www.silenttreatmentstudy.com/download/. Accessed 26 Aug 2017.

McComb S, Simpson V. The concept of shared mental models in healthcare collaboration. J Adv Nurs. 2014;70(7):1479–88.

Mitchell G. Selecting the best theory to implement planned change. Nurs Manag. 2013;20(1):32–7.

Mitchell L, Flin R, Yule S, Mitchell J, Coutts K, Youngson G. Evaluation of the scrub practitioners' list of intraoperative non-technical skills system. Int J Nurs Stud. 2012;49(2):201–11.

Mohammed S, Klimoski R, Rentsch JR. The measurement of team mental models: we have no shared schema. Organ Res Methods. 2000;3(2):123–65.

Nagpal K, Vats A, Lamb B, Ashrafian H, Sevdalig N, Vincent C, Moorthy K. Information transfer and communication in surgery: a systematic review. Ann Surg. 2010;252(2):225–39.

Neily J, Mills PD, Young-Xy Y, Carney BT, West P, Berger DH, Mazzia LM, Paull DE, Bagan JP. Association between implementation of a medical team training program and surgical mortality. JAMA. 2010;304(15):1693–700.

O'Daniel M, Rosenstein AH. Professional communication and team collaboration. In: Patient safety and quality: an evidence-based handbook for nurses. Rockville: Agency for Healthcare Research and Quality; 2008.

Parker SH, Yule S, Flin R, McKinley A. Surgeons' leadership in the operating room: an observational study. Am J Surg. 2012;204(3):347–54.

Pauley K, Flin R, Yule S, Youngson GG. Surgeon's intraoperative decision making and risk management. Am J Surg. 2011;202(4):375–81.

Pearson A, Vaughan B, Fitzgerald M. Nursing Models for Practice. Third edition. Butterworth-Heinemann, Oxford; 2005. https://trove.nla.gov.au/work/3557898?q&versionId=10529631+231608465+248182408

Powell SM, Hill RK. My copilot is a nurse–using crew resource management in the OR. AORN J. 2006;83(1):179–202.

Pratt SD, Sachs BP. Team training: classroom training vs. high-fidelity simulation. Agency for Healthcare Research and Quality. 2006.

Resnick M. The effect of affect: Decision making in the emotional context of health care. Symposium on Human Factors and Ergonomics in Healthcare. 2012.

Richardson LD, Irvin CB, Tamayo-Sarver JH. Racial and ethnic disparities in the clinical practice of emergency medicine. Acad Emerg Med. 2003;10(11):1184–8.

Riley W, Davis S, Miller K, Hansen H, Sainfort F, Sweet R. Didactic and simulation nontechnical skills team training to improve perinatal patient outcomes in a community hospital. Jt Comm J Qual Patient Saf. 2011;37(8):357–64.

Rivard PE, Rosen A, Caroll JS. Enhancing patient safety through organizational learning: are patient safety indicators a step in the right direction? Health Serv Res. 2006;41(4):1633–53.

Roes L, De Schepper S, Franck E. Eindverslag TETRA-project. Naar een veiligere patiënten-zorg: Crew Resource Management tijdens urgenties. Expertisecentrum Psychisch Welzijn in Patiëntenzorg, KdG Hogeschool, Antwerpen. 2017.

Salas E, Sims DE, Burke CS. Is there a "big five" in teamwork? Small Gr Res. 2005;36(5):555–99.

Schulz CM, Endsley MR, Kochs EF, Gelb AW, Wagner KJ. Situation awareness in anesthesia: concept and research. Anesthesiology. 2013;118(3):1–14.

Sevdalis N. Non-technical skills and the future of teamwork in healthcare settings. The Health Foundation. 2013.

Shaw EK, Howard J, West DR, Crabtree BF, Nease DE, Tutt B, Nutting PA. The role of the champion in primary care change efforts. J Am Board Fam Med. 2012;25(5):676–85.

Van Bogaert P, Meulemans H, Clarke S, Vermeyen K, Van de Heyning P. Hospital nurse practice environment, burnout, job outcomes and quality of care: test of a structural equation model. J Adv Nurs. 2009;65(10):2175–85.

Vandijck D, Bergs J, Vermeir P, Hellings J. Patiëntveiligheid in de ziekenhuissector: Wat kunnen we leren van de luchtvaartsector? Tijdschr voor Geneeskunde. 2015;71:1379–90.

Way L, Stewart L, Gantert W, Kingsway L, Crystine ML, Whang K, Hunter JG. Causes and prevention of laparoscopic bile duct injuries. Ann Surg. 2003;237(4):460–9.

Weaver SJ, Dy SM, Rosen MA. Team-training in healthcare: a narrative synthesis of the literature. BMJ Qual Saf. 2014;23(5):359–72.

Westli HK, Johnsen BH, Eid J, Rasten I, Brattebo G. Teamwork skills, shared mental models, and performance in simulated trauma teams: an independent group design. Scand J Trauma Resusc Emerg Med. 2010;18:47.

Wilson KA, Burke CS, Priest H, Salas E. Promoting health care safety through training high reliability teams. Qual Saf Health Care. 2005;14(4):303–9.

Wright S. Changing nursing practice. 2nd ed. London: Hodder Arnold; 1998.

Yule S, Flin R, Maran N, Rowley D, Youngson G, Paterson-Brown S. Surgeons' non-technical skills in the operating room: reliability testing of the NOTSS behavior rating system. World J Surg. 2008;32(4):548–56.

Yule S, Flin R, Paterson-Brown S, Maran N. Non-technical skills for surgeons in the operating room: a review of the literature. Surgery. 2006;139(2):140–9.

# Standardizing Care Processes Using Evidence-Based Strategies: Implementation of a Rapid Response System in Belgian Hospitals

Filip Haegdorens, Koenraad Monsieurs, and Peter Van Bogaert

**Abstract**

Since the turn of the millennium, the safety of hospital inpatients has become an important subject of research. Problems associated with in-hospital preventable deaths such as poor clinical monitoring, diagnostic errors, and inadequate therapy are most likely to occur in general wards. Studies demonstrate the presence of a substantial window between physiological instability and cardiac arrest where timely intervention could influence patient outcomes. Accordingly, the European Resuscitation Council has emphasized the importance of recognizing those at risk of cardiac arrest in the hope of preventing the need for resuscitation efforts through early treatment. However, in-hospital physiological instability is often missed, misinterpreted, and/or mismanaged by hospital staff. Moreover, a considerable number of preventable in-hospital deaths may be linked to poor practice and multiple failures of the various systems, reflecting environmental contexts of care that are discussed elsewhere in this book. This chapter describes five possible short-term outcomes that are influenced by patient and hospital characteristics as well as processes of care because of clinically deteriorating patient on the general wards. We propose the concept of rapid response system (RSS) as an umbrella term for all approaches aimed at improving detection and

F. Haegdorens (✉)
Emergency Department Antwerp University Hospital, Antwerp, Belgium

Nursing and Midwifery Sciences, Centre for Research and Innovation in Care (CRIC), Faculty of Medicine and Health Sciences, University of Antwerp, Antwerp, Belgium
e-mail: filip.haegdorens@uantwerpen.be

K. Monsieurs
Faculty of Medicine and Health Sciences, Antwerp University Hospital, Antwerp, Belgium

Emergency Department Antwerp University Hospital, Antwerp, Belgium

P. Van Bogaert
Nursing and Midwifery Sciences, Centre for Research and Innovation in Care (CRIC), Faculty of Medicine and Health Sciences, University of Antwerp, Antwerp, Belgium

interpretation of in-hospital clinical deterioration and enhancing communication between caregivers around deterioration and the initiation of an appropriate response in a timely manner. We describe and discuss the theoretical base and our experiences with implementing an RRS in Belgian hospitals within a randomized study design to study and improve outcomes. An evidence-based strategy was used to standardize care processes on general wards. During this research project, we identified barriers and facilitators at various levels that could have a possible impact on the adoption of a rapid response system on the general ward in acute hospitals. We formulate a conclusion based on previous studies and our research findings.

**Keywords**
Medical and surgical wards • Patient outcome • Deterioration • Cardiac arrest • Mortality • ICU admission • Rapid response system

## 11.1   Introduction

Since the turn of the millennium, the safety of hospital inpatients has become an important subject of research. Early and influential estimates published in the Institute of Medicine's report "To Err is Human" suggested that 7–14% of all hospitalized patients die each year as a result of medical errors (Kohn et al. 2000). These estimates were extrapolated from data from the Harvard Medical Practice Study. However, the use of outdated data and questionable methodology caused criticism and led to several studies around the world to reevaluate the magnitude of this problem (McDonald et al. 2000). Recent international studies suggest that 3 to 6% of all in-hospital deaths are either probably or definitely preventable—and can thus be attributed to systems of care (Hogan et al. 2012). Although the incidence of preventable in-hospital deaths may not be as high as previously assumed, harm from preventable problems in care is still substantial.

Problems associated with in-hospital preventable deaths are most likely to occur in general wards (Hogan et al. 2012). They involve poor clinical monitoring (31%), diagnostic errors (30%), and inadequate therapy (21%). A UK-based independent research organization (NCEPOD) retrospectively reviewed 585 records of patients who experienced a cardiac arrest (Findlay et al. 2012). They concluded that 62% of these patients showed physiological instability for longer than 6 h, 47% longer than 12 h, and 20% longer than 24 h prior to cardiac arrest. This demonstrates that there is a substantial window between physiological instability and cardiac arrest where timely intervention could influence patient outcomes. Over the last years, hospitals have dedicated much attention and resources in training their staff to adequately perform cardiopulmonary resuscitation. This is certainly a positive development, to be encouraged, embraced, and even enforced by governments and local authorities because it ensures that every hospitalized patient experiencing cardiac arrest receives the best care possible. Nonetheless, it is well known that survival until hospital discharge and favorable neurological outcomes in survivors of cardiac arrest are both low (Nolan et al. 2010). Accordingly, the European Resuscitation Council has emphasized the importance of recognizing those at risk of cardiac arrest in the hope of preventing the need for resuscitation efforts through early treatment. However, in-hospital physiological instability is often missed, misinterpreted, and/or mismanaged by hospital staff (Goldhill et al. 1999). A considerable number of preventable in-hospital deaths could be linked to poor practice and failures of the various systems, reflecting environmental contexts of care that are discussed elsewhere in this book (De Meester et al. 2013a).

## 11.2  Outcomes for Deteriorating Patients on the General Ward

The clinically deteriorating patient on the general ward has five possible short-term outcomes that are influenced by patient and hospital characteristics as well as processes of care (Fig. 11.1): (1) deterioration is detected and the patient receives prompt and adequate therapy on the general ward, (2) deterioration and even death are expected (in the case of terminal illness) and the patient receives end-of-life care on the general ward, (3) the patient is transferred to the intensive care unit (ICU), (4) the patient has a cardiac arrest and receives cardiopulmonary resuscitation (CPR), and (5) the patient dies unexpectedly. Possible long-term outcomes of the deteriorating patient are survival until hospital discharge, increased comorbidity at discharge, or in-hospital death. The first and second short-term outcomes, situations where deteriorating patients receive adequate and appropriate care outside the ICU, are obviously the most desirable since they do not consume additional hospital resources.

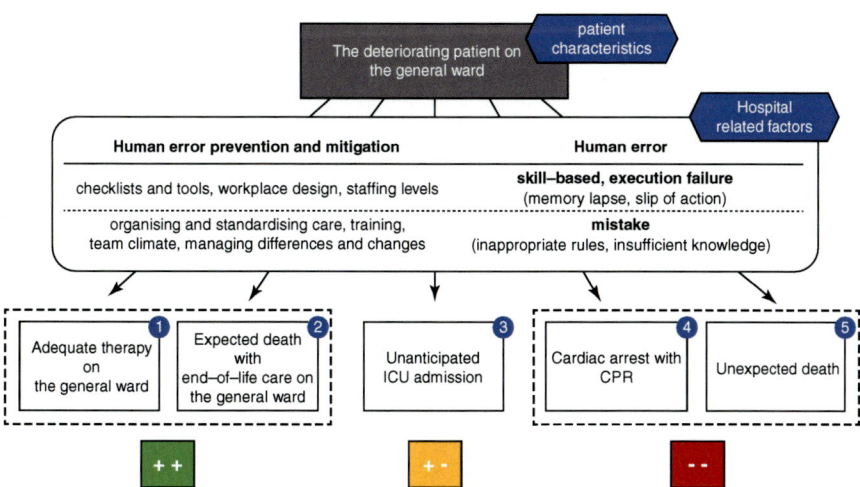

**Fig. 11.1**  Potential short-term outcomes of the deteriorating patient on the general ward

## 11.2.1 Unanticipated ICU Admissions

The ICU is a highly staffed unit within the acute hospital to care for patients with severe and life-threatening conditions. It is equipped with high-technology equipment and provides costly treatments and advanced life support for critically ill patients. Hospitalized patients are admitted to the intensive care unit (ICU) for a variety of reasons including conditions requiring respiratory, circulatory, neurological, and renal support and continuous monitoring of vital signs. An in-hospital ICU admission can be preplanned (e.g., postoperative management after major surgery) but is sometimes also unanticipated (e.g., following clinical deterioration of a patient on the general ward). Deteriorating patients who cannot be treated or monitored safely on a general ward but whose conditions are expected to improve definitely benefit from admission to an ICU.

Unanticipated ICU admissions have a significant impact on costs of care and tend to prolong hospital stay (Mercier et al. 2010). It is estimated that up to 9% of all admissions to the ICU are unanticipated and 56% of all unanticipated ICU admissions are preceded by an adverse event (Fig. 11.2) (Marquet et al. 2015). Furthermore, one in four unanticipated ICU admissions is associated with highly preventable adverse events such as incorrect drug therapy, complications from surgery, a delayed or wrong diagnosis, and a system issue related to hospital processes. This implies that some unanticipated admissions to the

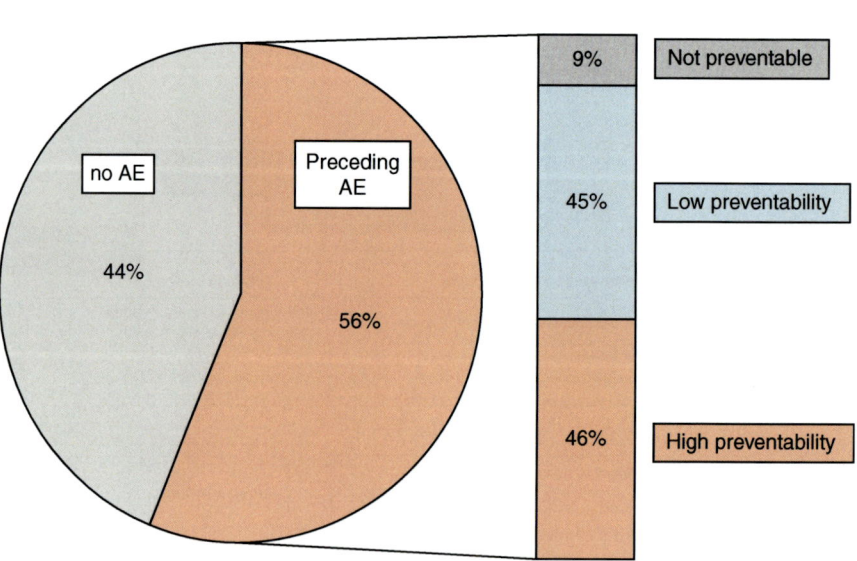

**Fig. 11.2** The preventability of unanticipated admissions to ICU. Data based on Marquet et al. (2015); *AE* adverse events

ICU could be prevented by system changes within hospitals. ICU admissions due to adverse events have a mean length of stay that ranges from 1.5 to 10.4 days and mortality percentages between 0 and 58% (Vlayen et al. 2012). This variability in data suggests that not all unanticipated transfers to the ICU should be considered as undesirable because some patients could benefit from a sudden transfer to a higher level of care. The third short-term outcome, where deteriorating patients are unanticipatedly admitted to the ICU, is therefore somewhat ambiguous. An example of a desirable but unanticipated ICU admission is the patient with a temporary need for respiratory support and continuous monitoring of vital signs. For this reason, researchers and hospital managers should be cautious when interpreting trends in unanticipated ICU admissions using hospital databases.

Because ICU beds are often a scarce and costly hospital resource, it is important that they be used in an efficient manner. A strong association has been found between the number of ICU beds available in a hospital and the processes of care for patients with sudden clinical deterioration (Stelfox et al. 2012). A lower probability of ICU admission and a higher probability of end-of-life care were noted as the number of ICU beds decreased. Hospital mortality was similar regardless of the number of ICU beds available. These results suggest that some patients experiencing deterioration do not necessarily need an upgrade of the level of care but rather would benefit from a change in medical therapy or even a shift to emphasize comfort at the end of life.

In patients where advanced medical care is considered futile, an upgrade to the intensive care unit is not always required or even appropriate since it could merely prolong the process of dying. Indeed, dying patients account for a significant proportion of hospital expenses for critical care (Khandelwal et al. 2015). It has been shown that terminally ill patients who receive advance care planning (e.g., do not resuscitate designations at hospital admission) or palliative care interventions resulted in a reduction of ICU admissions and the ICU length of stay. Hospitals where there are few or no mechanisms for engaging patients and families in advance care planning may therefore have higher proportions of unanticipated admissions to the ICU. If care systems were implemented to detect patient deterioration on the general ward, this could theoretically result in either an increase or decrease in ICU admissions. These systems could promote an early transfer to a higher level of care (e.g., a patient with an acute exacerbation of chronic obstructive pulmonary disease requiring invasive ventilation) or even prevent the unanticipated admission to the ICU by early treatment on the general ward (e.g., a patient with a rapidly diagnosed pyelonephritis who immediately receives antibiotics, thus avoiding sepsis). Hospitals implementing new systems to detect and respond to clinical deterioration should keep in mind that clinicians transfer patients to the ICU because they believe it is beneficial and is congruent with the patients' values and preferences. Clinicians should therefore prevent excessive use of ICU beds by (re)organizing care processes for situations where the likelihood of benefit from critical care is very slim to nonexistent.

## 11.2.2 Cardiac Arrest and Unexpected Death

The final two possible short-term outcomes for patients who experience clinical deterioration are cardiac arrest with cardiopulmonary resuscitation (CPR) and unexpected death. These are negative patient outcomes that hospital systems seek to minimize as much as possible. These two outcome indicators are not always clearly defined in the existing literature, making it difficult to interpret results (Maharaj et al. 2015). In-hospital cardiac arrests outside the ICU with cardiopulmonary resuscitation efforts occur in patients who experience an unforeseeable acute physiological collapse (e.g., cardiac arrhythmia) and in patients with unfolding deterioration where there has been no intervention or where interventions have been unsuccessful. When cardiac arrest is predictable but not preventable, all possible options should be discussed with the patient and his family to assist them in making an informed decision about CPR. When deteriorating patients are managed correctly, in-hospital cardiac arrest with CPR should be relatively rare and almost always unpredicted. In-hospital cardiac arrest rates reported in the literature range from one to five per 1000 admissions (Sandroni et al. 2007). In-hospital cardiac arrest with CPR can result in a return of spontaneous circulation (ROSC) or death. About 17.6% of all patients survive until hospital discharge after experiencing an in-hospital cardiac arrest (Meaney et al. 2010). International guidelines support performing immediate CPR with early defibrillation when appropriate because it is effective and improves survival rates (Nolan et al. 2010). We may assume that the deteriorating patient who died on the general ward after receiving CPR was supposedly in an earlier phase of deterioration compared to the patient who died unexpectedly without receiving CPR where possibly the deterioration was not even noticed. Furthermore, since early in-hospital CPR improves survival, every inpatient experiencing cardiac arrest should receive CPR when appropriate. For these reasons, death following resuscitation efforts should be differentiated from the fifth short-term outcome: "unexpected death." Unexpected death is defined in the literature as "all deaths without do-not-resuscitate (DNR) order in place" (Hillman et al. 2005). Since not all hospitals have adequate advanced care planning in place that ensures that every patient's resuscitation status is clear and correct, it is possible that this definition is imprecise. Some patients could therefore have died expectedly without a DNR order in place in a palliative or terminal care setting (Yuen et al. 2011). When studying the incidence of in-hospital unexpected death, it is important to choose a technically correct and unequivocal definition. Furthermore, there should be no overlap allowed between the outcomes of death after cardiac arrest with CPR and unexpected death so that results can be clearly interpreted.

## 11.2.3 Factors Associated with Outcomes in Deteriorating Patients

Serious adverse events such as unanticipated admissions to the ICU, cardiac arrest with CPR, and unexpected death have various attributing patient-related and hospital-related factors. When studying outcomes in hospitalized patients, especially across hospitals or units, and over time, it is important to account for factors that are known to affect patient outcomes but are not under the control of the hospital or its staff. This is a process known in the research literature as risk adjustment. We can assume that the patient case mix has an impact on commonly studied outcome indicators. An important type of adjuster that should be considered is the patient comorbidity score. Comorbidities are co-occurring chronic conditions that render patients more vulnerable to complications and introduce challenges in treatment selection and implementation. Comorbidities are associated with hospital mortality, resource utilization, and length of stay (Yang et al. 2010). These associations are found even after adjustment for demographic and clinical characteristics. The Charlson comorbidity index (CCI), one tool widely used internationally, is a useful instrument for measuring comorbid disease status in healthcare research (Christensen et al. 2011). Charlson et al. developed this index by assigning a weighted score to each of 19 common comorbidities (Charlson et al. 1994). High total Charlson comorbidity scores are an indicator of disease burden and are strong predictors of mortality. Various studies demonstrate consistently that the CCI is a valid prognostic tool and equal to more complex severity of illness scores (Christensen et al. 2011).

Various hospital-related factors may also influence the development of serious adverse events such as cardiac arrest with CPR or unexpected death. Hospitals are complex organizations with often strict hierarchical structures that encompass vast numbers of departments, people, and processes. Decisions made by managers about numbers and qualifications of nursing staff and other health professionals and staff members appear to influence patient outcomes in hospitals. A classic study by Aiken et al. documented a relationship between nurse staffing and nurses' education and 30-day inpatient mortality after adjusting for common hospital and patient characteristics. Improved hospital nurse staffing and education is associated with decreased risk of mortality. Similar findings have been reported in other studies (Estabrooks et al. 2005; Aiken et al. 2011). It is also notable that traditionally, hospital managers and clinicians have strong opinions regarding how things need to be done and how different healthcare professionals should work together. This sometimes results in care processes that have not been challenged in decades and do not necessarily reflect research evidence. The current healthcare quality movement has changed the way governments and organizations think about patient safety. Today, the emphasis is on the system of care delivery to prevent errors and even learn from them as they occur. It is well known that the system approach to human errors in healthcare compares quite favorable to approaches focusing on individuals (Reason 2000). The person approach, which has a long history and still predominates in medicine, focuses on the errors of individuals, whereas in the system approach, errors are seen as consequences of ineffective processes in the organization. Traditionally, the detection and escalation of deteriorating patients on the general ward are performed by nurses. The nurse acts as a safeguard for situations that are out of the ordinary. Multiple factors such as the clinical experience of the nurse, existing procedures, and team climate have an influence on this existing barrier against patient harm.

Intuition may play an important role in the decision-making of nurses, but it is a subjective concept that has limited usefulness (Douw et al. 2015). Citing intuition can reflect clinicians' inability to explain what they see is going on with patients ("this patient just does not look good"), or it may stand in for a process where subtle signs observed by experienced nurses and physicians are analyzed quickly. Even if (objective) vital signs are recorded in the deteriorating patient, the interpretation of them depends on the expertise of the nurse and physician. When a deteriorating patient is identified, nurses often have to decide what to do next, and precious time can be lost. Most hospitals have a clear procedure for patients experiencing cardiac arrest on the general ward (start basic life support and call resuscitation team). When dealing with deterioration, rules are often absent, very complicated, or unclear.

Human error influencing the detection and management of the deteriorating patient on the general ward can be divided into skill-based failures and mistakes. Skill-based failures are failures of execution and are termed as slips of action and lapses of memory (Reason 1995). These errors happen when an adequate plan is in place but the associated actions are not adequate (e.g., forgotten vital signs in a postoperative patient). Mistakes can be made when actions go as planned but the underlying plan is not adequate to achieve its intended goal. They can be subdivided into rule-based mistakes and knowledge-based mistakes. A rule-based mistake can, for instance, occur when an existing procedure is not followed or if (and this is often the case) the procedure is unworkable and therefore ignored. A typical example of an unworkable procedure is the cardiology patient who is admitted to a surgical ward because of hospital overcrowding. Nurses are often instructed to call a junior physician responsible for their ward when deterioration occurs. In this case, it could be a surgeon in training responding without sufficient experience to assess and treat the patient. Knowledge-based mistakes occur in novel situations where the problem must be resolved without preexisting solutions or rules. An example is the inexperienced nurse on her first night shift not detecting clinical deterioration in a patient because of a lack of knowledge related to pathophysiology.

Human error can be prevented and mitigated by reducing the chance of skill-based failures and mistakes. Checklists and tools can be used to support the recording of vital signs. The workplace should be designed with ergonomic considerations in mind, and staffing levels should be adequate so skill-based failures are reduced to a minimum. Protocols for care of the deteriorating patient keep differences in hospital and ward characteristics in mind, but there ought to be some hospital-wide procedures that are regularly updated. Furthermore, nurses and physicians need training in communication skills and how to effectively manage deteriorating patients. Clearly a system-based approach is necessary to ensure patient safety on the general ward.

## 11.3   Rapid Response System

Over the last 15 years, various initiatives to prevent serious adverse events such as unanticipated admissions to the ICU, cardiac arrest with CPR, and unexpected death have been proposed and studied by means of randomized clinical trials (NIfHaCE 2007). Studies have repeatedly showed deficiencies in the clinical monitoring of patients and lack of adequate response to those in need of treatment (Hillman et al. 2001; Jacques et al. 2006). Together these observations led to the development and evolution of the concept of the rapid response system (RRS).

An RRS is an umbrella term for all approaches aimed at improving detection and interpretation of in-hospital clinical deterioration and enhancing communication between caregivers around deterioration and the initiation of an appropriate response in a timely manner. Conceptually speaking, an RRS consists of (1) an afferent limb (processes for detecting a patient at risk) which triggers a response, (2) an efferent limb (actions and resources to resolve issues), (3) an administrative limb, and (4) a data acquisition point to improve the process. Researchers continue to work toward identifying the most useful processes in this system (Edelson and Churpek 2012).

## 11.3.1 Efferent Limb

Initiatives located in the efferent limb like the rapid response team (RRT), medical emergency team (MET), patient-at-risk team (PART), or critical care outreach service (CCOS) usually consist of an ICU or emergency department physician and/or critical care nurse(s) who respond to calls from the general ward if specialized help is needed (Jones et al. 2012). The scope and structure of a CCOS differ from other efferent limb initiatives. In many of the forms in which it has been implemented, it has been nurse-led and more proactive in nature, and team activities have included performing rounds to identify patients at risk. Some CCOSs concentrate largely on patients who are discharged from the ICU. Moderate quality of evidence shows that the incorporation of a RRT/MET/PART may improve survival and reduce cardiac arrest rates (McNeill and Bryden 2013). Evidence for the effectiveness of nurse or physician-led CCOSs remains equivocal (McGaughey et al. 2007).

## 11.3.2 The Afferent Limb

It would appear that the success of an RRT/MET/PART is determined in part by the way it is activated. To identify patients' clinical deterioration on the general ward (afferent limb), physiological "track-and-trigger" systems have been introduced to ensure that patients receive timely attention from specialized staff. These systems include the periodic observation of vital signs (track) with agreed criteria as to when to alert personnel who can offer more specialized care (trigger). A wide variety of track and trigger systems exist and can be categorized into single-, multiple parameter and aggregate weighted scoring systems. The latter, also commonly known as early warning scores (EWSs), appear to be the most effective to date (McNeill and Bryden 2013).

The effectiveness of EWSs may be due to it being relatively easy for clinicians using guidelines to place vital signs outside normal physiological limits into clear categories and combine information into in a weighted score that objectively estimates the risk of deterioration. EWSs avoid subjectivity in assessing and reporting the clinical status of the patient. In general, trends toward improved clinical outcomes have been observed after introduction of an EWS (Alam et al. 2014). However, the wide variability in the scoring systems and accompanying practice guidelines evaluated in the literature has made it impossible to draw broad conclusions. Therefore, the Royal College of Physicians in London published a recommendation to standardize the assessment of vital signs in the UK (RCoP 2012). It identified the National Early Warning Score (NEWS), a tool with better predictive power to identify patients at risk for cardiac arrest, unanticipated ICU admission, or death than 33 other EWSs (Smith et al. 2013). These findings were confirmed in subsequent studies (Jarvis et al. 2015; Abbott et al. 2015). However, it is worth mentioning that a scoring system with superior statistical properties does not necessarily result in better clinical outcomes when adopted in clinical settings. All scoring systems simply flag patients in need of clinical review and still require nurses and doctors to have clinical knowledge and insight into the scores in order to reach the correct decisions.

An aggregate root cause analysis of reports concerning serious adverse events (SAEs) on general wards across the UK in 2007 revealed that even when deterioration is recognized and assistance is sought, obtaining medical attention is sometimes delayed (NPSA 2007). Delays could reflect suboptimal interdisciplinary communication, since up to 65% of SAEs include communication as a contributing factor to the event (Haig et al. 2006). The introduction of a structured and standardized communication protocol could help nurses and doctors to communicate in a more effective and efficient way. Introducing the SBAR (situation, background, assessment, and recommendation) communication framework showed an increased perception of effective communication and collaboration in nurses (De Meester et al. 2013b). Additionally, an increase in unplanned ICU admissions and a decrease in unexpected deaths were found.

### 11.3.3 Evaluations to Date

To date the quality of research evidence on RRSs in relation to patient outcomes is poor (Edelson and Churpek 2012; Alam et al. 2014). Hospitals are nonetheless introducing different types of RRSs since preventable in-hospital SAEs are common and need to be addressed. There is no consensus on what the most effective strategy is to prevent SAEs. Numerous before-and-after studies have shown an improvement in patient outcomes after implementing some sort of EWS (afferent limb) (Alam et al. 2014). The use of different scores with different thresholds for activation and the poor or inadequate methodology makes it difficult to draw a general conclusion. Although an EWS seems a simple and easy-to-use tool, the coupled response strategy is not (Alam et al. 2014). Studies such as the MERIT RCT have been focusing on the effect of interventions on the efferent limb (Hillman et al. 2005). They used a single parameter triggering system which activated a doctor-led medical emergency team (MET). The MERIT trial investigators found no significant difference in unexpected death (death without DNAR code), cardiac arrest, or unplanned ICU admissions. Another RCT by Priestley et al. examined the effect of the phased introduction of a critical care outreach team (CCOT) in one general hospital on mortality (Priestley et al. 2004). The CCOT was activated in this study by a non-weighted multiple parameter score. This study suggested that the intervention reduced mortality in general hospital wards by 30% with statistical adjustment for time, gender, age, comorbidity, and ward type (odds ratio 0.70; 95% CI 0.50–0.97). Although numerous before-and-after studies and one RCT suggest an improvement in patient outcomes after implementing some sort of RRS, it is still unclear which components of the RRS are effective and how they should be implemented. A comprehensive approach for future research has been proposed including afferent as well as efferent interventions (McNeill and Bryden 2013). To address the need for research into the afferent loop of RRSs, in 2013 our research group started a multicenter, stepped wedge cluster randomized controlled trial in seven Belgian acute hospitals to investigate the effect of an evidence-based RRS on patient outcomes. The aim of this study was to ascertain the benefit of an evidence-based afferent limb strategy while ensuring an adequate and timely medical response (efferent limb) using existing hospital resources. Therefore, this study was named the Afferent Limb Ascertainment and Response Method (ALARM) intervention trial. The methodology behind the intervention and implementation strategy is explained in detail in the following section.

## 11.4   Intervention and Implementation Strategy

### 11.4.1 Intervention

A "whole system approach," where both afferent and efferent limbs of the response system are considered, should be adopted to ensure effectiveness of a rapid response system (McNeill and Bryden 2013). It is also clear that a comprehensive implementation strategy is needed to ensure adoption of this new intervention in routine clinical practice. In a research project funded by the Belgian government, we introduced and evaluated the impact of an RRS in seven Belgian acute hospitals. Our intervention was based on the latest available evidence and comprised an afferent and efferent limb. We introduced a standardized observation protocol where nurses were required to calculate the NEWS in all patients at ward admission and subsequently every 12 h. The NEWS resulted in four levels of clinical risk for deterioration: zero, low, medium, and high. The observation frequency required by the protocol corresponded to these four levels. A patient with zero risk had to be observed every 12 h, while a patient with a medium risk had to be observed every hour. In some cases, patients had a high baseline NEWS at admission (e.g., COPD patients with lower oxygen saturation). On doctor's orders in the patient record, deviations from these observation frequencies or call criteria were allowed (Fig. 11.3).

A standardized response strategy linked to the levels of clinical risk resulting from the NEWS was initiated. It listed interventions, who to contact including

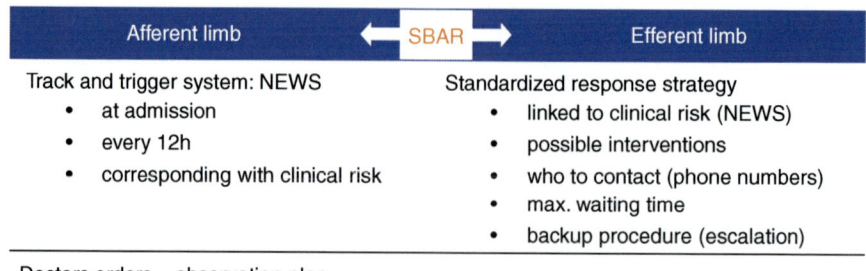

**Fig. 11.3** Intervention

phone numbers, a maximum waiting time for medical assistance, and a backup procedure if the regular medical response was late or unavailable. We did not include a rapid response team in our intervention because it required additional hospital resources that simply were not available. It was made clear to all clinicians that this system was in place to detect and respond to early deterioration and that when a patient was clinically unstable, the resuscitation team should be called. Because hospitals and even wards have different approaches when attending patients, we allowed some flexibility in defining the medical response strategy while still ensuring protocol adherence. To connect the afferent and efferent limbs, we emphasized a sound and clear communication technique using the SBAR (situation, background, assessment, and recommendation) communication method which is a standardized and concise way of communicating. When using SBAR, nurses are motivated to collect all relevant data concerning the patient including the vital signs and medical history before calling a physician. This ensures that no time is wasted and the patient is treated early.

## 11.4.2 Implementation Strategy

Compliance rates after translating scientific evidence into practice are often disappointingly low (Grol and Grimshaw 2003). A comprehensive and improved implementation strategy is necessary to achieve the adoption of new innovations in care (Huis et al. 2013). Plans to improve patient safety that prevent complications, morbidity, and mortality should therefore address barriers and facilitators for change. Researchers have recognized that every individual's decision concerning an innovation results from a specific process that occurs over time (Rogers 1995). Our intervention was based on Rogers "innovation-decision process" which describes five sequential stages (Fig. 11.4).

In the first stage (knowledge), individuals have three main concerns: "What is the innovation?," "How does it work?," and "Why does it work?." To answer these questions regarding our innovation, we started with a 4-h interactive training

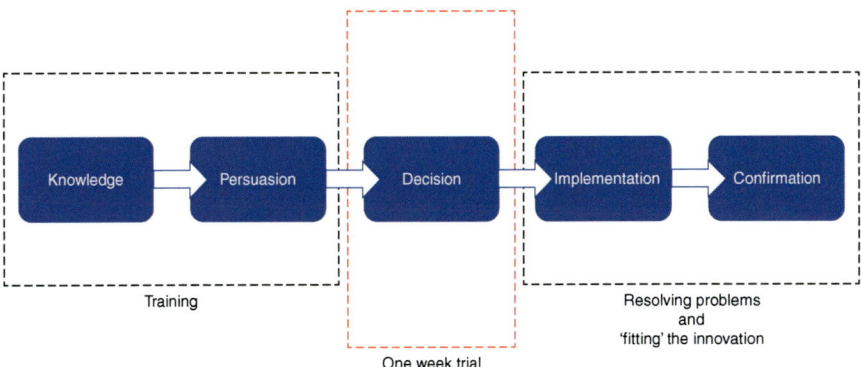

**Fig. 11.4** Innovation-decision process (Rogers 1995)

session for nurses and physicians concerning the measurement and interpretation of vital signs, clinical observation, communication skills when dealing with deteriorating patients, and practical tips and tricks in handling NEWS and SBAR. We started each session with a 20-min discussion about clinicians' own experiences concerning deteriorating patients on the general ward. Sometimes, when people were hesitant to share their stories, the trainers shared an impactful real-life example from their own experience. We assured participants that the training session was confidential and emphasized the importance of an open and nonpunitive climate when talking about local patient safety concerns. It is also important to mention that even though training sessions were given to multiple wards at the same time, clinicians were not hesitant to share problems they experienced on their own ward. This is because a feeling of solidarity was deliberately created by the trainers ("we're all experiencing the same problems across the country"). After this discussion, selective exposure (the avoidance of conflicting messages) was minimized because most clinicians perceived the innovation as relevant to their needs and consistent with their existing attitudes and beliefs. After this introduction, we explained using recent patient safety literature: the importance of patient monitoring, the crucial role of the nurse in detecting deterioration, and the problems regarding interdisciplinary communication. The strategy of the trainers was to link all theory with own examples and the experiences of participants shared at the beginning of the session. Active participation was stimulated by asking questions throughout the session. Subsequently, we explained our intervention ("how should we use it?") including possible issues that participants could experience during implementation. We allowed some time for questions and answers and provided social reinforcement by sharing success stories from other hospitals. We know that in this stage (persuasion), participants are mentally applying the innovation to their work environment ("what will be the advantages and disadvantages in my situation?") and a favorable or unfavorable attitude is formed toward the innovation.

The interactive training was always planned 2 weeks before the start of the intervention. It is known that most individuals will not adopt an innovation without trying it first. Therefore, we organized a "1-week trial" the week before the official start of the intervention. During this week nurses and physicians could test the innovation and make the necessary adjustments to their daily work routines. Interdisciplinary agreements concerning the efferent limb were proposed by a project manager (often a nurse or doctor in a management position) so that adaptations could still be made considering local habits and practicalities. This was done to ensure maximum "fit" of our standardized intervention with hospital- and ward-specific characteristics. It also empowered clinicians and avoided early rejection of the intervention because of the possible incompatibility with ward and hospital resources. We explained that this was a dynamic process because changes could still be made throughout the study period. This pragmatic implementation strategy helped individuals and care teams to adjust to the innovation and resolve possible problems. When teams put an innovation into use, the implementation stage is reached. The new idea is now actually in use on the general ward. Problems concerning the usage of the innovation could crop up at this stage. We therefore organized monthly meetings with all project managers of all participating hospitals so they could ask for help and exchange ideas with their peers. On the wards, we asked for two volunteers to act as project nurses who could resolve small problems themselves or escalate bigger problems to their hospital project managers. The last step in the innovation-decision process is the confirmation stage where individuals or care teams seek reinforcement for the innovation decision already made. It is important that, if work environments change, innovations are positioned to so that adaptation can take place to these new situations to avoid rejection.

Because of the importance of team performance when introducing an innovation to improve patient safety issues, we applied a literature-based state-of-the-art strategy supplemented with interventions based on theory around social influence and leadership (Table 11.1) (Huis et al. 2013).

## 11.5   Barriers and Facilitators Influencing RRS Adoption

During this research project, we could differentiate barriers and facilitators at three levels that could have a possible impact on the adoption of an RRS on the general ward in acute hospitals (Fig. 11.5).

In this research project, we experienced a fair number of problems before but mostly during implementation of the RRSs. Adoption was sometimes very difficult or even impossible when clinicians perceived the innovation as "extra work without any benefit." This happened predominantly on wards where nurses complained about staffing levels due to absence of colleagues on sick leave without replacements. We also noticed that while they were always invited, few physicians attended the interactive training sessions. This led to limited awareness of the problem among physicians and appeared to undermine motivation to participate in the study. Compliance to our protocol was also difficult on wards with a negative social climate where there was inadequate support from ward managers. On one occasion a ward manager was not convinced of the usefulness of the intervention and therefore did not accommodate our request to bring the intervention to the unit. There were hospitals where they were not prepared to collect data concerning processes and

**Table 11.1** State-of-the-art strategy

| Education |
|---|
| • Training based on the innovation-decision process |
| • Written protocol available on every ward |
| • Online educational material on a central website with the possibility for self-assessment |
| Reminders |
| • Posters explaining the intervention |
| • Publications in hospital magazines |
| • General reminders and support by ward and hospital management |
| Feedback |
| • Process indicators on a performance dashboard (maintained by the project manager, ward manager, or project nurses) |
| Facilities and products |
| • Screening for, and if necessary, adaptation of facilities and products (e.g., every nurse received a personal watch to measure the respiratory rate) |
| *Team and leaders-directed strategy* |
| Setting norms and targets within the team |
| • Team meeting together with the project manager (2 weeks after the intervention) to set norms and targets and to solve problems |
| • Nurses address each other in the case of non-compliance to the innovation |
| Getting active commitment of the ward management |
| • The ward manager designated patient safety as a priority |
| • The ward manager supports the team and project nurses |
| • Process indicators are discussed in the team by the ward manager |
| Modeling by informal leaders |
| • Two volunteers become a project nurse on their own ward supported by ward management and the project manager |
| • They address problems and manage the practicalities during and after implementation of the innovation on their own ward |

A state-of-the-art strategy supplemented with interventions based on social influence and leadership based on Huis et al. (2013)

RRS adoption

| | Barriers | Facilitators |
|---|---|---|
| Health care professional | • Perceived increased workload<br>• Low nurse staffing<br>• Limited awareness of the problem | • Sense of responsibility<br>• The need for unambiguous rules |
| Team | • Non–supportive (in)formal leaders<br>• Hierarchic strutures<br>• Negative social climate | • Supportive (in)formal leadres<br>• Recent incidents (urgency)<br>• Evaluating team performance |
| Organisation | • Top–down leadership<br>• Not measuring patient outcomes or processes<br>• Logistical problems | • Accreditation<br>• Safety and health management system<br>• Supportive medical and nursing leader |

**Fig. 11.5** Barriers and facilitators possibly influencing adoption of an RRS

patient outcomes because of the workload involved. Logistical problems (e.g., monitors to check vital signs not available) were not common but did result into the dropout of one hospital.

Fewer problems to implement the RRS were seen when unit clinicians took on responsibility and had the motivation to make the project move forward. A good example of this was seen in a nurse manager who struggled daily with deteriorating patients on her ward without finding a comprehensive solution to her ongoing problem. She lost valuable time every day in supporting her staff to improve their practice, with the intention of saving patient lives, and was therefore very eager to implement our innovation. We also noticed that the intervention led to clear agreements and rules where they were vague or nonexistent before. Some ward managers really needed the 1-week trial period to adjust their daily work routines to new practices. The supportive role of (in)formal leaders facilitated the adoption of our intervention. Some project managers took ward managers or even project nurses to our monthly meetings in order to empower their employees. Because of the occurrence of a recent serious adverse event on one of the wards, adoption went fast without any significant problems. Clinicians were still traumatized about what happened, and they wanted safety measures in place so it would not happen again. In wards where the performance of the team was measured (e.g., current observation frequency vs. their goal), people felt more motivated to improve.

Project managers let us know that sometimes an ongoing accreditation process was the driving motor behind the successes they booked. Every hospital had a safety and health management system in place, but some hospitals used the systems in place to evaluate the effectiveness of the RRS, and it motivated them to continue forward because they noticed changes in care and outcomes. It came as no surprise that when organizations had supportive medical and nursing leaders, the adoption was less problematic.

## Conclusion

In this chapter, we reviewed key concepts and important research findings around the issue of identifying and responding to clinical deterioration and then discussed the implementation of a rapid response system in Belgian hospitals using an evidence-based strategy to standardize care processes on general wards. The implementation of a new care process into a dynamic and continuously changing organization is a challenging process influenced by numerous factors. First, before changing practice it is important to clearly define associated process and outcome indicators. We know that commonly used indicators could be imprecise and difficult to collect. Especially mortality, an often-used and seemingly evident patient outcome indicator, is sometimes difficult to interpret in the existing literature. Second, not only outcome indicators should be collected but also factors contributing to these outcomes. This is of importance when hospitals compare results before and after an intervention because of the possible influence of time. Third, more high-quality research is needed since much of the existing evidence about the effectiveness of RRSs is of poor methodological quality. To date, we do not know which components of the RRS are effective and how it should be implemented. Lastly, we proposed an RRS with an evidence-based afferent limb and a pragmatic efferent limb including a state-of-the-art implementation strategy supplemented with interventions based on social influence and leadership. The crucial factor of our implementation strategy is the flexibility to adapt to different and changing environmental conditions. A one-size-fits-all approach would likely be less effective because of the considerable differences between hospitals and even general wards.

*This chapter is a part of a doctoral project supervised by Koenraad Monsieurs and Peter Van Bogaert and funded by the Belgian Federal Government.*

## References

Abbott TE, Vaid N, Ip D, et al. A single-centre observational cohort study of admission National Early Warning Score (NEWS). Resuscitation. 2015;92:89–93.

Aiken LH, Cimiotti JP, Sloane DM, et al. Effects of nurse staffing and nurse education on patient deaths in hospitals with different nurse work environments. Med Care. 2011;49:1047–53.

Alam N, Hobbelink EL, van Tienhoven AJ, et al. The impact of the use of the Early Warning Score (EWS) on patient outcomes: a systematic review. Resuscitation. 2014;85:587–94.

Charlson M, Szatrowski TP, Peterson J, et al. Validation of a combined comorbidity index. J Clin Epidemiol. 1994;47:1245–51.

Christensen S, Johansen MB, Christiansen CF, et al. Comparison of Charlson comorbidity index with SAPS and APACHE scores for prediction of mortality following intensive care. Clin Epidemiol. 2011;3:203–11.

De Meester K, Van Bogaert P, Clarke SP, et al. In-hospital mortality after serious adverse events on medical and surgical nursing units: a mixed methods study. J Clin Nurs. 2013a;22:2308–17.

De Meester K, Verspuy M, Monsieurs KG, et al. SBAR improves nurse-physician communication and reduces unexpected death: a pre and post intervention study. Resuscitation. 2013b;84:1192–6.

Douw G, Schoonhoven L, Holwerda T, et al. Nurses' worry or concern and early recognition of deteriorating patients on general wards in acute care hospitals: a systematic review. Crit Care. 2015;19:230.

Edelson DP, Churpek MM. Sifting through the heterogeneity of the rapid response system literature. Resuscitation. 2012;83:1419–20.

Estabrooks CA, Midodzi WK, Cummings GG, et al. The impact of hospital nursing characteristics on 30-day mortality. Nurs Res. 2005;54:74–84.

Findlay GP, Shotton H, Kelly K, et al. Time to intervene? A review of patients who underwent cardiopulmonary resuscitation as a result of an in-hospital cardiorespiratory arrest: a report by the national confidential enquiry into patient outcome and death. 2012.

Goldhill DR, White SA, Sumner A. Physiological values and procedures in the 24 h before ICU admission from the ward. Anaesthesia. 1999;54:529–34.

Grol R, Grimshaw J. From best evidence to best practice: effective implementation of change in patients' care. Lancet. 2003;362:1225–30.

Haig KM, Sutton S, Whittington J. SBAR: a shared mental model for improving communication between clinicians. Jt Comm J Qual Patient Saf. 2006;32:167–75.

Hillman KM, Bristow PJ, Chey T, et al. Antecedents to hospital deaths. Intern Med J. 2001;31:343–8.

Hillman K, Chen J, Cretikos M, et al. Introduction of the medical emergency team (MET) system: a cluster-randomised controlled trial. Lancet. 2005;365:2091–7.

Hogan H, Healey F, Neale G, et al. Preventable deaths due to problems in care in English acute hospitals: a retrospective case record review study. BMJ Qual Saf. 2012;21:737–45.

Huis A, Schoonhoven L, Grol R, et al. Impact of a team and leaders-directed strategy to improve nurses' adherence to hand hygiene guidelines: a cluster randomised trial. Int J Nurs Stud. 2013;50:464–74.

Jacques T, Harrison GA, McLaws ML, et al. Signs of critical conditions and emergency responses (SOCCER): a model for predicting adverse events in the inpatient setting. Resuscitation. 2006;69:175–83.

Jarvis S, Kovacs C, Briggs J, et al. Aggregate National Early Warning Score (NEWS) values are more important than high scores for a single vital signs parameter for discriminating the risk of adverse outcomes. Resuscitation. 2015;87:75–80.

Jones D, Drennan K, et al. Rapid Response Team composition, resourcing and calling criteria in Australia. Resuscitation. 2012;83:563–7.

Khandelwal N, Kross EK, Engelberg RA, et al. Estimating the effect of palliative care interventions and advance care planning on ICU utilization: a systematic review. Crit Care Med. 2015;43:1102–11.

Kohn LT, Corrigan JM, Donaldson MS. To Err is Human: building a safer health system. Washington, DC: National Academies Press; 2000.

Maharaj R, Raffaele I, Wendon J. Rapid response systems: a systematic review and meta-analysis. Crit Care. 2015;19:254.

Marquet K, Claes N, De Troy E, et al. One fourth of unplanned transfers to a higher level of care are associated with a highly preventable adverse event: a patient record review in six Belgian hospitals. Crit Care Med. 2015;43:1053–61.

McDonald CJ, Weiner M, Hui SL. Deaths due to medical errors are exaggerated in Institute of Medicine report. JAMA. 2000;284:93–5.

McGaughey J, Alderdice F, Fowler R, et al. Outreach and Early Warning Systems (EWS) for the prevention of intensive care admission and death of critically ill adult patients on general hospital wards. Cochrane Database Syst Rev. 2007;3:CD005529.

McNeill G, Bryden D. Do either early warning systems or emergency response teams improve hospital patient survival? A systematic review. Resuscitation. 2013;84:1652–67.

Meaney PA, Nadkarni VM, Kern KB, et al. Rhythms and outcomes of adult in-hospital cardiac arrest. Crit Care Med. 2010;38:101–8.

Mercier E, Giraudeau B, Giniès G, et al. Iatrogenic events contributing to ICU admission: a prospective study. Intensive Care Med. 2010;36:1033–7.

NIfHaCE. NICE clinical guideline 50 Acutely ill patients in hospital: recognition of and response to acute illness in adults in hospital. London: National Institute for Health and Clinical Excellence; 2007.

Nolan JP, Soar J, Zideman DA, et al. European Resuscitation Council Guidelines for Resuscitation 2010 Section 1. Executive summary. Resuscitation. 2010;81:1219–76.

NPSA. Recognising and responding appropriately to early signs of deterioration in hospitalised patients. London: National Patient Safety Agency; 2007.

Priestley G, Watson W, Rashidian A, et al. Introducing critical care outreach: a ward-randomised trial of phased introduction in a general hospital. Intensive Care Med. 2004;30:1398–404.

RCoP. National Early Warning Score (NEWS): Standardising the assessment of acute-illness severity in the NHS. Report of a working party in the Royal College of Physicians 2012.

Reason J. Understanding adverse events: human factors. Qual Saf Health Care. 1995;4:80–9.

Reason J. Human error: models and management. BMJ. 2000;320(7237):768.

Rogers EM. Diffusion of innovations. 4th ed. New York: Free Press; 1995.

Sandroni C, Nolan J, Cavallaro F, et al. In-hospital cardiac arrest: incidence, prognosis and possible measures to improve survival. Intensive Care Med. 2007;33:237–45.

Smith GB, Prytherch DR, Meredith P, et al. The ability of the National Early Warning Score (NEWS) to discriminate patients at risk of early cardiac arrest, unanticipated intensive care unit admission, and death. Resuscitation. 2013;84:465–70.

Stelfox HT, Hemmelgarn BR, Bagshaw SM, et al. Intensive care unit bed availability and outcomes for hospitalized patients with sudden clinical deterioration. Arch Intern Med. 2012;172:467–74.

Vlayen A, Verelst S, Bekkering GE, et al. Incidence and preventability of adverse events requiring intensive care admission: a systematic review. J Eval Clin Pract. 2012;18:485–97.

Yang Y, Yang KS, Hsann YM, et al. The effect of comorbidity and age on hospital mortality and length of stay in patients with sepsis. J Crit Care. 2010;25:398–405.

Yuen JK, Reid MC, Fetters MD. Hospital do-not-resuscitate orders: why they have failed and how to fix them. J Gen Int Med. 2011;26:791–7.

# Interprofessional Collaboration and Communication

12

Martijn Verspuy and Peter Van Bogaert

**Abstract**

Interprofessional collaboration is crucial in hospitals because healthcare teams face challenges, such as complexity of clinical practice, high variation in clinical demand, ever-changing teams, and heavy workload. Moreover, communication between professionals does not always flow as it should. Ineffective or absent interprofessional collaboration has a negative impact on patient outcomes, such as medication errors, failure to rescue, increased hospital-acquired infection rates, and extended lengths of stay. Ineffective collaboration between healthcare workers was linked to two out of every three sentinel events (severe adverse events) reported to the Joint Commission's databases. Developing effective teams and redesigned systems is vital to achieving safer, timelier, more patient-centered, effective, efficient, and equitable patient care. We can look at the Interprofessional Education Collaborative or IPEC competency framework for the competencies teams need to master to achieve role clarity, clear communication, and excellent teamwork and create a climate of mutual respect and shared values. The TeamSTEPSS educational intervention package can be used for improving team performance. In order to ensure the best possible patient outcomes, a smooth flow of collaboration and communication in the triangle between clinical nurses, nurse managers, and physicians can overcome turbulence and uncertainty in healthcare settings.

M. Verspuy (✉)
Nursing Department, Antwerp University Hospital, Antwerp, Belgium

Nursing and Midwifery Sciences, Centre for Research and Innovation in Care (CRIC), Faculty of Medicine and Health Sciences, University of Antwerp, Antwerp, Belgium
e-mail: martijn.verspuy@uza.be

P. Van Bogaert
Nursing and Midwifery Sciences, Centre for Research and Innovation in Care (CRIC), Faculty of Medicine and Health Sciences, University of Antwerp, Antwerp, Belgium

© Springer International Publishing AG 2018
P. Van Bogaert, S. Clarke (eds.), *The Organizational Context of Nursing Practice*,
https://doi.org/10.1007/978-3-319-71042-6_12

**Keywords**

Interprofessional collaboration • Communication • Patient-centered care • System design • Clinical nurse-nurse manager-physician triangle • Patient safety • IPEC competency framework

## 12.1 Introduction

The World Health Organization described interprofessional collaboration as "multiple health care workers from different professional backgrounds, provide comprehensive services by working with patients, their families, caregivers and community to deliver highest quality of care across different settings" (Hopkins 2010, p. 7). Interprofessional collaboration on nursing wards has been defined simply as "clinical nurses, nurse managers and physicians working together, sharing responsibilities for solving problems, and making decisions to formulate and carry out plans for patient care" (Baggs et al. 1997).

Interprofessional collaboration is especially crucial in hospitals, where healthcare teams face a number of challenges, such as complexity of clinical practice, high variation in clinical demand, ever-changing teams, and heavy workloads. When interdisciplinary teams experience collaboration at its best, the quality of care improves. The Robert Wood Johnson Foundation has stated that interprofessional collaboration contributes to the use of individual and collective skills and experience of team members, allowing them to function more effectively and deliver a higher level of care than when each would work alone. Clinical nurses, nurse managers, and physicians make up the largest group of healthcare providers, and all confront complex problems on a daily basis (Keenan et al. 1998). However, communication between professions does not always flow as it should. An increasing volume of literature reports that an ineffective or a lack of interprofessional collaboration has a negative impact on patient outcomes, such as medication errors, failure to rescue, increase of infection rates, and extended length of stay (Martin et al. 2010). The Joint Commission (Commission 2016) reported in 2015 that two out of three reported incidents were based on ineffective collaboration between healthcare workers. In acute care settings, effective interprofessional collaboration is important to address challenges in healthcare such as increased complexity of clinical practice and heavy workloads. Increased perceived workloads affect the quality of care and nurse well-being, and heavy workloads may affect patient safety because they restrict the ability of healthcare workers to communicate effectively with each other.

In sum, improving interprofessional collaboration and communication is vital to improve patient outcomes and nurses' work environment. The aim of this chapter is to explore the collaboration and communication in the triangle linking clinical nurses, nurse managers, and physicians on medical and surgical wards and to present strategies discussed in the literature for improving collaboration and communication as an organizational and interdisciplinary means of ensuring high-quality patient outcomes.

### 12.1.1  Definition

A wide variety of definitions of collaboration can be found in the literature; this heterogeneity in the use of terms creates complications in comparing research studies. Authors use terms such as multidisciplinary, interprofessional, teamwork, interdisciplinary, and joined-up thinking interchangeably. Mahler et al. (2014) explain how choice of terminology can be influenced by the researcher's native language. Nevertheless, in order to compare study results and interventions across studies, an unambiguous definition of interprofessional collaboration is essential.

## 12.2  Competencies for Interprofessional Collaboration

In order to ensure high-quality interprofessional collaboration, healthcare workers need to develop a set of competencies. The *Core Competencies for Interprofessional Collaborative Practice*, developed by US experts representing a variety of health professions, is a framework consisting of five domains (Panel IECE 2011): (1) communication, (2) teams and teamwork, (3) roles and responsibilities, (4) leadership, and (5) values and ethics. Definitions of the domains and their relationships to collaboration are depicted in Fig. 12.1.

An interesting challenge arises around managing the confidentiality of the practitioner-patient relationship when professional borders fade and teams function as units. Patients discuss a great deal of personal and sometimes very private

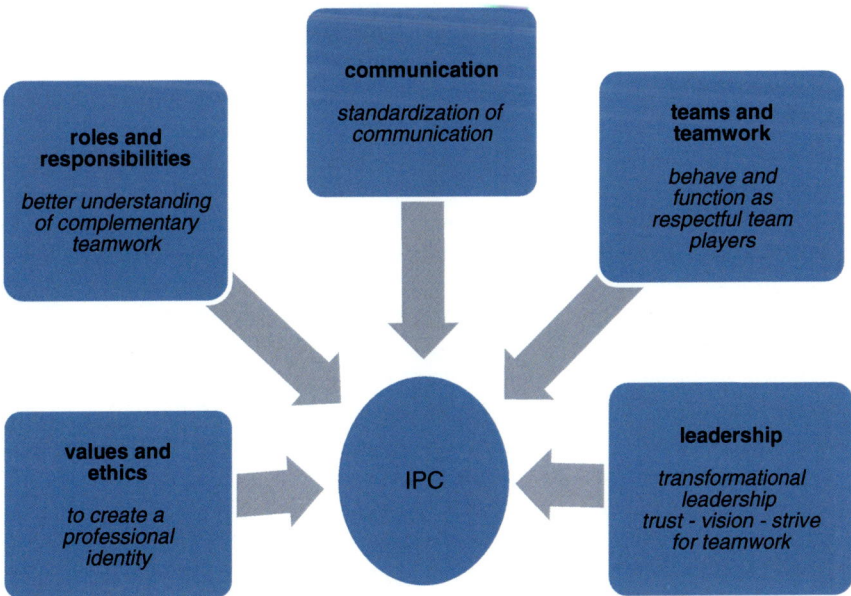

**Fig. 12.1**  Competency framework

information with health professionals. It sometimes happens that patients explicitly request that specific pieces of information not be shared with the rest of the healthcare team. Careful consideration must be given to the benefits as well as risks and harms of withholding potentially important information from team members from an ethical standpoint.

## 12.3 Interprofessional Collaboration Triangle of Clinical Nurses, Nurse Managers, and Physicians on Medical and Surgical Nursing Wards

When physicians and nurses cooperate interprofessionally, the effectiveness of care increases. Since physicians and nurses can be supportive of each other in carrying out tasks and can share expertise and experiences, this can increase patient safety and improve patient outcomes (Martin et al. 2010; Ontario RNAo 2013). In addition, improved interprofessional collaboration has been linked with reduced lengths of stay, lower mortality rates, and fewer referrals to the intensive care unit (Epstein 2014; Martin et al. 2010; Baggs et al. 1997). In the literature, interprofessional collaboration is also associated with benefits for caregivers. High-quality interprofessional collaboration between clinical nurses and physicians is typically related to increases in job satisfaction, greater commitment to teams, reductions in turnover, greater use of evidence in care, higher patient centeredness, and superior clinical outcomes (Galletta et al. 2016; Ontario RNAo 2013) as well as higher patient satisfaction (Ontario RNAo 2013). Cummings and colleagues have found in their research that failures of nurses and physicians to work as interprofessional teams have also been linked to increases in patient mortality (Cummings 2013).

Physicians, nurse managers, and clinical nurses often have completely different visions of interprofessional collaboration, in part because they see collaboration through their own roles and responsibilities (House and Havens 2017; Muller-Juge et al. 2013, 2014). Clinical nurses, nurse managers, and physicians also tend to hold different opinions regarding nurses' autonomy, shared decision-making, team roles, and interdependency (Muller-Juge et al. 2013). Studies have shown that the experience of interprofessional collaboration differs among physicians, nurse managers, and clinical nurses (Bowles et al. 2016; Collette et al. 2017). Some studies have shown that clinical nurses have more positive views of interprofessional collaboration than physicians (Caricati et al. 2016) because of different vantage and mental models and perceptions of interprofessional collaboration (Muller-Juge et al. 2013; Matziou et al. 2014). Another study showed that nurse involvement in ward rounds may have a positive influence on nurse-physician collaboration that in turn leads to a more open communication and shared decision-making processes (Caricati et al. 2016) and contribute to emergence of shared mental models (Henkin et al. 2016). Heavy workloads for clinical nurses and physicians combined with an absence of nurses on ward rounds were described as barriers to interprofessional collaboration (Suarez et al. 2017).

Clinical nurse, nurse manager, and physician communication has yet other impacts. Good communication occurs when messages are clear and communicated in a respectful way. Yet communication between the different disciplines sometimes is ineffective, and physicians, nurse managers, and clinical nurses may not exchange sufficient information for safe care delivery. Hierarchies can also constitute a barrier to communication. As mentioned earlier, clinical nurses, nurse managers, and physicians each have different roles to fulfill. Sometimes these roles lead to conflicts. The CanMEDS model contains seven roles: (medical) expert, communicator, collaborator, leader, health advocate, scholar, and professional; in order to ensure a high quality of care, healthcare workers need to manage these seven roles. In daily practice role conflicts occur. Health professionals can define and locate problems within their specific roles/competencies (Kassam et al. 2016).

Clinical nurses, nurse managers, and physicians tend to work next to each other instead of with each other. It is important for healthcare leaders to endorse a common vision of interprofessional collaborative practice. This is especially true for particularly nurse managers, who can have a pivotal role in providing the means to achieve effective communication and interprofessional collaboration (Manojlovich and Talsma 2007). Skills in communication, quality improvement, and collaboration are needed to build interpersonal trust, create a common vision, and achieve the synergies possible with teamwork (Ontario RNAo 2013).

Successful nurse managers, who focus on people and relationships as well as on shared decision-making and social capital within the team (Van Bogaert et al. 2013), tend to manage units where there is less emotional exhaustion, better teamwork with physicians and others , higher job satisfaction and other employee outcomes, and superior clinical outcomes (Cummings et al. 2010; Ontario RNAo 2013). These relationships also function in the reverse direction—teams that communicate well and collaborate effectively will often stimulate transformational leadership (Ontario RNAo 2013). The nurse manager must reach some degree of resolution between proximity to and distance from clinical practice. The nurse manager adopts a role as a mediator and balances attention to oversight of nursing care and attention to leadership (Sorensen et al. 2011) and faces barriers in doing so: fluctuating team capacity, high workloads, lack of time, and insufficient support. As a consequence, difficulties are experienced in adequately monitoring the clinical process and achieving goals (Rankin et al. 2016). Ultimately, nurse managers are ideally leaders of the nursing team who establish and support a culture of open feedback with a view to continuous quality improvement. Often nurse managers serve as intermediaries between clinical nurses and physicians to discuss issues regarding collaboration and patient care. Balancing between those two pursuits—being a leader and being a quality manager at the same time—is seen as a real challenge (Carlin and Duffy 2013; Eggenberger 2012; McCallin and Frankson 2010; Rankin et al. 2016; Sorensen et al. 2011), and how best to juggle these functions has not always been clear for nurse managers (Eggenberger 2012; McCallin and Frankson 2010). Role ambiguity can be an explanatory factor for experiencing difficulties in carrying out the job of a nurse manager. Feelings of overwork, powerlessness, and frustration can also be the result of perceiving high expectations from others and an overload of tasks (McCallin and Frankson 2010). In a Belgian study, one out of every six nursing unit managers demonstrated high to very high levels of emotional exhaustion; however, two out of three showed high to very high work engagement. Hierarchical regression models showed that role conflict and role meaningfulness, along with various job and organizational characteristics, were strong predictors of nursing unit managers' work-related stress and well-being. The authors concluded that the next challenge is to develop appropriate interventional strategies to support nursing unit managers and their teams in daily practice in delivering the best and safest possible patient care (Van Bogaert et al. 2014).

The main goal of every healthcare team should be to achieve an excellent interprofessional collaborative patient-centered practice. The next section of this chapter will describe systems to improve interprofessional collaboration and patient safety. The conditions for implementing interprofessional collaboration have been widely described and discussed, but the literature describing how to translate them as completely as possible into practice is rather sparse.

The trick is not to be bound by any one strategy but to blend to context.

(Charles Vincent, 2016)

## 12.4    Systems to Improve Interprofessional Collaboration: Clinical Microsystems, Human Factors Engineering Model SEIPS 2.0, and TeamSTEPPS

This section presents three frameworks that can be used to improve interprofessional collaboration and improve quality of care.

### 12.4.1 Clinical Microsystems

Clinical microsystems are the building blocks of a healthcare system. Nelson and colleagues describe a healthcare clinical microsystem as:

> a small group of people (including healthcare professionals and care-receiving patients and their families) who work together in a defined setting on a regular basis (or as needed) to create care for discrete subpopulations of patients. As a functioning unit it has clinical and business aims, linked processes and a shared information environment, and it produces performance outcomes. Microsystems evolve over time and are embedded in larger organisations. As a living, complex, adaptive system, the microsystem has many functions, which include (1) to do the work associated with core aims, (2) to meet member needs, and (3) to maintain itself over time as a functioning clinical unit (Nelson et al. 2007).

Each element of the term "clinical microsystem" has particular significance. *Clinical* refers to the type of work that is the true priority of healthcare. *Micro* refers to the smallest replicable unit of healthcare delivery (e.g., nursing ward). A *system* is a unit that has a common goal and consists of people, processes, technologies, and patterns of information that interact and is dynamic such as SEIPS. It is the place where patients, families, and caregivers meet. Therefore, clinical microsystems always have a patient at their centers. Deming, White, and Donabedian all addressed similar clusters of ideas, but one person can be designated as the founding father of the clinical microsystem: James Brian Quinn. Quinn focused his attention on excellent organizations and the reasons why they were so successful. He discovered that all these organizations had one thing in common: they focused on the smallest replicable units within their organizations. Research performed on complex and adaptive systems has shown that every complex system has structures, processes, patterns, and outcomes (Nelson et al. 2007). The anatomy of clinical microsystems is based on these elements. In fact, the writers in the clinical microsystems have gone even further and developed the well-known 5Ps: *purpose, patients, professionals, processes*, and *patterns*. In order to improve clinical microsystems, it is vital that caregivers have a rich knowledge of the physiology of their microsystem. Nelson et al. (2007) described this as the "anatomy and physiology" model that can be used to make a systematic assessment of the performance of the microsystem and formulate recommendations for improvement and innovation. Key elements linked to the success of clinical microsystem can be divided in five groups: leadership, performance, staff, patients, and information and technology.

### 12.4.1.1 How Can Clinical Microsystems Improve Patient Safety and Ameliorate Interprofessional Collaboration?

The clinical microsystems approach can be combined with conceptual and practical frameworks to evaluate and improve the delivery of care. Interprofessional collaboration in clinical microsystems is critical to an efficient and safe working climate. It is crucial that clinical nurses, physicians, and patients work together in order to have a shared care plan. This can only happen when healthcare workers (e.g., clinical nurses, nurse managers, and physicians) respect each other's roles and responsibilities, communicate effectively, and have a shared vision of patient-centered care. Creating a safe working climate is essential to function as a high interdependence team. Therefore, clinical microsystems have six principles in order to achieve this level of safety (Nelson et al. 2007).

1. When an error occurs the focus will be on the system and looking for multiple contributing factors instead of seeing errors as individual problems. In that way the system can be improved/redesigned.
2. Microsystems need to include safety principles in their daily routines and simulate error-prone situations that occur on a regular or non-regular basis so that teams know how to respond consistently. Teams that are skilled and trained have better outcomes in acute care settings.
3. Design systems that contain opportunities to identify, prevent, absorb, and mitigate errors. Transparency of data is essential. Make sure that every team member has the knowledge to interpret data. Apply simple, understandable, and standardized protocols. Make sure that the system is designed to absorb errors before they reach the patient.

4. Create a culture where clinical nurses, nurse managers, and physicians report errors, near misses, and adverse events and consider them as opportunities to learn.
5. Listen to patients and involve them in creating a safe climate. Give patients and their families the opportunity to provide feedback about safety matters on nursing wards.
6. As mentioned, patient-centered care—with integrated practices from human factors engineering—is the key to success in a clinical microsystem.

Clinical microsystems are primarily a theoretical idea; because microsystems are so complex and different professionals are involved in them, conducting replicable research on them is very difficult. Quality improvement projects are often not published in peer-reviewed journals because they are conducted using an iterative and empiric process, and therefore they are not evaluated using controlled designs. However, the strength of clinical microsystems is that there are constant opportunities for quality improvement drawing upon their teams' in-depth understandings of processes, structures, and team composition—clinical nurses, nurse managers, and ward physicians can be constantly engaged in quality measurement and improvement on a daily basis. This is important because often, externally driven quality improvement goals are not reached.

In 2000, the National Health Service (NHS) initiated an improvement project to evaluate the potential for clinical microsystems to improve the performance of the UK healthcare system (Williams et al. 2009). Semi-structured interviews were held to evaluate the role of clinical microsystems in daily work. Respondents in settings where clinical microsystems approach were implemented unanimously stated that they experienced better team cohesiveness, mutual support, and communication that led to identifying areas of strengths and opportunities to improve. Another benefit was an increase of empowerment in frontline staff clinical nurses, who were given a platform to take an active role in quality improvement on their nursing wards. Improvements in role clarity were also mentioned. Higgins and Cole-Poklewski (2010) used a qualitative approach to studying the impact of the clinical microsystems model on nursing wards. After conducting interviews they concluded that after implementing the clinical microsystems model, clinical nurses experienced an increase of productivity and that satisfaction levels remained strong. Most of these outcomes have been evaluated qualitatively or subjectively (i.e., are "soft" outcomes) and mostly directed to two Ps: people and processes. What about the "hard" evidence regarding clinical microsystems?

Samiei et al. (2011) describe the implementation of the clinical microsystem model at Cooley Dickinson Hospital in Northampton, Massachusetts (USA), a 140-bed community hospital that received the Patient Safety Excellence Award in 2015 and 2016. After implementing the clinical microsystems model, this hospital found a significant drop in the volume of patient bedside calls (−75%). A reduction in patient room turnover time (from 34 to 18 min) and a drop in staff overtime hours were further noted. Data showed reductions on monthly rates of surgical site infections, central line-associated bloodstream infections, and catheter-associated urinary tract infections from 4.1 to 1.3 infections per month. The mean acute care inpatient mortality rate declined from 2.47% to 1.65%. Also, falls in acute care areas dropped from a 12-month average of 12.5% to 11.8%. Berry et al. (2009) described how clinical microsystems thinking was able to improve clinical outcomes in coronary artery bypass graft (CABG) patients. They conducted a pre- and post-intervention study. The 30-day clinical outcomes showed a decrease of ICU readmissions from 2.9% to 0.9% and a decrease in blood product usage from 23.4% to 16.2%. The frequency and length of readmissions also fell.

A study by Varkey et al. (2008) showed how clinical microsystems thinking can influence nurse work environments. They conducted a 1-year follow-up after implementing the principles of high-performing microsystems in the Department of Preventive, Occupational, and Aerospace Medicine at the Mayo Clinic in Rochester, MN (USA). Their survey showed an increase in involvement in work decisions (+25%), opportunities to expand skills (+17%), and increased perceptions of the institution's interest in employee well-being by 17%. Research suggests a positive impact of clinical microsystems on interprofessional collaboration and communication and patient outcomes. As mentioned, clinical nurses have reported a higher-quality collaboration and improved quality of care after implementing the clinical microsystems model.

But how do teams achieve this? The challenge is to match resources to tasks, in part by having healthcare teams work interprofessionally to achieve high standards of care. In order to get a balanced system, it is essential to "understand" the work environment. Therefore, human factors engineering (HFE) principles can be applied to explore the challenges faced in work environments. In addition, the TeamSTEPPS initiative can be used to raise the collaborative skills of team members. HFE and TeamSTEPPS will be discussed in the next paragraphs.

## 12.4.2  Human Factors Engineering Model SEIPS 2.0

Human factors engineering in healthcare has been described as a method of improving patient safety (Carayon et al. 2006) and focuses on three principles (Dul et al. 2012).

1. *System orientation:* Performance results from interactions of elements of a system where each person is just one component. Because of this, healthcare organizations need to replace a blame-the-person culture to a more system-based approach.
2. *Person centeredness:* Where people, whether patients or healthcare workers, have a central place and systems are designed to support them and fit with their capabilities, limitations, and needs.
3. *Design-driven improvements:* Purposeful adjustments are made to work structures and processes to improve patient, healthcare worker, and organizational outcomes.

Version 2.0 of the SEIPS model is, like the original model, based on a structural understanding of sociotechnical work systems that engage in processes and generate outcomes. It has the same structure as Donabedian's structure-process-outcome model (Donabedian 1988) and also the input-transformation-output framework of Karsh et al. (2006). The SEIPS model 2.0 includes also different feedback loops; therefore, it is adjustable over time.

The SEIPS 2.0 model consists of three parts (left, middle, right). The left part of the model represents the work system, where people occupy a central place. It is important to clarify that the model proposes that systems support people and not replace them or compensate for their weaknesses. In SEIPS 2.0, people can be healthcare workers, patients, or interprofessional teams. Holden and colleagues recommended that both patients and healthcare workers be considered together under the "people" component (Holden et al. 2013). According to the Institute of Medicine's Committee on Quality of Health Care in 2000, system design should also take into account patient characteristics, including patient preferences, goals, and needs. The model also includes tasks, tools and technologies, organization, and internal and external environments.

- Tasks are specific actions within the work processes.
- Tools and technologies are objects that people use to fulfill their task.
- Organization refers to the structures within the organization such as time, work space, resources, and activities.
- Organization factors have both social (e.g., culture) and technical (e.g., technical infrastructure) as well as social-technical (e.g., leadership) characteristics (Holden et al. 2013).
- Internal environment deals with lighting, noise, temperature, and layout. External environmental factors include socioeconomic and political factors outside the organization, for example (Holden et al. 2013).

In the SEIPS 2.0 model, all the components interact with each other, potentially at the same time. This can make it really difficult to truly understand the system and renders system improvement a real challenge. Focusing on system interactions is the key element of human factors engineering. In the words of Holden and colleagues, "*while all components of the work system potentially interact, only a subset of all possible interactions is actually relevant in a given work process or situation*" (Holden et al. 2013). In daily practice, it is important to measure and evaluate your system design and check where there are potential aspects to improve. These aspects can change over time. Interprofessional teams need to adapt different work system configurations in order to address the challenges in healthcare. By using the SEIPS 2.0 model in everyday practice, it is possible to compare teams/wards to understand the best configurations for achieving the highest quality of care.

Work processes in the SEIPS 2.0 model are divided into physical, cognitive, and social/behavioral performance processes. There are also three types of engagement in terms of which individuals are actively committed to performing various tasks. *Professional work* is undertaken by nurses, nurse managers, and physicians directly involved in delivering care. *Patient work* is patient engagement in the plan of care (e.g., medication management, symptom monitoring). Patients who are actively engaged in their care tend to show better outcomes (Ontario RNAo 2013). In *professional-patient work*, professionals and patients collaborate in order to achieve the goals.

The right side of the SEIPS model consists of outcomes at the patient, professional, and organizational levels. Proximal outcomes are the immediate result of work system processes, while distal outcomes are outcomes that emerge over time. Adaptations are required in order to redesign the processes and achieve the best outcomes.

### 12.4.2.1 SEIPS 2.0 Model in Practice

As mentioned, HFE can guide a wide scope of improvement initiatives. Here we will focus on interprofessional collaboration, patient safety, and work environments on medical and surgical wards. The SEIPS model explains how work systems influence processes and outcomes. Although there is some empirical evidence of direct effects of HFE factors on work environments and patient safety in medical and surgical wards, there have been relatively few studies. De Vries et al. (2010) developed the SURPASS checklist based on HFE principles, to improve safety of patients on surgical clinical pathways. Significant drops in complication rates after surgery (15.4% vs. 10.6% $p < 0.001$) and in-hospital mortality (1.5% vs. 0.8%, $p < 0.003$) were shown after implementation of the SURPASS checklist. In a demonstration of the usefulness of HFE in increasing efficiency of task completion, Rousek and Hallbeck (2011) introduced an efficient "code" cart medication drawer that resulted in faster medication administration during resuscitation efforts ($p = 0.005$). Applying HFE to the design of medical equipment, for instance, patient-controlled analgesia (PCA) pumps, has been linked with faster programming times ($p < 0.0.25$), lower mental workload ($p = 0.025$), and fewer errors ($p < 0.05$) (Lin et al. 1998).

Rozenbaum et al. (2013) redesigned medication rooms on nursing wards in order to improve patient safety. An interesting finding in their work was that safety indicators that were fully system design-dependent (organization, internal environment, and tools and technologies) showed a higher level of improvement ($p < 0.0001$) than indicators that were behavior-dependent where differences over time were not significant. Examples of system design-dependent indicators included separation of medications and pharmacy-printed labels for each drug compartment, storing high-risk medications in an area separate from other intravenous drugs, clearing work surfaces of unnecessary equipment, and storing equipment for medication administration in the medication room. Behavior-dependent indicators included storage of leftover portions of tablets in drug compartments, recording the dates of opening bottles, storing only drugs in refrigerators, and cleaning and leaving equipment in a ready-to-use state, which relate the work system components of tasks and person(s). These results indicate that system redesign is only one piece of the puzzle. Behavior change is required to create well-organized, efficient, and safe work environments.

Clinical nurses, nurse managers, and physicians are regularly confronted with unbalanced work environments, where demands exceed resources. Clinical nurses, nurse managers, and physicians are not able to meet patients' needs. Imbalances in responsibilities, severe time pressures, lack of training opportunities, and absence of supervision are hallmarks of dysfunctional work environments. Multiple impacts of poor work environments on nurse well-being have been noted. In unbalanced work environments, nurses report higher workloads and decreased social capital and decision latitude. There is also an adverse impact on emotional exhaustion, depersonalization, and personal accomplishment. Higher workloads have negative impacts on how nurses assessed the quality of care and on the adequacy and efficacy of clinical nurses. They also affect nurses' feelings of frustration (Van Bogaert et al. 2017). A study by Kramer and Schmalenberg (2008) identified the characteristics of balanced nursing work environments: *work with other clinical nurses who are clinically competent, collegial/collaborative nurse-physician and interdisciplinary relationships, autonomy, clinical decision-making, supportive nurse managers, control of nursing practice, support for education, perception that staffing is adequate, and creating a culture in which concern for patients is paramount.* Clinical nurses, nurse managers, physicians, and directors have shared responsibilities to achieve a balanced work environment and must have clear understandings of each other's roles and shared mental models, be supportive, give feedback, and communicate in a respectful and clear manner. All aspects of the work system are connected such that interventions addressing one aspect influence others. Clearly interprofessional collaboration can have impacts on the sequencing of tasks. It is also possible that internal environmental barriers directly influence organization of care, which can lead to ineffective processes on nursing wards and a negative impact on patient, professional, and organizational outcomes. This means that assessment of multiple aspects of the work environment is needed for a thorough view of systems.

### 12.4.3 TeamSTEPPS

TeamSTEPPS resulted from a joint research and development project by the US Agency for Healthcare Research and Quality (AHRQ) and the Department of Defense (DoD) to improve team performance in care delivery. Team Strategies and Tools to Enhance Performance and Patient Safety (TeamSTEPPS) was released in 2006 (King et al. 2008). As mentioned earlier, physicians, clinical nurses, nurse managers, and other healthcare workers must coordinate their work with each other to deliver safe and efficient patient care. Members of these three groups work together but have different backgrounds and in the case of clinical nurses and physicians come from different disciplines and diverse educational programs. Because patient-centered care is founded on interprofessional collaboration, good teamwork is essential to ensure patient safety. In effective teams, roles and responsibilities of each team member are clear, and therefore fewer mistakes are made.

TeamSTEPPS is built upon assumptions about the importance of shared knowledge, skills, and attitudes and evidence originating from research on aviation teams. Key skills include leadership, maintaining a positive group climate, anticipating and planning, managing workload distribution, communicating, and giving and receiving feedback. The following competencies, identified in research findings, serve as the basis for the TeamSTEPPS initiative:

1. Team leadership
2. Mutual performance monitoring
3. Backup behavior
4. Adaptability
5. Teams/collective orientation
6. Mutual trust
7. Closed-loop communication

Adaptability and flexibility are skills every team member should have. The philosophy is that clinical nurses, nurse managers, and physicians must leverage them when they face unpredictable situations. TeamSTEPPS instructs team members to monitor the performance of others and provide assistance, plan and organize team roles, and communicate on an efficient and effective way. Leadership, communication, situation monitoring, and mutual support used together result in better outcomes in terms of knowledge, performance, and attitude outcomes.

The TeamSTEPPS curriculum is intended to be provided to the interprofessional care team. Possible barriers to implementing TeamSTEPPS include a lack of information sharing, hierarchical team structures, lack of coordination and follow-up with co-workers, varying communication styles, lack of role clarity, strong distractions, and a lack of physician engagement. In order to tackle these barriers, King and colleagues suggest a number of tools and strategies. One of the most vital aspects of collaboration is communication. It is an absolute must to communicate effectively and clearly to all participants—the situation, background, assessment, and recommendation (SBAR) technique is useful in this respect. In order to arrive at a more systematic approach to the daily management of nursing wards and collaboration on particular nursing wards, daily huddles can be implemented to keep team members informed and help them review their work and make plans. With information from huddles in hand, team members get a clear understanding of what is happening on their units and can plan their work.

As mentioned, clinical nurses and nurse managers face a lot of daily challenges. One of them is getting an overview of the current state of the work environment (e.g., nursing ward). The STEP tool can be used to such a picture. STEP is a mnemonic for status of the patient, team members, environment, and progress toward the goal. Important in teamwork is mutual support. Every team member needs to assist each other, give feedback and be assertive, and name behavior that inflicts patient safety. If teams manage to implement these tools and strategies, mutual trust, team performance, and patient safety increase. Also teams show a higher degree of adaptation to changes and shared mental models.

The process of implementation of the TeamSTEPPS initiative is based on Kotter's model of organizational change (Kotter 1996). In a shift toward a culture of safety, the first phase is to determine organizational readiness. Organizations need to identify opportunities for improvement that can be realized by interprofessional collaborative practice. In the second phase, planning and implementation of the TeamSTEPSS initiative can take place. TeamSTEPSS is designed to be adaptable to a wide variety of healthcare facilities. In the third and final phase, organizational improvements, e.g., team performance, clinical processes, and outcomes, need to be evaluated, improved if necessary, and sustained.

### 12.4.3.1 Effect of TeamSTEPPS on Interprofessional Collaboration and Patient Safety

Study results show that the TeamSTEPPS initiative has a positive impact on interprofessional collaboration and patient safety. For instance, Vincent (2016) points out that after implementing TeamSTEPPS in one operating room suite, the number of adverse patient harm-related events (APHRE) dropped by more than 10%. Weaver et al. (2010) performed a multilevel evaluation after implementing TeamSTEPPS and found a large number of significant improvements. After training the TeamSTEPPS initiative, 81% felt more confident to work as an effective team member. There was also an increase in willingness to speak up and participate in briefings and a higher frequency of contingency plan discussion. A significant increase in standardized handovers was also reported. MANOVAs revealed improvements in a number of teamwork domains: communication, mutual support, situation monitoring, and leadership. Improvements were also seen on the following areas of the Agency for Healthcare Research and Quality's hospital survey on patient safety culture: teamwork within units, feedback and communication about error, communication openness, and overall patient safety grades. Stead et al. (2009) reported improvements of role clarity, team behavior, and team performance after redesigning interprofessional team meetings. Cima et al. (2009) showed reduction of retained foreign objects in surgical patients after implementing the TeamSTEPPS initiative. Although they provided few specifics, authors from Mountain View Hospital in Madras, Oregon (USA), reported that TeamSTEPPS training resulted in improved communication during critical situations; inclusion of patients and families in team huddles and care planning; reduction in or prevention of medication errors, procedural errors, and supply shortages; and also increases in patient satisfaction and staff satisfaction (Coburn and Gage-Croll 2011). To summarize, after reviewing the literature, we found that the TeamSTEPPS initiative had positive effects on many aspects of interprofessional collaboration and patient safety.

## 12.5    The Umbrella as a Model for Achieving Excellent Interprofessional Collaborative Patient-Centered Care.

We view patient-centered care as an umbrella intended to protect patients—who are the center of the umbrella (or the handle). The collaborative triangle of clinical nurses, nurse managers, and physicians forms the shaft that connects the clinical microsystem to the patient. To prevent patients from harm, work systems where tasks and resources are balanced form the stretchers or fabric—and incorporate features of HFE, TeamSTEPPS, and collaborative competencies. Weaknesses in any of

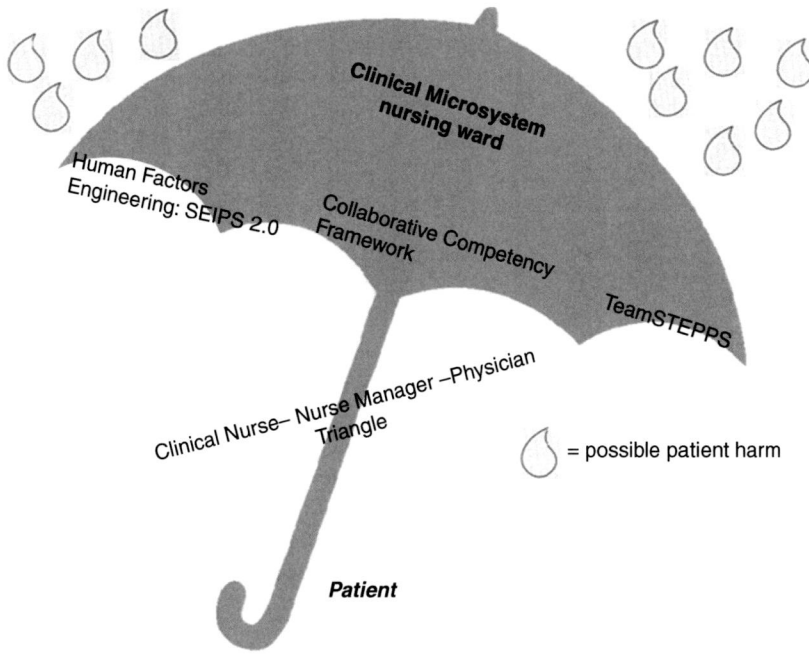

**Fig. 12.2** The umbrella model: excellence in interprofessional collaborative patient-centered care

the stretchers risk rain or harm reaching the patient, which is what we wish to avoid at all times (Fig. 12.2).

## 12.6 Conclusions and Recommendations for Further Research

In the hospital setting, interprofessional collaboration is crucial as healthcare teams face a number of challenges. Clinical nurses, nurse managers, and physicians make up the majority of healthcare providers, and they daily confront complex problems with challenging solutions. However, collaboration and communication between these professions do not always unfold as it should. Ineffective or lack of interprofessional collaboration has a negative impact on patient outcomes. Therefore, systems must be designed to strengthen interprofessional collaborative practice. The IPEC competency framework should be applied by clinical nurses, nurse managers, and physicians in order to achieve role clarity, clear communication, and excellent teamwork and create a climate of mutual respect and shared values. Clinical microsystems, human factors engineering, and TeamSTEPPS have proven their values in daily practice. These models respond to the challenges clinical nurses, nurse managers, and physicians face every day, continuously improving their interprofessional collaborative triangle and patient outcomes.

Redesigning systems at the unit level offers the possibility to improve interprofessional collaboration between clinical nurses, nurse managers, and physicians, and it can also lead to an increase in patient empowerment and patient outcomes. Further research is needed to clarify the expectations and experiences of clinical nurses, nurse managers, and physicians on nursing wards regarding interprofessional collaboration in order to arrive at clarity in roles and responsibilities and shared mental models and decision-making processes. Research on system design provides an opportunity to understand interactions within systems in order to improve quality of care and patient outcomes.

## 12.6.1 An Ongoing Research Project

Our current research project focuses on interprofessional collaboration between clinical nurses, nurse managers, and physicians on medical and surgical wards and how this triangle of collaborative relationships is associated with patient outcomes and nurses' work environments. We are examining the hypothesis that optimization of interprofessional collaboration and communication between clinical nurses, nurse managers, and physicians on medical and surgical wards will improve nurse work environments and patient outcomes.

The following research questions will be addressed:

1. How do clinical nurses perceive their work environments, and how does the nurse work environment relate to objectively measured outcome variables?
2. How does interprofessional collaboration occur on surgical and medical wards? What are clinical nurses', nurse managers', and physicians' perceptions and expectations regarding interprofessional collaboration?
3. What is the effect on interprofessional collaboration as well as perceived workload and patient outcomes of the implementing interventions based on insights from our research data and review of the literature?

This research project consists of three phases. The first phase is to measure the perceived nurse work environment based on approaches from the 10-year program of research discussed in earlier chapters in this volume, with objective variables such as staffing measured in terms of nurse to patient ratios and nursing hours per patient day. In terms of measures of care, we will examine nurse-sensitive outcomes such as hospital-acquired pressure ulcers, central line-associated bloodstream infection, catheter-associated urinary tract infections, and falls with injury. We will also measure the number of serious adverse events (unexpected hospital mortality, unplanned ICU transfer, and cardiac arrest calls). These measures of quality indicators directly linked to patient care will be presented in statistical process control charts. The nurse work environment will be measured longitudinally. In addition, we will use the NASA Task Load Index to measure various types of nurse workload such as mental demand, physical demand, temporal demand, performance, effort, and frustration. The second phase involves a qualitative exploration of interprofessional collaboration on medical and surgical wards. Semi-structured interviews with clinical nurses, nurse managers, and physicians will be conducted with the goal to describe and compare perceptions, expectations, and values related to interprofessional collaboration on medical and surgical wards. In the third phase, we will implement two radical interventions to improve interprofessional collaboration and organizational structure at the nursing ward and improve patient empowerment on two nursing wards. A radical intervention is one that has a dramatic impact that creates new and unique work systems and structures through redesign; it changes components and how they interact and work together. Radical innovations often come with a higher degree of risk and resistance. On the other hand, they can also result in greater rewards in the form of improved nurse work environments and patient outcomes. On four other nursing wards, we will implement specific incremental interventions to improve interprofessional collaboration (e.g., structured interdisciplinary bedside rounds (SIBR)). Incremental interventions improve existing structures and processes through changes over time, which can improve adaptation and lower the risk of resistance and failure. Both the radical and incremental interventions will be developed with thorough literature searches. After implementation, we will repeat measures of the nurse work environment and will evaluate changes in outcome indicators (nurse-sensitive outcomes and serious adverse events) through statistical process control charts.

*The chapter is a part of doctoral project supervised by Sven Francque, PhD, MD, chair of the Gastroenterology Department at the Antwerp University Hospital, and Peter Van Bogaert.*

# References

Baggs JG, Schmitt MH, Mushlin AI, Eldredge DH, Oakes D, Hutson AD. Nurse-physician collaboration and satisfaction with the decision-making process in three critical care units. Am J Crit Care. 1997;6(5):393–9.

Berry SA, Doll MC, McKinley KE, Casale AS, Bothe A Jr. ProvenCare: quality improvement model for designing highly reliable care in cardiac surgery. Qual Saf Health Care. 2009;18(5):360–8. https://doi.org/10.1136/qshc.2007.025056.

Bowles D, McIntosh G, Hemrajani R, Yen MS, Phillips A, Schwartz N, Tu SP, Dow AW. Nurse-physician collaboration in an academic medical centre: the influence of organisational and individual factors. J Interprof Care. 2016;30(5):655–60. https://doi.org/10.1080/13561820.2016.1201464.

Carayon P, Hundt AS, Karsh BT, Gurses AP, Alvarado CJ, Smith M, Brennan PF. Work system design for patient safety: the SEIPS model. Qual Saf Health Care. 2006;15(Suppl 1):i50–8. https://doi.org/10.1136/qshc.2005.015842.

Caricati L, Mancini T, Sollami A, Bianconcini M, Guidi C, Prandi C, Silvano R, Taffurelli C, Artioli G. The role of professional and team commitments in nurse-physician collaboration. J Nurs Manag. 2016;24(2):E192–200. https://doi.org/10.1111/jonm.12323.

Carlin A, Duffy K. Newly qualified staff's perceptions of senior charge nurse roles. Nurs Manag. 2013;20(7):24–30. https://doi.org/10.7748/nm2013.11.20.7.24.e1142.

Cima RR, Kollengode A, Storsveen AS, Weisbrod CA, Deschamps C, Koch MB, Moore D, Pool SR. A multidisciplinary team approach to retained foreign objects. Jt Comm J Qual Patient Saf. 2009;35(3):123–32.

Coburn AF, Gage-Croll Z. Improving hospital patient safety through teamwork: the use of TeamSTEPPS in critical access hospitals. Challenge. 2011;5:7.

Collette AE, Wann K, Nevin ML, Rique K, Tarrant G, Hickey LA, Stichler JF, Toole BM, Thomason T. An exploration of nurse-physician perceptions of collaborative behaviour. J Interprof Care. 2017;31(4):470–8. https://doi.org/10.1080/13561820.2017.1301411.

Commission J. Sentinel Event Data Root Causes by Event Type 2004–2015. 2016. http://www.jointcommission.org/assets/1/18/Root_Causes_by_Event_Type_2004-2015.pdf. Accessed 18 Mar 2016.

Cummings GG. Nursing leadership and patient outcomes. J Nurs Manag. 2013;21(5):707–8. https://doi.org/10.1111/jonm.12152.

Cummings GG, MacGregor T, Davey M, Lee H, Wong CA, Lo E, Muise M, Stafford E. Leadership styles and outcome patterns for the nursing workforce and work environment: a systematic review. Int J Nurs Stud. 2010;47(3):363–85. https://doi.org/10.1016/j.ijnurstu.2009.08.006.

de Vries EN, Prins HA, Crolla RMPH, den Outer AJ, van Andel G, van Helden SH, Schlack WS, van Putten MA, Gouma DJ, Dijkgraaf MGW, Smorenburg SM, Boermeester MA. Effect of a comprehensive surgical safety system on patient outcomes. N Engl J Med. 2010;363(20):1928–37. https://doi.org/10.1056/NEJMsa0911535.

Donabedian A. The quality of care: how can it be assessed? JAMA. 1988;260(12):1743–8. https://doi.org/10.1001/jama.1988.03410120089033.

Dul J, Bruder R, Buckle P, Carayon P, Falzon P, Marras WS, Wilson JR, van der Doelen B. A strategy for human factors/ergonomics: developing the discipline and profession. Ergonomics. 2012;55(4):377–95. https://doi.org/10.1080/00140139.2012.661087.

Eggenberger T. Exploring the charge nurse role: holding the frontline. J Nurs Adm. 2012;42(11):502–6. https://doi.org/10.1097/NNA.0b013e3182714495.

Epstein NE. Multidisciplinary in-hospital teams improve patient outcomes: a review. Surg Neurol Int. 2014;5(Suppl 7):S295–303. https://doi.org/10.4103/2152-7806.139612.

Galletta M, Portoghese I, Carta MG, D'Aloja E, Campagna M. The effect of nurse-physician collaboration on job satisfaction, team commitment, and turnover intention in nurses. Res Nurs Health. 2016;39(5):375–85. https://doi.org/10.1002/nur.21733.

Henkin S, Chon TY, Christopherson ML, Halvorsen AJ, Worden LM, Ratelle JT. Improving nurse-physician teamwork through interprofessional bedside rounding. J Multidiscip Healthc. 2016;9:201–5. https://doi.org/10.2147/jmdh.s106644.

Higgins J, Cole-Poklewski T. Case management reform: an illustrative study of one hospital's experience. Prof Case Manag. 2010;15(2):79–89. https://doi.org/10.1097/NCM.0b013e3181d2106a.

Holden RJ, Carayon P, Gurses AP, Hoonakker P, Hundt AS, Ozok AA, Rivera-Rodriguez AJ. SEIPS 2.0: a human factors framework for studying and improving the work of healthcare professionals and patients. Ergonomics. 2013;56(11). https://doi.org/10.1080/00140139.2013.838643.

Hopkins D. Framework for action on interprofessional education & collaborative practice (WHO/HRH/HPN/10.3). Geneva: World Health Organization; 2010. http://apps.who.int/iris/bitstream/10665/70185/1/WHO_HRH_HPN_10.3_eng.pdf.

House S, Havens D. Nurses' and physicians' perceptions of nurse-physician collaboration: a systematic review. J Nurs Adm. 2017;47(3):165–71. https://doi.org/10.1097/nna.0000000000000460.

Institute of Medicine Committee on Quality of Health Care in America. In: Kohn LT, Corrigan JM, Donaldson MS, editors. To Err is Human: Building a Safer Health System. Washington, DC: National Academies Press (US); 2000. https://doi.org/10.17226/9728.

Karsh BT, Holden RJ, Alper SJ, Or CKL. A human factors engineering paradigm for patient safety: designing to support the performance of the healthcare professional. Qual Saf Health Care. 2006;15(Suppl 1):i59–65. https://doi.org/10.1136/qshc.2005.015974.

Kassam A, Cowan M, Donnon T. An objective structured clinical exam to measure intrinsic CanMEDS roles. Med Educ Online. 2016;21:31085. https://doi.org/10.3402/meo.v21.31085.

Keenan GM, Cooke R, Hillis SL. Norms and nurse management of conflicts: keys to understanding nurse-physician collaboration. Res Nurs Health. 1998;21(1):59–72.

King HB, Battles J, Baker DP, Alonso A, Salas E, Webster J, Toomey L, Salisbury M. Advances in patient safety. Rockville: Agency for Healthcare Research and Quality; 2008.

Kotter JP. Leading change. Brighton: Harvard Business School Publishing; 1996.

Kramer M, Schmalenberg C. Confirmation of a healthy work environment. Crit Care Nurse. 2008;28(2):56–63.

Lin L, Isla R, Doniz K, Harkness H, Vicente KJ, Doyle DJ. Applying human factors to the design of medical equipment: patient-controlled analgesia. J Clin Monit Comput. 1998;14(4): 253–63.

Mahler C, Gutmann T, Karstens S, Joos S. Terminology for interprofessional collaboration: definition and current practice. GMS Z Med Ausbildung. 2014;31(4):40. https://doi.org/10.3205/zma000932.

Manojlovich M, Talsma A. Identifying nursing processes to reduce failure to rescue. J Nurs Adm. 2007;37(11):504–9. https://doi.org/10.1097/01.NNA.0000295608.94699.3f.

Martin JS, Ummenhofer W, Manser T, Spirig R. Interprofessional collaboration among nurses and physicians: making a difference in patient outcome. Swiss Med Wkly. 2010;140:w13062. https://doi.org/10.4414/smw.2010.13062.

Matziou V, Vlahioti E, Perdikaris P, Matziou T, Megapanou E, Petsios K. Physician and nursing perceptions concerning interprofessional communication and collaboration. J Interprof Care. 2014;28(6):526–33. https://doi.org/10.3109/13561820.2014.934338.

McCallin AM, Frankson C. The role of the charge nurse manager: a descriptive exploratory study. J Nurs Manag. 2010;18(3):319–25. https://doi.org/10.1111/j.1365-2834.2010.01067.x.

Muller-Juge V, Cullati S, Blondon KS, Hudelson P, Maitre F, Vu NV, Savoldelli GL, Nendaz MR. Interprofessional collaboration on an internal medicine ward: role perceptions and expectations among nurses and residents. PLoS One. 2013;8(2):e57570. https://doi.org/10.1371/journal.pone.0057570.

Muller-Juge V, Cullati S, Blondon KS, Hudelson P, Maitre F, Vu NV, Savoldelli GL, Nendaz MR. Interprofessional collaboration between residents and nurses in general internal medicine: a qualitative study on behaviours enhancing teamwork quality. PLoS One. 2014;9(4):e96160. https://doi.org/10.1371/journal.pone.0096160.

Nelson EC, Batalden PB, Godfrey MM. Quality by design: a clinical microsystems approach. San Francisco: Jossey-Bass; 2007.

Ontario RNAo. Developing and Sustaining Interprofessional Health Care: Optimizing patients/clients, organizational, and system outcomes. Ontario: RNAo; 2013.

Panel IECE. Core competencies for interprofessional collaborative practice: report of an expert panel. Interprofessional Education Collaborative Expert Panel. 2011.

Rankin J, McGuire C, Matthews L, Russell M, Ray D. Facilitators and barriers to the increased supervisory role of senior charge nurses: a qualitative study. J Nurs Manag. 2016;24(3):366–75. https://doi.org/10.1111/jonm.12330.

Rousek JB, Hallbeck MS. Improving medication management through the redesign of the hospital code cart medication drawer. Hum Factors. 2011;53(6):626–36. https://doi.org/10.1177/0018720811426427.

Rozenbaum H, Gordon L, Brezis M, Porat N. The use of a standard design medication room to promote medication safety: organizational implications. Int J Qual Health Care. 2013;25(2):188–96. https://doi.org/10.1093/intqhc/mzt005.

Samiei VAI, Sharifa Ezat WP, Alsheikh HI, Kari HA, Saleh M, Sengee G, Waruegh N. Clinical microsystem approach-A method for health care improvement. Malays J Publ Health Med. 2011;11(1):16–28.

Sorensen EE, Delmar C, Pedersen BD. Leading nurses in dire straits: head nurses' navigation between nursing and leadership roles. J Nurs Manag. 2011;19(4):421–30. https://doi.org/10.1111/j.1365-2834.2011.01212.x.

Stead K, Kumar S, Schultz TJ, Tiver S, Pirone CJ, Adams RJ, Wareham CA. Teams communicating through STEPPS. Med J Aust. 2009;190(11):128.

Suarez M, Asenjo M, Sanchez M. Job satisfaction among emergency department staff. Australas Emerg Nurs J. 2017;20(1):31–6. https://doi.org/10.1016/j.aenj.2016.09.003.

Van Bogaert P, Adriaenssens J, Dilles T, Martens D, Van Rompaey B, Timmermans O. Impact of role-, job- and organizational characteristics on Nursing Unit Managers' work related stress and well-being. J Adv Nurs. 2014;70(11):2622–33. https://doi.org/10.1111/jan.12449.

Van Bogaert P, Kowalski C, Weeks SM, Van Heusden D, Clarke SP. The relationship between nurse practice environment, nurse work characteristics, burnout and job outcome and quality of nursing care: a cross-sectional survey. Int J Nurs Stud. 2013;50(12):1667–77. https://doi.org/10.1016/j.ijnurstu.2013.05.010.

Van Bogaert P, Peremans L, Van Heusden D, Verspuy M, Kureckova V, Van de Cruys Z, Franck E. Predictors of burnout, work engagement and nurse reported job outcomes and quality of care: a mixed method study. BMC Nurs. 2017;16:5. https://doi.org/10.1186/s12912-016-0200-4.

Varkey P, Karlapudi SP, Hensrud DD. The impact of a quality improvement program on employee satisfaction in an academic microsystem. Am J Med Qual. 2008;23(3):215–21. https://doi.org/10.1177/1062860608314957.

Vincent TD. Implementation of TeamSTEPPS in the operating room a quality improvement project. graduate theses, dissertations, and capstones. Bellarmine University; 2016.

Weaver SJ, Rosen MA, DiazGranados D, Lazzara EH, Lyons R, Salas E, Knych SA, McKeever M, Adler L, Barker M, King HB. Does teamwork improve performance in the operating room? A multilevel evaluation. Jt Comm J Qual Patient Saf. 2010;36(3):133–42.

Williams I, Dickinson H, Robinson S, Allen C. Clinical microsystems and the NHS: a sustainable method for improvement? J Health Organ Manag. 2009;23(1):119–32. https://doi.org/10.1108/14777260910942597.

# Stress Resistance Strategies

# 13

Nina Geuens, Erik Franck, and Peter Van Bogaert

**Abstract**

The psychological syndrome of burnout is of key importance to nurse managers, given that it is a widespread problem, with anywhere from 10–78% of European and American nurses considering themselves to be "burned out." Reviewing the literature on the consequences of burnout for individual nurses, patients, teams, and healthcare organizations, it is evident that burnout has a prominent concern for the nursing profession.

One of the most comprehensive models that describes the development of burnout is the vulnerability-stress model. This model addresses the interactions between various factors that render individuals susceptible to burnout and various situational stressors; it implies an inverse relationship between these two types of influences.

Numerous studies have described vulnerability and situational risk factors for burnout independently. However, even though vulnerability and stressors can be considered to be conceptually distinct constructs, their ability to predict burnout is limited when examined in isolation of each other.

N. Geuens (✉)
Centre of Expertise Psychological Wellbeing in Patient Care, Karel De Grote University College, Antwerp, Belgium

Nursing and Midwifery Sciences and Centre, Research and Innovation in Care (CRIC), Faculty of Medicine and Health Sciences, University of Antwerp, Antwerp, Belgium
e-mail: nina.geuens@kdg.be

E. Franck
Nursing and Midwifery Sciences and Centre, Research and Innovation in Care (CRIC), Faculty of Medicine and Health Sciences, University of Antwerp, Antwerp, Belgium

Karel De Grote University College, Antwerp, Belgium

P. Van Bogaert
Nursing and Midwifery Sciences and Centre, Research and Innovation in Care (CRIC), Faculty of Medicine and Health Sciences, University of Antwerp, Antwerp, Belgium

© Springer International Publishing AG 2018
P. Van Bogaert, S. Clarke (eds.), *The Organizational Context of Nursing Practice*,
https://doi.org/10.1007/978-3-319-71042-6_13

Considering the wide array of consequences of burnout and the long period from onset of stressors to emergence of the syndrome, prevention is an appropriate goal. Preventive measures should include joint individual and organizational interventions to effectively reduce stress and burnout and increase resilience in healthcare workers. Additionally, preventive measures should reflect the complexity of this syndrome, be well-thought out, and devote special attention to the discrepancy between individual and situational factors. Well-designed, multicomponent prevention programs show promise in reducing burnout and its negative consequences.

**Keywords**
Nurse burnout • Vulnerability • Stressor • Prevention • Personality

## 13.1 Impact of Burnout

Burnout is a psychological syndrome that may develop as a result of exposure to chronic occupational stress. The psychological syndrome of burnout encompasses three dimensions: (1) emotional exhaustion, which refers to feeling depleted of all resources and overwhelmed, emotionally speaking and experiencing extreme emotional and/or physical fatigue; (2) depersonalization, which entails tendencies to maintain distance between oneself and one's work, expressed by treating patients as objects and assuming an indifferent and cynical attitude toward them; and (3) reduced personal accomplishment, which refers to feelings of incompetence and lack of personal achievement in the job (Maslach 1998; Peng et al. 2016).

The body of evidence on burnout in the nursing population is extensive and still growing at a steady pace. Healthcare managers are eager to know more about the psychological syndrome of burnout given that it is a widespread problem with anywhere from 10–78% of European and American nurses considering themselves to be "burned out" (Aiken et al. 2012). The consequences of this psychological syndrome are significant. Individual nurses suffering from burnout may experience psychological distress, somatic complaints, insomnia, substance use or abuse, and lower job satisfaction (Aiken et al. 2002; Birkmeyer et al. 2004; Jackson and Maslach 1982; Vahey et al. 2004). However, destructive impacts of burnout do not stop at the individual. They have a ripple effect that spreads to patients, nursing teams, and healthcare organizations as a whole.

Research suggests that nurses influence patient satisfaction through the affective nature of their interactions with patients (Leiter et al. 1998) and that nursing care accounts for 45% of the variance in the overall quality of care ratings (Carey and Seibert 1993). As a consequence, symptoms of nurse burnout such as depersonalization and emotional exhaustion can affect patient satisfaction and patient safety (Gravlin 1994; Laschinger et al. 2006; Leiter et al. 1998; Vahey et al. 2004). Nurses with symptoms of burnout also tend to report worse perceptions of quality of care (Van Bogaert et al. 2010). Additionally, emotional exhaustion has been associated with patient safety indicators such as errors, adverse events, and standardized mortality ratios (Rothschild et al. 2005; Welp et al. 2014).

Perhaps some of these associations relate to the association of burnout with decreased job performance by nurses. Nurse burnout appears to cause a reduction in empathy, compassion, and caring (Firth-Cozens and Cornwell 2009; Keidel 2002). Several researchers have reported linking nurse burnout to various types of neglect of work (Basar and Basim 2016; Reader and Gillespie 2013). Neglect can take the form of inattentive behavior, a lack of caring behavior, or absences from work and can go as far as psychological inattention and abandonment (Farrell 1983). Nurses neglecting their work may extend their breaks, work slowly, talk on the phone, chat without purpose, daydream, occupy themselves with non-work-related subjects and activities, ignore patients' requests, and overlook issues and problems in their work (Basar and Basim 2016). Because patient care constitutes the vital part of nurses' work, neglect of patient care by nurses may have severe and even irreversible consequences (Basar and Basim 2016), such as emotional harm (from loss of dignity and feeling uncared for), and even put patients at risk for injuries or death (Reader and Gillespie 2013). In research studies, emotionally exhausted clinicians have been found to be less vigilant and to demonstrate less motivation to work safely, both of which increase likelihood of errors (Halbesleben and Rathert 2008; Nembhard and Edmondson 2006).

Patients may experience negative consequences from direct contact with individual nurses suffering from burnout; however, team factors may also be involved. For instance, Welp et al. (2016) suggested that the negative effect of emotional exhaustion on patient safety is mediated by the influence of emotional exhaustion on effective teamwork. Emotionally exhausted clinicians are less able to participate in the teamwork, necessary to maintain patient safety (Welp et al. 2016). In addition, Bakker et al. (2005) presented data consistent with burnout as a contagious phenomenon that could be transferred from one nurse to another either consciously or unconsciously (Bakker et al. 2005). Thus, burnout is not only a problem for individual nurses but for the entire nursing team and even the whole healthcare organization.

From an economic perspective, the effect that reduced patient satisfaction and safety may have on patient loyalty is only one of the potential threats that nurse burnout poses to the organization financially speaking (Aiken et al. 2012). Burnout has also been linked with substantially increased costs due to reduced engagement, increased absenteeism, and excess nurse turnover (Aiken et al. 2012; Leiter and Maslach 2009; Van Bogaert et al. 2009). Indeed, impending resignations and unexpected resignations can result in substantial costs to healthcare organizations in terms of lost productivity, along with costs of recruiting and training replacement nurses (Basar and Basim 2016; Yavas et al. 2013).

Taking all of these considerations together, it is clear that burnout has extensive influences on the nursing profession. The impacts of burnout call for interventions to protect the well-being of individual nurses, patients, and healthcare organizations. However, to design and implement effective interventions, a thorough understanding of the development of this complex psychological syndrome is in order. The vulnerability-stress model can provide such a comprehensive framework.

## 13.2    Vulnerability-Stress Model

That not all individuals who experience significant stress develop a disorder—such as burnout from work stress—has led to the recognition that vulnerability processes are of importance (Ingram and Luxton 2005). One of the most comprehensive models to describe the development of burnout is the vulnerability-stress model. This model states that all people have some level of predisposing factors (vulnerability or diathesis) for any given mental disorder. However, each individual appears to develop stress-related disorders after experiencing different levels of stress; the "breaking point" seems to depend on the interaction between the degree of vulnerability and the number and severity of precipitating environmental events (stressors) experienced by the individual. According to the model, vulnerability has a trait like nature and resides within the person. It tends to be stable but can change. Vulnerability factors may include but are not necessarily limited to genetic factors, biological processes, cognitive structures, maladaptive ways of interacting with others, insecure attachment styles, and deficits in emotional regulation (Hankin and Abela 2005). Situational stressors, on the other hand, tend to be life events (major or minor) that disrupt mechanisms that maintain stable individual physiological, emotional, and/or cognitive functions (Ingram and Luxton 2005). For instance, one major category of stress is significant life events (stressors) that are interpreted by a person as undesirable (vulnerability) (Ingram and Luxton 2005; Lazarus and Folkman 1984; Monroe and Simons 1991). The phrase "interpreted as undesirable" suggests an important role of appraisal processes in determining which events are perceived as stressful (Monroe and Simons 1991). Even though some events are universally appraised as unpleasant and stressful—such as being fired—individual differences determine the degree of perceived/experienced stress. By a similar token, events that are perceived as stressful by some individuals may be perceived as either not stressful or minimally stressful by others (Ingram and Luxton 2005). Therefore, stressors are by definition not purely "external" to the individual. Furthermore, vulnerable individuals also play a role in creating their own stressors (Depue and Monroe 1986; Hammen 1991; Hammen 1992; Ingram et al. 1998; Monroe and Simons 1991). For example, people with neurotic personality traits are more likely to perceive their work environment or work-related events as negative, while other coworkers might not perceive those same circumstances as disruptive. As such, vulnerability created by neuroticism can influence the nature of the stressors to which a nurse is exposed, how those events are perceived, and the coping or defenses used to cope with them—which in combination may precipitate burnout (Alarcon et al. 2009; Cañadas-De la Fuente et al. 2015; Geuens et al. 2017b; Ingram and Luxton 2005; Swider and Zimmerman 2010).

Because the vulnerability-stress model addresses interactions between individual susceptibilities and situational stressors, it can be used to predict who might develop a disorder like burnout and who is less likely to do so (Ingram and Luxton

2005; Monroe and Hadjiyannakis 2002; Monroe and Simons 1991). The model implies an inverse relationship between factors whereby greater presence of one factor (more vulnerability or more stressors) lowers the levels of the other factor needed to bring about the disorder. Consequently, the number and/or intensity of stressors that might trigger the development of the disorder can be counterbalanced or compensated for by the level of vulnerability and vice versa (Ingram and Luxton 2005). Simply put, burnout can arise in an individual confronted by relatively few stressors if they have limited resilience (higher vulnerability). Conversely, high resilience (lower vulnerability) may mean that individuals resist burnout in all but situations of very greatest stressors. Therefore, a person with high stress resilience may not develop burnout easily, but can also become susceptible if stressors pile up. According to the vulnerability-stress model, burnout develops when the experienced stressors outweigh the personal resilience (Ingram and Luxton 2005). However, in a vulnerability-stress model, individuals with high vulnerability are no more likely to develop burnout or its symptoms in the absence of stressors (Hankin and Abela 2005).

A cognitive vulnerability-stress model incorporates the notion that when confronted by stressful life events, latent negative self-schemas incorporating dysfunctional attitudes about the self are activated in an automatic, repetitive, unintended, and difficult-to-control manner (Clark et al. 1999). This leads to specific negative cognitions (automatic thoughts), including negative views of oneself (lower levels of self-esteem) that result in sadness and other depressive symptoms (Beck 1979; Beck 2002; Clark et al. 1999). In the absence of stressful life events, these negative schemas remain latent and less consciously accessible, and do not directly bias the information processing system (Haaga et al. 1991).

The vulnerability-stress model has been studied in relation to depression, suicidal behavior, schizophrenia, substance use, personality disorders, anxiety disorders, and eating disorders (Hankin and Abela 2005). It can also be applied to burnout. Burnout as a psychological syndrome shows similarities with the aforementioned psychopathologies, since not all individuals exposed to the same stressors (even if major stressors) develop burnout, and vulnerability plays an important role in predisposing some individuals to burnout (Ingram and Luxton 2005).

It should be noted that the interaction between stressors and vulnerability might not be static and can change over time. The diathesis (or individual vulnerability/susceptibility) may increase or decrease so that the number and severity of stressors needed to trigger burnout may decrease or increase, respectively. This idea, the so-called kindling phenomenon (Post 1992), illustrates the dynamic character of the interaction between stressors and vulnerability. Repeated occurrences of a disorder may cause neuronal changes that result in more sensitivity to stress. The kindling hypothesis proposes that vulnerability may change so that more or less stress becomes necessary to activate vulnerability factors (Ingram and Luxton 2005; van Heeringen 2012).

## 13.3    Individual and Situational Correlates of Burnout

In the literature, numerous factors have been described as causes of burnout. When applying the vulnerability-stress model, these causes can be categorized into (1) individual vulnerability factors, including personality, behavior, and coping, and (2) situational stressors, including team stressors, organizational stressors, and personal issues or circumstances.

### 13.3.1 Individual Vulnerabilities

In terms of individual vulnerability, several studies point to psychological variables and have found that certain personality traits may promote the development of burnout and, in contrast, that others may protect against the development of the disorder (Cañadas-De la Fuente et al. 2015). The five-factor model of personality has been widely studied in relation to burnout (Hoekstra et al. 2012). This model defines five interdependent groups of personality traits referred to as "the Big Five": neuroticism (level of emotional instability), extraversion (level of sociability), openness (level of intellectual curiosity and esthetic sensibility), agreeableness (level of orientation toward others), and conscientiousness (level of self-control and self-determination) (Graziano and Eisenberg 1997; Hoekstra et al. 2012). Several researchers established that the burnout dimensions of emotional exhaustion and depersonalization were negatively related to emotional stability (the opposite of neuroticism), agreeableness, conscientiousness, and extraversion (Alarcon et al. 2009; Cañadas-De la Fuente et al. 2015). In contrast, personal accomplishment was positively related to emotional stability, agreeableness, conscientiousness, extraversion, and openness to experience (Alarcon et al. 2009). In agreement with these findings, Geuens et al. (2017b) found a strong association between neuroticism and the three burnout dimensions of emotional exhaustion, depersonalization, and personal accomplishment in a sample of nurses. Several explanations for neuroticism as a risk factor for burnout have been described (Geuens et al. 2017b). Armon et al. (2012) state that certain personality traits may predispose individuals to experience stressors more intensely, thus potentially stimulating burnout (Armon et al. 2012), and neuroticism is characterized by a tendency to negatively interpret events and show negative emotions such as anxiety, depression, and frustration (Cañadas-De la Fuente et al. 2015; Hoekstra et al. 2012). Therefore, people with higher levels of neuroticism tend to use coping strategies based on avoidance and distraction (Bakker et al. 2006).

Additionally, coping strategies have also been identified as correlates of burnout. Passive avoidant and emotional coping strategies, especially when used alone or as dominant modes of coping, have been found to be ineffective in dealing with stress. Active problem-focused coping, on the other hand, was found to be related to lower levels of emotional exhaustion and depersonalization and to higher personal accomplishment (Adriaenssens et al. 2015; Maslach et al. 2001; Semmer and Schabracq 2003; Shimizutani et al. 2008; Shirey 2006).

Furthermore, Geuens et al. (2017b) study found that interpersonal behavior in nurses predicted all three burnout dimensions. For example, emotional exhaustion and depersonalization were lower in nurses with scores suggesting greater orientation toward friendliness or cooperative behavior. There are several possible explanations for this finding. First of all, friendly behavior from nurses can stimulate friendly behavior in patients given that friendliness seems to provoke similar responses in others (Locke 2010) Additionally, it is plausible that friendly behavior from nurses can increase patients' satisfaction with nursing care, which in turn can improve the nurse-patient relationship and increase nurse job satisfaction and reduce symptoms of burnout. Second of all, in healthcare teams, friendly behavior evokes similar responses from colleagues and may assist with creating social support and a positive work atmosphere, which in turn can augment job satisfaction and reduce burnout symptoms. After all, workers are more likely to be able to cope with work pressures when they feel they have friends at work (Eurofound 2012).

Not surprisingly, lack of flexibility, stubbornness, judgmental behavior, and difficulties in adapting to new situations have been suggested as potential correlates of burnout (Walsh et al. 1998).

### 13.3.2  Situational Stressors

In terms of situational stressors at the level of teams, researchers have described poor nurse-physician relationships, weak management at the unit level, conflictual nurse-nurse relationships, and horizontal violence as important determinants of nurse burnout (Taylor and Barling 2004; Van Bogaert et al. 2013). García-Izquierdo and Ríos-Rísquez (2012) presented results suggesting that interpersonal conflicts are related to emotional exhaustion and depersonalization and inversely related to personal accomplishment (García-Izquierdo and Ríos-Rísquez 2012). At the organizational level, stressors such as job complexity, work overload, recurrent night duty, hospital management and organizational support or issues with management and the system, organizational culture, reward, the number of patients per nurse, inadequate resources and services, and aggressive (or criminal) patients have been identified as potential causes of burnout (Garrosa et al. 2008; Jourdain and Chenevert 2010; Ksiazek et al. 2011; Lasebikan and Oyetunde 2012; Maslach et al. 2001; Melchior et al. 1997; Van Bogaert et al. 2010; You et al. 2013). Additionally, personal circumstances related to social support, lifestyle, and economic and social context in one's private life may also be predictors of burnout (Manzano-García and Ayala 2017).

### 13.3.3  Combining Individual Vulnerabilities and Situational Stressors

Geuens et al. (2017a) used the broad framework of a vulnerability-stress model in their qualitative study. They explored vulnerability factors and stressors experienced by Flemish hospital nurses that they perceived as contributing to burnout (Geuens et al. 2017a). Results suggested that the development of nurse burnout was linked to a discrepancy between "being passionate about doing well or being good"—an individual factor—and issues around "teamwork," "managers," and "work and personal circumstances," situational stressors. The authors argued that nurse burnout is not caused by individual or situational factors separately but a mismatch between these two factors. For instance, when there is a discrepancy between valuing doing one's job well and the values or behavior of one's manager. All the nurses in this study stated that unit managers and upper-level managers were some of the most important stressors because they felt hindered by them from doing their job well by providing insufficient support, managing situations incompetently, behaving inappropriately or unfairly, and failing to focus on caring. These behaviors often caused nurses to feel as if they were not being heard and were powerless. Because they counted strongly on feeling valued, almost all nurses were frustrated by the lack of appreciation, rewards, and caring for the employees demonstrated by their managers (Geuens et al. 2017a).

Individual factors act as modulators between the situational stressors experienced by the nurse and their consequent psychological correlates. The degree of stress perceived by the individual increases or decreases according to their personality traits and/or their personal values, consequently affecting the origin and development of burnout (Manzano-García and Ayala 2017). Recent studies have continued to confirm the influence of a combination of situational stressors and individual vulnerability as they describe the role of core self-evaluations (CSEs) and organizational factors in the development of nurse burnout (Best et al. 2005; Peng et al. 2016). Core self-evaluations consist of a combination of (1) self-esteem, (2) generalized self-efficacy, (3) neuroticism, and (4) locus of control (Bono and Judge 2003). These core self-evaluations (CSEs) are fundamental, essential evaluations that individuals hold about themselves, the world, and others. As such, CSEs influence people's appraisal of themselves, the world, and others, on a subconscious level. Appraisals of specific situations—such as the evaluation of one's work or colleague's—are affected by these deeper and more fundamental self-appraisals, even though most people are not aware of the influence their CSEs have on their perceptions or behavior as they occur (Bono and Judge 2003; Judge et al. 1997). A recent study suggested that CSEs are at the root of stress and strain processes or loss cycles, ultimately influencing feelings of burnout because of more unfavorable experiences with organizational factors linked with more avoidance and rumination coping and less problem-focused coping (Geuens et al. 2018).

### 13.3.4 Summary

To summarize, numerous studies have described vulnerabilities and situational risk factors for burnout independently of each other. However, even though vulnerability and stressors can be considered to be conceptually distinct, separately, their relevance to describe key aspects of burnout is limited (Ingram and Luxton 2005; Manzano-García and Ayala 2017). Manzano-García and Ayala (2017) suggest that individual and situational risk factors do not occur in isolation and may in fact be associated with each other (Manzano-García and Ayala 2017). Therefore, both types of factors should be studied together, and their interactions deserve further explorations.

## 13.4 Interventions

When considering interventions to address burnout, many authors advocate preventive measures (Awa et al. 2010; Oginska-Bulik 2006). After all, burnout is characterized by a long lag or lead-in period where psychological and physical effects tend to stay invisible until quite a late stage, and once a stressed individual becomes physically and/or psychologically unwell, it can take a long time to recover (Wright 2014). Therefore, it is important to intervene to arrest the progress of the syndrome early in the process.

Programs for preventing burnout can either be person-directed (individuals/ groups), organization-directed, or a combination of both. Person-directed prevention programs usually emphasize cognitive behavioral measures aimed at enhancing job competence and personal coping skills, development of social supports, or instruction and practice in different kinds of relaxation exercises. On the other hand, organization-directed prevention efforts usually involve restructuring work, evaluation practices, and supervision to decrease job demands or increase workers' sense of control or their level of participation in decision-making (Awa et al. 2010).

In developing preventive approaches, because intertwined individual and situational factors cause nurse burnout, it is important to blend individual and organizational interventions to reduce stress and burnout and increase resilience (Awa et al. 2010). After all, if attention is confined to changing work environments to reduce stressors, some individuals may still experience high levels of burnout because of their vulnerabilities (Alarcon et al. 2009). Therefore, it is important to simultaneously enhance nurses' self-awareness of their vulnerabilities and reflect on how they think about stressful situations and why situations cause them concern, as well as what they can do to improve them (including learning to accept certain circumstances) (Wright 2014).

When developing preventive measures for healthcare organizations, it is important to provide ample time for exploring and addressing the complex range of causal factors involved. Preventive measures should reflect this complexity, be carefully planned, and devote special attention to the discrepancy between individual and situational factors (Geuens et al. 2017a). First of all, it is important to explore which individual and organizational factors form a source of stress in a specific organization and need to be addressed so that appropriate organizational interventions can be developed alongside appropriate individual interventions. The individual intervention should aim to create overall self-awareness with special attention being devoted to issues related to the organizational stressor. For example, if a healthcare organization distributes questionnaires and results suggest certain nurse manager behaviors are an organizational stressor as well as high levels of neurotic personality traits among the staff. This would suggest that stress caused by possible deficiencies in nurse manager leadership skills is being aggravated by the negative thinking that staff appear to be predisposed toward. Based on these results, the healthcare organization can aim to develop the nurse manager's leadership skills (in terms of social support, coaching, transparent communication, and provision of opportunities for innovation and quality assurance) (Adriaenssens et al. 2015) through training and guidance. The individual intervention to complement this organizational intervention can focus on changing the perception of the individuals within the team by creating self-awareness, encouraging open communication between all members of the team—including the nurse manager—and addressing neurotic behavior, perhaps by stimulating optimism.

Positive psychology approaches posit that the negative effects of stressors related to work environment and daily life can be avoided, at least partially, by enhancing individuals' awareness of their personal strengths, such as optimism, hardy personality, and emotional intelligence so that positive emotions act as a shock absorber in the event of adversity (Manzano-García and Ayala 2017). Practically speaking, this can be achieved either through cognitive behavioral therapy-based guidance, workshops, or the more cost-effective alternative: e-learning or online self-help, for instance (Ruotsalainen et al. 2015). With this individually oriented intervention, the organization offers training possibilities and resources and provides the individual nurses with the opportunity to develop personal "bottom-up" approaches to prevent burnout that are under their own control (Demerouti 2015).

A recent study describes the effects of an individualized e-learning program designed to prevent stress and burnout in nurses (Geuens et al. In press). This evidence-based online program is rooted in cognitive behavioral therapy (CBT) and aims to increase self-awareness and resilience to stress and burnout. It is intended specifically for nurses and was codeveloped by nurses and research experts. An e-learning program overcomes several barriers to using CBT strategies to reduce burnout (Ruotsalainen et al. 2015). CBT is commonly offered through individual or group therapy sessions and is therefore not easily accessible, tends to be expensive, and has a restricted outreach. Costs to train an entire nursing staff within an organization using this method can be extensive. To reduce costs, several nurses can be selected for this traditional delivery. However, it is preferable to equip all employees within an organization with the necessary skills to deal with stress and prevent burnout. Providing an online intervention may offer a suitable and effective strategy for reaching a large target group in the workplace. In particular, online self-help interventions are potentially more affordable and accessible, as opposed to face-to-face interventions which use up resources such as therapists' time (Bolier et al. 2014; Muñoz 2010). In addition, nurses can use self-help interventions at their convenience, at their own pace, and in the privacy of their own homes (Bolier et al. 2014). Furthermore, online self-help interventions can apply a stepped-care principle, according to which nurses start with the least restrictive technique in terms of costs and personal inconvenience and only move to a more intensive treatment when they do not seem to benefit from the basic first-line intervention (Bower and Gilbody 2005). As such, limited financial resources can be optimized. Furthermore, online interventions have been proven to be effective within nursing workplaces in terms of favoring participation, consistency, transfer and retention of information, time use, and accessibility (Franck and Langenkamp 2000; Jeffries 2001; Masys 2002; McDaniel et al. 1997; Wolford and Hughes 2001). The study aims to investigate the effect of this individualized e-learning program to prevent stress and burnout in nurses and explain these effects through a mixed method research with an explanatory sequential design (Geuens et al. In press).

To complement other interventions, healthcare organizations can actively screen for burnout risk in terms of vulnerabilities and situational stressors in order to target preventive efforts at the employees who need them most (Geuens et al. 2017a). Additionally, special attention should be paid to addressing the lingering taboo around burnout, which creates shame and impedes healing. If individuals aren't afraid to admit they experience stress in certain situations (since no one is immune to stress), steps can be taken to offer them adequate support.

Finally, as part of this complex intervention, healthcare organizations should be prepared to meet additional requests of nurses concerning self-development by providing supervision, professional guidance, the possibility to partake in additional workshops, and/or adequate referral. After all, once self-awareness has been raised, individuals are often stimulated to continue discovering and developing themselves. When no follow-up is provided by the organization, this might stunt the individual's personal growth and induce more frustration.

Awa et al. (2010) suggest in their review that a combination of both person- and organization-directed interventions promotes longer-lasting benefits of 12 months or more. Refresher courses or booster interventions might enhance these effects even further (Awa et al. 2010). Consequently, well-designed, multicomponent prevention programs for burnout have great promise to enhance nurse well-being, patient satisfaction, and patient safety, as well as reduce absenteeism, nurse turnover, and recruitment difficulties.

### Conclusion

The summation of the causal factors and their interaction depicts the complexity of the burnout construct and places the individual prolonged stress experience within a larger organizational context of people's relation to their work. Therefore, more research should be devoted to studying both factors simultaneously in order to explore these interactions even further.

Furthermore, it is important to prevent burnout to limit the multitude of negative effects it causes. In the development of preventive measures, tailored organizational interventions should be harmonized with simultaneous individual interventions to create self-awareness and increase resilience. Interventions must respect the complexity of the psychological process, be carefully planned, and devote special attention to the relationship between individual vulnerabilities and situational factors. Finally, healthcare organizations should anticipate additional requests for self-development and actively screen for nurses at risk for burnout based on vulnerabilities and experienced situational stressors.

*This chapter is a part of a doctoral project supervised by Erik Franck and Peter Van Bogaert.*

# References

Adriaenssens J, De Gucht V, Maes S. Determinants and prevalence of burnout in emergency nurses: a systematic review of 25 years of research. Int J Nurs Stud. 2015;52:649–61.

Aiken LH, Clarke SP, Sloane DM, Sochaliski J, Silber JH. Hospital nurse staffing and patient mortality, nurse burnout, and job dissatisfaction. J Am Med Assoc. 2002;288:1987–93.

Aiken LH, et al. Patient safety, satisfaction, and quality of hospital care: cross sectional surveys of nurses and patients in 12 countries in Europe and the United States. BMJ. 2012;344:e1717. https://doi.org/10.1136/bmj.e1717.

Alarcon G, Eschleman KJ, Bowling NA. Relationships between personality variables and burnout: a meta analysis. Work Stress. 2009;23:244–63.

Armon G, Shirom A, Melamed S. The big five personality factors as predictors of changes across time in burnout and its facets. J Pers. 2012;80:403–27.

Awa WL, Plaumann M, Walter U. Burnout prevention: a review of intervention programs. Patient Educ Couns. 2010;78:184–90. https://doi.org/10.1016/j.pec.2009.04.008.

Bakker AB, Le Blanc PM, Schaufeli WB. Burnout contagion among intensive care nurses. J Adv Nurs. 2005;51:276–87. https://doi.org/10.1111/j.1365-2648.2005.03494.x.

Bakker AB, Van Der Zee KI, Lewig KA, Dollard MF. The relationship between the big five personality factors and burnout: a study among volunteer counselors. J Soc Psychol. 2006;146:31–50. https://doi.org/10.3200/SOCP.146.1.31-50.

Basar U, Basim N. A cross-sectional survey on consequences of nurses' burnout: moderating role of organizational politics. J Adv Nurs. 2016;72:1838–50. https://doi.org/10.1111/jan.12958.

Beck AT. Cognitive therapy of depression. New York: Guilford Press; 1979.

Beck AT. Cognitive models of depression. In: Clinical advances in cognitive psychotherapy: theory and application, vol. 14. New York: Springer; 2002. p. 29–61.

Best RG, Stapleton LM, Downey RG. Core self-evaluations and job burnout: the test of alternative models. J Occup Health Psychol. 2005;10:441.

Birkmeyer JD, Dimick JB, Birkmeyer NJ. Measuring the quality of surgical care: structure, process, or outcomes? J Am Coll Surg. 2004;198:626–32. https://doi.org/10.1016/j.jamcollsurg.2003.11.017.

Bolier L, Ketelaar SM, Nieuwenhuijsen K, Smeets O, Gärtner FR, Sluiter JK. Workplace mental health promotion online to enhance well-being of nurses and allied health professionals: a cluster-randomized controlled trial. Internet Interventions. 2014;1:196–204. https://doi.org/10.1016/j.invent.2014.10.002.

Bono JE, Judge TA. Core self-evaluations: a review of the trait and its role in job satisfaction and job performance. Eur J Personal. 2003;17:S5–S18.

Bower P, Gilbody S. Stepped care in psychological therapies: access, effectiveness and efficiency narrative literature review. Br J Psychiatry. 2005;186:11–7.

Cañadas-De la Fuente GA, Vargas C, San Luis C, García I, Cañadas GR, De la Fuente EI. Risk factors and prevalence of burnout syndrome in the nursing profession. Int J Nurs Stud. 2015;52:240–9. https://doi.org/10.1016/j.ijnurstu.2014.07.001.

Carey RG, Seibert JH. A patient survey system to measure quality improvement: questionnaire reliability and validity. Med Care. 1993;31:834–45.

Clark DA, Beck AT, Alford BA. Scientific foundations of cognitive theory and therapy for depression. New York: Wiley; 1999.

Demerouti E. Strategies used by individuals to prevent burnout. Eur J Clin Investig. 2015;45:1106–12. https://doi.org/10.1111/eci.12494.

Depue RA, Monroe SM. Conceptualization and measurement of human disorder in life stress research: the problem of chronic disturbance. Psychol Bull. 1986;99:36.

Eurofound (2012) Fifth European Working Conditions Survey Luxembourg.

Farrell D. Exit, voice, loyalty, and neglect as responses to job dissatisfaction: a multidimensional scaling study. Acad Manag J. 1983;26:596–607.

Firth-Cozens J, Cornwell J. The point of care. Enabling compassionate care in acute hospital settings. London: The King's Fund; 2009.

Franck LR, Langenkamp ML. Mandatory education via the computer: cost-effective, convenient, and creative. J Nurs Prof Dev. 2000;16:157–63.

García-Izquierdo M, Ríos-Rísquez MI. The relationship between psychosocial job stress and burnout in emergency departments: an exploratory study. Nurs Outlook. 2012;60:322–9.

Garrosa E, Rainho C, Moreno-Jiménez B, Monteiro MJ. The relationship between job stressors, hardy personality, coping resources and burnout in a sample of nurses: a correlational study at two time points. Int J Nurs Stud. 2008;47:205–15. https://doi.org/10.1016/j.ijnurstu.2009.05.014.

Geuens N, Van Bogaert P, Franck E. Vulnerability and stressors for burnout within a population of hospital nurses: a qualitative phenomenological study. in press. 2017a.

Geuens N, Van Bogaert P, Franck E. Vulnerability to burnout within the nursing workforce–the role of personality and interpersonal behaviour. J Clin Nurs. 2017b.

Geuens N, Franck E, Daemen C, Van Bogaert P. The effect of an individualized e-learning program to prevent stress and burnout in nurses – a mixed method intervention study. In preparation for publication.

Geuens N, Franck E, Vlerick P, Verheyen H, Van Bogaert P. Exploring nurse burnout through a combination of individual vulnerability and organizational stressors - the influence of core-self evaluations, organizational factors, and coping. In submisson October 10th 2017.

Gravlin GL. The relationships among nurse work satisfaction, burnout, and patient satisfaction with nursing care. New York: Columbia University Teachers College; 1994.

Graziano WG, Eisenberg NH. Agreeableness: a dimension of personality. In: Hogan R, Johnston J, Briggs S, editors. Handbook of personality psychology. San Diego: Academic Press; 1997. p. 795–824.

Haaga DA, Dyck MJ, Ernst D. Empirical status of cognitive theory of depression. Psychol Bull. 1991;110:215–36.

Halbesleben JR, Rathert C. Linking physician burnout and patient outcomes: exploring the dyadic relationship between physicians and patients. Health Care Manag Rev. 2008;33:29–39.

Hammen C. Generation of stress in the course of unipolar depression. J Abnorm Psychol. 1991;100:555.

Hammen C. Cognitive, life stress, and interpersonal approaches to a developmental psychopathology model of depression. Dev Psychopathol. 1992;4:189–206.

Hankin BL, Abela JRZ. Development of psychopathology: a vulnerability-stress perspective. Thousand Oaks: Sage Publications; 2005.

Hoekstra HA, Ormel J, de Fruyt F. NEO-PI-R en NEO-FFI handleiding. Amsterdam: Hogrefe; 2012.

Ingram RE, Luxton DD. Vulnerability-stress models. In: Hankin BL, JRZ A, editors. Development of psychopathology: a vulnerability-stress perspective. Thousand Oaks: Sage Publications; 2005.

Ingram RE, Miranda J, Segal ZV. Cognitive vulnerability to depression. New York: Guilford Press; 1998.

Jackson SE, Maslach C. After-effects of job-related stress: families as victims. J Occup Behav. 1982;3:63–77.

Jeffries PR. Computer versus lecture: a comparison of two methods of teaching oral medication administration in a nursing skills laboratory. J Nurs Educ. 2001;40:323–9.

Jourdain G, Chenevert D. Job demands-resources, burnout and intention to leave the nursing profession: a questionnaire survey. Int J Nurs Stud. 2010;47:709–22. https://doi.org/10.1016/j.ijnurstu.2009.11.007.

Judge TA, Locke EA, Durham CC. The dispositional causes of job satisfaction: a core evaluations approach. Res Organ Behav. 1997;19:151–88.

Keidel GC. Burnout and compassion fatigue among hospice caregivers. Am J Hosp Palliat Med. 2002;19:200–5.

Ksiazek I, Stefaniak TJ, Stadnyk M, Ksiazek J. Burnout syndrome in surgical oncology and general surgery nurses: a cross-sectional study. Eur J Oncol Nurs. 2011;15:347–50. https://doi.org/10.1016/j.ejon.2010.09.002.

Laschinger S, Heather K, Leiter MP. The impact of nursing work environments on patient safety outcomes: the mediating role of burnout engagement. J Nurs Adm. 2006;36:259–67.

Lasebikan VO, Oyetunde MO. Burnout among nurses in a nigerian general hospital: prevalence and associated factors. ISRN Nurs. 2012;2012:402157. https://doi.org/10.5402/2012/402157.

Lazarus RS, Folkman S. Stress, appraisal and coping. New York; Springer; 1981.

Leiter MP, Maslach C. Nurse turnover: the mediating role of burnout. J Nurs Manag. 2009;17:331–9. https://doi.org/10.1111/j.1365-2834.2009.01004.x.

Leiter MP, Harvie P, Frizzell C. The correspondence of patient satisfaction and nurse burnout. Soc Sci Med. 1998;47:1611–7.

Locke KD. Circumplex measures of interpersonal constructs. In: Handbook of interpersonal psychology. New York: Wiley; 2010. p. 313–24. https://doi.org/10.1002/9781118001868.ch19.

Manzano-García G, Ayala J-C. Insufficiently studied factors related to burnout in nursing: results from an e-Delphi study. PLoS One. 2017;12:e0175352. https://doi.org/10.1371/journal.pone.0175352.

Maslach C. A multidimensional theory of burnout. In: Cooper CL, editor. Theories of organizational stress. Oxford: Oxford University Press; 1998. p. 68–85.

Maslach C, Schaufeli WB, Leiter MP. Job burnout. Annu Rev Psychol. 2001;52:397–422.

Masys DR. Effects of current and future information technologies on the health care workforce. Health Aff. 2002;21:33–41.

McDaniel AM, Matlin C, Elmer PR, Paul K, Monastiere G. Computer use in staff development. A national survey. JNSD. 1997;14:117–26.

Melchior ME, van den Berg AA, Halfens R, Huyer Abu-Saad H, Philipsen H, Gassman P. Burnout and the work environment of nurses in psychiatric long-stay care settings. Soc Psychiatry Psychiatr Epidemiol. 1997;32:158–64.

Monroe SM, Hadjiyannakis K. The social environment and depression: focusing on severe life stress. In: Gotlib IH, Hammen CL, editors. Handbook of depression. New York: Guilford Press; 2002.

Monroe SM, Simons AD. Diathesis-stress theories in the context of life stress research: implications for the depressive disorders. Psychol Bull. 1991;110:406.

Muñoz RF. Using evidence-based internet interventions to reduce health disparities worldwide. J Med Internet Res. 2010;12(5):172–80.

Nembhard IM, Edmondson AC. Making it safe: the effects of leader inclusiveness and professional status on psychological safety and improvement efforts in health care teams. J Organ Behav. 2006;27:941–66. https://doi.org/10.1002/job.413.

Oginska-Bulik N. Occupational stress and its consequences in healthcare professionals: the role of type D personality. Int J Occup Med Environ Health. 2006;19:113–22.

Peng J, Li D, Zhang Z, Tian Y, Miao D, Xiao W, Zhang J. How can core self-evaluations influence job burnout? The key roles of organizational commitment and job satisfaction. J Health Psychol. 2016;21:50–9.

Post RM. Transduction of psychosocial stress into the neurobiology. Am J Psychiatry. 1992;149:999–1010.

Reader TW, Gillespie A. Patient neglect in healthcare institutions: a systematic review and conceptual model. BMC Health Serv Res. 2013;13:156.

Rothschild JM, et al. The critical care safety study: the incidence and nature of adverse events and serious medical errors in intensive care. Crit Care Med. 2005;33:1694–700.

Ruotsalainen JH, Verbeek JH, Mariné A, Serra C. Preventing occupational stress in healthcare workers. Cochrane Database Syst Rev. 2015;4:CD002892.

Semmer N, Schabracq M. Individual differences, work stress and health. Handb Work Health Psychol. 2003;2:83–120.

Shimizutani M, Odagiri Y, Ohya Y, Shimomitsu T, Kristensen TS, Maruta T, Iimori M. Relationship of nurse burnout with personality characteristics and coping behaviors. Ind Health. 2008;46:326–35. https://doi.org/10.2486/indhealth.46.326.

Shirey MR. Stress and coping in nurse managers: two decades of research. Nurs Econ. 2006;24:193.

Swider BW, Zimmerman RD. Born to burn-out: a meta-analytic path model of personality, job burn-out, and work outcomes. J Vocat Behav. 2010;76:487–506.

Taylor B, Barling J. Identifying sources and effects of carer fatigue and burnout for mental health nurses: a qualitative approach. Int J Ment Health Nurs. 2004;13:117–25.

Vahey DC, Aiken LH, Sloane DM, Clarke SP, Vargas D. Nurse burnout and patient satisfaction. Med Care. 2004;42:II57–66. https://doi.org/10.1097/01.mlr.0000109126.50398.5a.

Van Bogaert P, Meulemans H, Clarke S, Vermeyen K, Van de Heyning P. Hospital nurse practice environment, burnout, job outcomes and quality of care: test of a structural equation model. J Adv Nurs. 2009;65:2175–85.

Van Bogaert P, Clarke S, Roelant E, Meulemans H, Van de Heyning P. Impacts of unit-level nurse practice environment and burnout on nurse-reported outcomes: a multilevel modelling approach. J Clin Nurs. 2010;19:1664–74. https://doi.org/10.1111/j.1365-2702.2009.03128.x.

Van Bogaert P, Clarke S, Willems R, Mondelaers M. Nurse practice environment, workload, burn-out, job outcomes, and quality of care in psychiatric hospitals: a structural equation model approach. J Adv Nurs. 2013;69:1515–24. https://doi.org/10.1111/jan.12010.

van Heeringen K. Stress–diathesis model of suicidal behavior. In: Dwivedi Y, editor. The neurobiological basis of suicide. Boca Raton: CRC Press/Taylor & Francis; 2012.

Walsh M, Dolan B, Lewis A. Burnout and stress among A&E nurses. Emerg Nurse. 1998;6:23–30.

Welp A, Meier LL, Manser T. Emotional exhaustion and workload predict clinician-rated and objective patient safety. Front Psychol. 2014;5:1573.

Welp A, Meier LL, Manser T. The interplay between teamwork, clinicians' emotional exhaustion, and clinician-rated patient safety: a longitudinal study. Crit Care. 2016;20:110.

Wolford RA, Hughes LK. CE test: using the hospital intranet to meet competency standards for nurses. J Nurses Staff Dev. 2001;17:188–9.

Wright K. Alleviating stress in the workplace: advice for nurses. Nurs Stand. 2014;28:37–42. https://doi.org/10.7748/ns2014.01.28.20.37.e8391.

Yavas U, Karatepe OM, Babakus E. Who is likely to quit nursing jobs? A study in the Turkish Republic of Northern Cyprus. Health Mark Q. 2013;30:80–96. https://doi.org/10.1080/07359 683.2013.758017.

You LM, et al. Hospital nursing, care quality, and patient satisfaction: cross-sectional surveys of nurses and patients in hospitals in China and Europe. Int J Nurs Stud. 2013;50:154–61. https://doi.org/10.1016/j.ijnurstu.2012.05.003.

# Part III

# Perspectives

# Future Steps in Practice and Research

14

Peter Van Bogaert and Sean Clarke

**Abstract**

The concepts at the heart of this book originated more than 35 years ago and stemmed from repeated observations of a single troublesome phenomenon: cyclical nurse shortages in hospitals. Inquiries to deal with nurse workforce problems occurred alongside growing research findings suggesting that clinical nurses and other professionals were at risk of mutating from enthusiastic workers engaged with their clients to becoming emotionally drained, cynical, and insecure—the phenomenon known as burnout. The journey of this research field—reflected in the progression of the chapters in this book—has led to a variety of studies attempting to address both phenomena by focusing on the organizational contexts of nursing practice. Each of the chapters in this book offers findings and insights that we have synthesized into four recommendations for future steps in practice and another four recommendations for future steps in research. Connecting all of these recommendations is an emphasis on continuous improvement and change processes embedded in the organizational context of nursing practice, the need to draw on relevant empirical research, and the imperative for research and practice in this field to guide and inspire each other.

P. Van Bogaert (✉)
Nursing and Midwifery Sciences, Centre for Research and Innovation in Care (CRIC), Faculty of Medicine and Health Sciences, University of Antwerp, Antwerp, Belgium
e-mail: peter.vanbogaert@uantwerpen.be

S. Clarke
William F. Connell School of Nursing, Boston College, Chestnut Hill, MA, USA
e-mail: clarkese@bc.edu

© Springer International Publishing AG 2018
P. Van Bogaert, S. Clarke (eds.), *The Organizational Context of Nursing Practice*,
https://doi.org/10.1007/978-3-319-71042-6_14

## 14.1  Understanding and Consequences of the Buildup Evidence

The ideas and concepts discussed in this book originated more than 35 years ago and stemmed from the observation of a troublesome phenomenon—cyclical shortages of hospital nurses that were becoming increasingly untenable. The documentation by researchers more than four decades ago of a phenomenon in nurses and other human service professionals whereby enthusiastic workers in constant contact with service users become emotionally drained, cynical, and unconfident in their abilities was another critical base for research in this area. The chapters in this book trace a path through concepts and research findings that address both phenomena by focusing on the organizational contexts of nursing practice. Over the past 2 decades, both nurse shortages and burnout have attracted a great deal of attention from many researchers who have generated a body of knowledge to assist clinicians and leaders to provide organizational support to nurses on the front lines of practice. Various strategies are now available that can prevent or remedy organizational contexts that undermine clinical nurses' and clinical teams' abilities to provide exemplary patient care.

Each author reviewed ideas, findings, and insights that serve as building blocks for the creation of adaptive and resilient practice environments where there is an awareness of challenges and the necessity of improvement through cyclical processes (see the chapters Learning and Innovation in Healthcare-Based Teams; Project Management and PDSA-based projects). Supporting outcome-driven and development-oriented processes in the practice environments of clinical teams is as challenging as it is essential: carefully accumulated evidence generated in our 10-year research program has revealed that it is the Achilles heel of hospitals and long-term facilities' practice environments. At the heart of practice environments are the alignment of goals across various levels of hospital management, organizational supports, as well as skillful nursing management at the unit level and strong interprofessional relations between nurses and physicians. In their roles and as members of the healthcare worker contingents of their facilities, executives and managers, nurse leaders and nurse managers, physicians, other healthcare workers, and of course clinical nurses, all bear responsibilities for creating clinical microsystems aligned with the social and economic realities faced by healthcare institutions and systems and ultimately societies. Alignment of goals implies functioning that considers and respects the dynamics at each level within an organization.

The evidence has shown extensive variability across teams within and between healthcare organizations. Differences in team performance are often symptoms of problems rather than problems in and of themselves. They tend to arise unconsciously from the dynamics of certain cultures and subcultures whose origins and impacts should be understood before attempts are made to change them. Acting before understanding reflects a distressingly common and troublesome top-down approach found in the DNA of many hospitals and long-term facilities. Nonetheless, positive deviations were carefully identified and reported by the Magnet Hospital Original study and later practice environment studies and have provided a guide for constructive and sustainable change. Leaders at Antwerp University Hospital, the academic health sciences center that has served as the setting for research projects in the program discussed throughout the book, were inspired by research on the Magnet recognition program suggesting that it was possible to transform hospitals from hierarchical and departmental organizations to flat and interprofessional ones that were more adaptive and versatile. They hoped that a series of initiatives involving practice environments and processes to improve quality could answer many current and future challenges in healthcare. Three of the forces of magnetism—promotion of unit decision-making processes, participative management style, and focus on interprofessional relationships—guided this transformation process. A large-scale improvement project developed by the NHS, the Productive Ward—Releasing Time to Care™ program, appears to develop the necessary processes within hospitals and clinical teams (see chapter Productive Ward—Releasing Time to Care™: A Ward-Based QI Intervention). Our ground-level experiences and our own and others' research findings alike all point to improvements following adoption of the productive ward model as well as weaknesses that are consistent with the broader findings in our research program.

Studies have repeatedly identified vulnerabilities of clinical teams to poor performance because of imbalances between the demands of care and of improvement needs on one hand and social capital, nurses' decision latitude, and workload management or aspects of empowerment on the other. The latter elements are the basic drivers mediating the relationship between how hospital and clinical teams are managed and clinical nurses' professional well-being. They influence the capacity of individual nurses as well as teams. Findings from qualitative studies focusing on these empowering features mirror models developed from quantitative approaches and provide additional insights regarding organizational vulnerabilities. A reactive organizational context where participants are not fully aware of the climate and (sub)cultures at various levels together with a lack of goal alignment and a top-down approach undermines social capital and decision latitude within clinical teams. Demands likely are unbalanced, which creates a toxic and unhealthy work environment that can only be compensated by the good will and energy of individuals at all levels, but not as a mutually supportive, well-organized, and focused system (Box 14.1).

---

**Box 14.1 Key Messages**
- Previous chapters reviewed knowledge and insights regarding the building blocks of adaptive and resilient practice environments based on an awareness of challenges and the need for mechanisms for improvement through cyclical processes (ambidexterity).
- The evidence indicates key vulnerabilities or Achilles heels in hospitals and long-term facilities that undermine favorable practice environments. It also demonstrates the need to align goals across various management levels identified by hospital management and provide organizational support as well as nurse management at the unit level along with support for positive interprofessional relations between nurses and physicians.
- Alignment of goals is a mutual process that considers and respects the dynamics at each level within an organization.

We offer four recommendations for future directions in practice and four recommendations for future research. Connecting all these recommendations is an emphasis on continuous improvement and change processes embedded in the organizational context of nursing practice, the need to draw on relevant empirical research, and the imperative for research and practice in this field to guide and inspire each other.

## 14.2    Future Steps in Practice

1. We recommend that clinicians and leaders work to strengthen interprofessional collaboration among clinical nurses, physicians, and other healthcare workers, directed at meeting the needs of patients and their families (see the chapters on Compassionate Care and Interdisciplinary Collaboration and Communication) as aligned and mutual goals at all levels in hospitals/long-term facilities, instead of managerial approaches and theory. Development of evidence-based interprofessional practice models and models of care can guide bottom-up approaches supported by hospital governance structures and policies (see the chapter Transformation to an Excellent Nursing Organization: A Chief Nursing Officers' Vision and Experience). Team resource management is an excellent example of the creation of an organizational context addressing the needs of professionals and patients in the most critical of clinical circumstances, where technical skills are not enough to achieve positive outcomes (see chapter Team Resource Management and Quality of Care). Moreover, in TRM, an awareness of weaknesses in clinical critical processes guides an emphasis on nontechnical skills and accurate collaboration and communication, rather than a reliance on traditions that perpetuate ineffective collaboration and communication, a lack of feedback regarding outcomes, or, even worse, the "blame culture" so clearly identified by the patient safety movement. Comparable initiatives that have attracted ongoing scientific interest and have been widely adopted have included rapid response systems and standardized clinical communication (SBAR) procedures—not as templates or scripts but as guides for information exchange and care practices in interdisciplinary contexts (see the chapter on Standardizing Care Processes Using Evidence-Based Strategy: Implementation of a Rapid Response System in Belgian Hospitals).

   Healthcare teams are larger and more dispersed in time and space than ever, and there are various types of teams. Thomas (2012) discussed the strengths, weaknesses, future use, and research needs of three approaches to improve teamwork in healthcare: (1) comprehensive generic curricula developed from successes in commercial aviation and military such as crew resource management (CRM) and the TeamSTEPPS approach developed by the Agency of Healthcare Research and Quality (AHRQ); (2) brief team training curricula for specific tasks and activities such as training for surgery, resuscitations, hand-off/sign-out procedures, and multidisciplinary daily rounds; and (3) quality improvement efforts that require teamwork such as checklists for prevention of postoperative complications, catheter-associated bloodstream infections, and ventilator-associated pneumonias. Depending on their purposes, resources, and the particularities of their circumstances, leaders in their healthcare organizations can choose one or more of these approaches to support interprofessional teamwork to achieve better outcomes.

2. A very worthy goal in our view is the creation of a proactive, adaptive, ambidextrous, and resilient organizational context for interprofessional practice that focuses on the needs of patients and their families as the conditions that professionals need to perform at their best, as opposed to initiatives with narrow themes and purposes, such as burnout prevention and enhancement of patient safety. Symptoms or feelings of burnout are potentially the result of an imbalance between the demands being placed on individual professionals or teams and the supports they are receiving organizationally speaking. Understanding individual vulnerabilities through a stress-diathesis model can promote awareness and assist in identification of chronically reactive and unhealthy practice environments and individual coping strategies that can potentially lead to nurse burnout (see the chapter on Stress Resistance Strategies). Understanding *the cycles of loss cycles and motivation/gain* connected with particular organizational contexts of nursing practice that shape team dynamics and collaborations can inform improvements systematically.

   Researchers and commentators in the patient safety movement have extensively discussed how discrete organizational flaws cause inconsistencies in the quality and safety of care with negative effects on both patients and healthcare workers. The lack of clear goals at all levels and within clinical processes as well as excessive distances between frontline workers (the so-called sharp end) and managers and the conditions managers influence (the so-called blunt end) leads to both distinct organizational and process flaws and poor safety culture. Focusing only on the more visible sharp end or active failure allows latent conditions in systems to remain undetected, and the accumulation of latent flaws makes systems prone to accidents and errors in the future (Page, and Work Environment for Nurses and Patient Safety Board; Health Care Services, Institute OM 2004). Therefore, the solution is in our view not a single shot and top-down approach to focus on a patient safety emphasizing, for instance, safety incident reporting systems. As Hudson (2017) points out, in a true safety culture, the value systems associated with safety and safe working have to be fully internalized as beliefs, almost to the point they are invisible. The entire suite of approaches used by the organization at all levels uses must be safety-based. Hudson describes five stages in an evolutionary model of safety culture from pathological ("who cares as long as we're not caught?"), reactive ("we do a lot every time we have an accident"), calculative ("we have systems in place to manage all hazards"), proactive ("we work on the problems that we still find"), and finally to generative ("safety is how we do business around here").

3. We propose that healthcare organizations and systems pursue comprehensive and continuous support of interprofessional teams in their daily work and of the development of *processes* that meet patients and frontline workers' needs, a *focus on exemplary outcomes* and *healthy work environments*. We further suggest that these approaches be embedded and ingrained in institutional governance, policy, and structure. Evidence suggests that these organizational features fit together to create mutually reinforcing gain cycles, a dynamic also uncovered by our studied models and findings. Based on these insights, unit-level awareness of vulnerable and critical clinical processes with a potential for error through a patient safety reporting and learning system and focus on nurse-sensitive patient outcomes owned and directed

by clinical teams and supported by the hospital governance and policy was set up in the study hospital. At the Antwerp University Hospital and in other institutions, it is clear that constant realignment of the patient safety agenda is needed and that initiatives are often more successful at the clinical team level than when treated as a top-down hospital management alone (see chapter Reporting and Learning Systems for Patient Safety). To move patient safety forward, we need to evolve at all organizational levels from awareness through knowledge and ultimately to firm attitudes as described by Rogers (2003) work *Diffusion of Innovations*.

4. Fourthly, while there are many commonalities across healthcare organizations and lessons that can be transferred across organizations, it is critical to understand and accept various dynamics and particularities or idiosyncrasies in organizations as learning opportunities to guide cyclical improvement processes. It is clear that improving organizational contexts of nursing and interprofessional practice is ill-suited to typical top-down and theory-based "one-size-fits-all" approaches at hospitals, facilities, and at the level of clinical teams (see chapter Transformation to an Excellent Nursing Organization: A Chief Nursing Officers' Vision and Experience). Each initiative will produce improvements and weaknesses that will point to opportunities to standardize and stimulate future initiatives, respectively. Of prime importance to the interprofessional clinical teams in doing the work on the ground are a range of stakeholders and partners interested in advancing the broader goals of exemplary and excellent patient care in a realistic manner based on resources (see chapters Learning and Innovation in Healthcare-Based Teams, Project Management, and PDSA-Based Projects) (Box 14.2).

---

**Box 14.2 Key Messages**

- We recommend strengthening *interprofessional collaboration*, focused on clinical nurses and physicians as well as on other healthcare workers, with the aims on patients' needs and their families as *aligned and mutual goals* at all levels in hospitals/long-term facilities, instead of decontextualized managerial approaches based on theory alone.
- A most relevant goal in our view is to create an organizational context of interprofessional practice that is *proactive and adaptive, ambidextrous, and resilient*. Such a context promotes range of programs that focus on patient and family needs and what professionals need to address to the best of their abilities, as opposed to narrower and unconnected projects to prevent burnout and to enhance patient safety.
- We propose *comprehensive and continuous approaches* that support interprofessional teams in their daily work be *embedded and ingrained* in institutional governance, policy, and structure. As a result, adequate processes meet patients and frontline workers' needs, focusing exemplary outcomes and healthy work environments, avoiding the temptation to rely on single-shot solutions.
- We recommend understanding and accepting dynamics in healthcare organizations as an opportunity to learn and as a guide for cyclical improvement processes, rather than attempting to force top-down and theory-based one-size-fits-all approaches on practice settings.

## 14.3 Future Steps in Research

1. Much research in this field has common characteristics—and therefore suffers from the same weaknesses. Over the last 35 years, research has been driven by empirical findings rather than theoretical or conceptual frameworks. Because we study settings where management decisions have real consequences for both professionals and patients, careful and thoughtful preparation for research studies drawing on both theory and consultation of a range of stakeholders including patients is preferable and to be recommended. Extensive use of surveys has yielded findings that have been replicated, but the surveys and results have also raised many questions, not the least of which relate to linguistic and cultural differences in the societies and healthcare systems that raise questions of comparability of cross-national results (Squires et al. 2013). As stated in the previous section, "one-size-fits-all" projects are a questionable approach; this is as true in research as in organizational development and quality improvement. Studies finding associations between measures of organizational context as experienced by professionals and "hard" patient outcomes have been limited. Research by Aiken and colleagues (and studies with designs building on their best-known work) has collected data from patients and nurses to investigate how nursing practice environment characteristics affected patient and nurse outcomes across hospitals but cannot link individual patients with the nurses involved in their treatment (Aiken et al. 2012). Therefore, in our view, use of electronic health records to match nurses and units to patients in large-scale data analyses and intervention studies including longitudinal follow-up with well-established instruments will be helpful. Furthermore, as we have seen in the research program at the University of Antwerp and Antwerp University Hospital, mixed method approaches such as explanatory sequential study designs combining quantitative and qualitative studies have special potential for explaining and interpreting complex phenomena embedded in context (Van Bogaert et al. 2017).
2. While considerably more complex and expensive than their cross-sectional counterparts, longitudinal study designs that test more comprehensive models and associations at various levels within organizations hold great potential for extending well-known and extensively replicated cross-sectional findings. Longitudinal studies also hold great potential for evaluating organizational interventions and better understanding dynamics in hospitals as well as in clinical teams. As Khamisa et al. (2013) discuss in their systematic review of specific factors contributing to burnout and the outcomes of burnout in terms of nurses' health, only a handful of studies have confirmed three-way relationships between work-related stressors, burnout, job satisfaction, and general health. The authors suggest that better understanding the complexity of these interrelationships between these variables may require simultaneous exploration of all of them. As well, whenever practical, future studies should build in identification of hospitals/facilities and/or clinical teams to enable multilevel analyses.

   We also strongly suggest that research in this area be extended to primary and community care (and to the interconnections between acute hospital care and care of patients in other settings), given the transition from institutionally based care to primary and community care around the world (Hall 2014). These health systems trends are a response to evolving conditions in industrialized societies such as the increased prevalence of chronic conditions, imperatives to control healthcare costs, and calls from a range of stakeholders to provide person-centered care emphasizing goal-oriented rather than problem-oriented/provider-centered care (Reuben and Tinetti 2012). Moreover, the role of clinical nurses in primary and community care is expanding and in the opinion of many should be better integrated in interprofessionally speaking (Bodenheimer and Bauer 2016), which provides further justification for expansion of the study of work environments for nurses outside hospitals. In addition, Thomas (2012) suggested that future studies could evaluate feasibility and sustainability of strategies to support teams, including team-related curricula in nursing and medical schools.

Tsakitzidis et al. (2015) concluded that in spite of the success of the Interprofessional Collaboration in Healthcare (IPCIHC) module as evaluated by its participants from the undergraduate programs at the University of Antwerp, there are still great challenges ahead in educating future healthcare providers to enact positive behaviors in interprofessional collaboration. Interprofessional collaboration (IPC) is a model of working together that considers the opportunities and challenges of involvement with members of other healthcare disciplines in order to address the needs of clients, families, and populations in an integrated and cohesive manner. These and other authors suggest that research is needed to investigate the effectiveness of educational programs on improving the quality and safety of practice.

3. More scientific projects on the outcomes of clinical nurses' cognitive and physical workloads and work demands in the contexts of work environments are needed. Such studies could provide vital insights into achieving a healthy nurse workforce and fostering excellent quality and safety of care, taking stress-diathesis and systems models into account. Members of clinical teams often deal with long work hours as well as frequent direct, personal, and emotional contact with a large number of patients with varied and complex needs. Besides the need to address what might be considered "soft" (human relations) issues such as nurses' and clinical teams' social capital and decision latitude through supportive leadership at the hospital and unit levels, more insight and knowledge regarding "hard" constraints (inescapable realities) such as dealing with heavy workloads seems essential. Studies that investigate performance under high work volumes and variable complexity have often revealed coping mechanisms such as selection, optimization, and compensation strategies (so-called SOC models) that support decision-making and ability to perform well (Baethge et al. 2016). Such models suggest that nurses need to use their individual resources more efficiently and adaptively to set priorities and focus on fewer but more relevant goals, pursue these goals in an optimal way, and apply compensatory strategies for dealing with contingencies. We therefore believe that more studies in the future will be based on insights and knowledge from systems approaches such as *human factors and ergonomics* (Carayon 2011) and the notion of *high reliability organizations* (Oster and Braaten 2016), even though these approaches are driven by a difficult blend of theory and empirical findings and sometimes

lack clear data for the intuitive conclusions they reach. We expect that more studies in the future will address the cognitive capacities and limitations of individual nurses, as well as the level of multitasking required of nurses and clinical teams (Compernolle 2014). The fit between humans (clinical nurses and teams as well as patients) and the systems in which they come together will be increasingly important, given that systems are highly dynamic, variable, and complex. There will be continued study of how certain *technologies* can support clinical practice (for instance, decision support within electronic patient records) (Zahabi et al. 2015) and evaluations of institutional embedded continuous improvement and change processes requiring close collaboration between healthcare organizations and researchers.

4. Leaders in government and the business world, as well as researchers and journalists, are expressing concerns about how new technologies (robotics), informatics, and social media are transforming personal and professional life throughout society. Many commentators warn of the potential disruptive impact of mass automation of routine work on daily life and life in workplaces, yet others point out the opportunities artificial intelligence will provide (Special Report Artificial Intelligence 2016). Progressive trends driven by technology, informatics, and social media are indeed creating new and interwoven problems in people's personal and work lives that we do not fully understand. We would urge research initiatives to address the issues of work environments, communication, and other concepts explored in this book in the context of emerging technologies.

We should hasten to mention that technologies will also open the door to new research initiatives harnessing the potential of huge quantities of real-world data (so-called Big Data). Although most researchers and practitioners know the limitations of retrospective and/or cross-sectional data well and are eager for alternatives, we must confront the twin realizations that prospective predictive models can at times provide excellent guidance for decisions and that their findings must be questioned carefully. Data quality is a critical vulnerability in much traditional research that has serious impacts on the strength of the conclusions that can be drawn. However, in "Big Data" research, complete data regarding entire populations, even if they are flawed, rough approximations of measures of concepts of true interest and affected by consistent biases, are an important part of the paradigm, as is the search for finding useful correlations without an attempt to track causality. Alemayehu and Berger (2016) argue that the digital data era is poised to impact and revolutionize the development and targeting of new medical treatments. As massive quantities of real-world data become ubiquitous, they will be routinely used in healthcare decision-making. This will require understanding limitations and associated challenges and genuinely collaborative efforts among pertinent disciplines including statisticians, computer scientists, and software engineers. We can expect these approaches to data to change clinical practice; we probably can expect that they will influence the next generation of work environment research as well (Box 14.3).

**Box 14.3 Key Messages**

- Because research studies in this field are conducted in "live" "real-life" settings where there are serious consequences for professionals and recipients of care, careful and well-thought empirical projects developed in close collaboration with all stakeholders including patients are preferable to studies that are narrow and investigator-focused.
- We propose stronger emphasis in future research on longitudinal study design and careful tests of more comprehensive models and associations at different organizational levels to extend cross-sectional findings as well as to better understand certain interventions or dynamics in hospitals and clinical teams. We further recommend further extending research in this field to clinical teams and/or programs in primary and community care.
- Research studies of clinical nurses' cognitive and physical workloads and work demands in the context of different types of psychosocial practice environments (e.g., interprofessional, supportive, and empowering) are recommended to provide insights into achieving a healthy nurse workforce and excellence in quality and safety of care, considering stress-diathesis models and the roles of nurses' personal vulnerabilities.
- Progress and trends driven by new technologies, informatics, and social media will create new and interwoven problems in people's personal and work lives. They will also create new possibilities in empirical research in the form of electronic Big Data and real-world data of unprecedented scale and comprehensiveness.

# References

Aiken LH, Sermeus W, Van den Heede K, Sloane DM, Busse R, McKee M, Bruyneel L, Rafferty AM, Griffiths P, Moreno-Casbas MT, Tishelman C, Scott A, Brzostek T, Kinnunen J, Schwendimann R, Heinen M, Zikos D, Sjetne IS, Smith HL, Kutney-Lee A. Patient safety, satisfaction, and quality of hospital care: cross sectional surveys of nurses and patients in 12 countries in Europe and the United States. BMJ. 2012;344:e1717.

Alemayehu D, Berger ML. Big data: transforming drug development and health policy decision making. Health Serv Outcome Res Methodol. 2016;16(3):92–102.

Baethge A, Müller A, Rigotti T. Nursing performance under high workload: a diary study on the moderating role of selection, optimization and compensation strategies. J Adv Nurs. 2016;72(3):545–57.

Bodenheimer T, Bauer L. Rethinking the primary care workforce—an expanded role for nurses. N Engl J Med. 2016;375(11):1015–7.

Carayon PE. Handbook of human factors and ergonomics in health care and patient safety. 2nd ed. Boca Raton: CRC Press; 2011.

Compernolle T. Brainchains: discover your brain, to unleash its full potential in a hyperconnected, multitasking world. Brussels: Compublications; 2014.

Hall P. Making primary care people-centred: a 21th century blueprint. Lancet. 2014;384(9953):1501–2.

Hudson P. Safety management and safety culture. The long, hard and winding road. Centre for Safety Research. Leiden University The Netherlands. Retrieved July 31th 2017. http://www.caa.lv/upload/userfiles/files/SMS/Read%20first%20quick%20overview/Hudson%20Long%20Hard%20Winding%20Road.pdf.

Khamisa N, Peltzer K, Oldenburg B. Burnout in relation to specific contributing factors and health outcomes among nurses: a systematic review. Int J Environ Res Public Health. 2013;10:2214–40. https://doi.org/10.3390/ijerph10062214.

Oster C, Braaten JE. High reliability organizations: a healthcare handbook for patient safety & quality. Sigma Theta Tau: Indianapolis; 2016.

Page AE, Work Environment for Nurses and Patient Safety Board; Health Care Services, Institute OM. Keeping patients safe: transforming the work environment of nurses. Washington, DC: National Academies Press; 2004.

Reuben DB, Tinetti ME. Goal-oriented patient care—an alternative health outcomes paradigm. N Engl J Med. 2012;366(9):777–9.

Rogers EM. Diffusion of innovations. 5th ed. New York: Free Press; 2003.

Special Report Artificial Intelligence. The return of the machinery question. 2016. The Economist June 25th 2016.

Squires A, Aiken LH, van den Heede K, Sermeus W, Bruyneel L, Lindqvist R, Schoonhoven L, Stromseng I, Busse R, Brzostek T, Ensio A, Moreno-Casbas M, Rafferty AM, Schubert M, Zikos D, Matthews A. A systematic survey instrument translation process for multi-country, comparative health workforce studies. Int J Nurs Stud. 2013;50(2):264–73.

Thomas EJ. Republished editorial: improving teamwork in healthcare: current approaches and the path forward; 2012.

Tsakitzidis G, Timmermans O, Callewaert N, Truijen S, Meulemans H, Royen P. Participant evaluation of an education module on interprofessional collaboration for students in healthcare studies. BMC Med Educ. 2015;15(1):188.

Van Bogaert P, Peremans L, Van Heusden D, Verspuy M, Kureckova V, Van de Cruys Z, Franck E. Predictors of burnout, work engagement and nurse reported job outcomes and quality of care: a mixed method study. BMC Nurs. 2017;16:5.

Zahabi M, Kaber DB, Swangnetr M. Usability and safety in electronic medical records interface design: a review of recent literature and guideline formulation. Hum Factors. 2015;57(5):805–34.

# General Conclusions

# 15

Peter Van Bogaert and Sean Clarke

Life in healthcare organizations mirrors conditions in society and the economy more broadly. To establish and build their market positions, businesses constantly adapt to persuade customers of the merits of their offerings, especially that their offerings represent good value for money. Markets are constantly in transformation, and thus businesses are forced to develop appropriate organizational governance mechanisms, policies, and structures in addition to attracting talented, well-trained knowledge workers. Hierarchical structures and command-and-control leadership styles are poorly suited to the need for constant transformation, but this does not mean that structural chaos and blurring of roles is preferable. Rather, the survival of organizations in conditions of turbulence requires alignment of company goals with leadership capacity at all levels and adapting roles from the boardroom down to the frontline workers closest to customers protecting everyone's contributions and performance to create resilient companies. In addition, cross-functional management and a dedicated learning strategy have proven to be among the best innovations in the history of successful businesses that bring the core of various professional departments together to create new products and services that push back boundaries. Key recent examples include the cell phone and later the smartphone.

Parallel trends can be found in healthcare organizations confronting constant transformations due to social and economic realities and the needs of patients and their families. As populations age and chronic illness burden increases and technologies are becoming more and more widely disseminated, more care is provided in primary and community settings instead of inpatient hospitals. If current trends

P. Van Bogaert (✉)
Nursing and Midwifery Sciences, Centre for Research and Innovation in Care (CRIC), Faculty of Medicine and Health Sciences, University of Antwerp, Antwerp, Belgium
e-mail: peter.vanbogaert@uantwerpen.be

S. Clarke
William F. Connell School of Nursing, Boston College, Chestnut Hill, MA, USA
e-mail: clarkese@bc.edu

© Springer International Publishing AG 2018
P. Van Bogaert, S. Clarke (eds.), *The Organizational Context of Nursing Practice*,
https://doi.org/10.1007/978-3-319-71042-6_15

continue, hospitals will become more and more highly technologically driven institutions where lengths of stay are very short. Leadership is not explicitly discussed in the majority of the chapters in this book chapters, but is present throughout implicitly. This is because of the steadily expanding need for frontline care providers to not only have a voice in care but to be involved in decision-making in resilient and high-performing interprofessional teams. Nurse managers' and executives' leadership will be more important than ever to support quality of care. Moreover, healthcare organizations have the unique positions to create governance and policy and appropriate structures to maximize the present and future capacities and abilities of healthcare workers such as clinical nurses, nurse managers, and leaders as well as physicians and other healthcare workers to solve and find answers for continuous changing needs of patients and their families regardless of place, time, or circumstances.

This book was inspired by concepts closely influenced by and developed from what was going on in the society from the late 1970s and early 1980s up to the present day. Researchers internationally documented these trends carefully and generated a body of knowledge to better understand and intervene in the realities of providing the best care to patients and their families on a daily basis as well as professionals' psychosocial environments and well-being. Evidence generated by our 10-year research program led us to bring various co-authors together to present and discuss interconnected topics related to improving practice through interventions addressing the organizational contexts of nursing care. Five chapters were based on insights from developing and conducting research projects (Learning and Innovation in Healthcare-Based Teams; Team Resource Management; Standardizing Care Processes Using Evidence-Based Strategy: Implementation of a Rapid Response System in Belgian Hospitals; Interdisciplinary Collaboration and Communication; Stress-Resistance Strategies)—in the case of the last three research projects, we expect new evidence in the near future. Two chapters (Project Management and PDSA-Based Projects; Reporting and Learning Systems for Patient Safety) were based on ongoing projects at the major hospital studied, Antwerp University Hospital, in its journey to become a mature and self-conscious healthcare organization meeting the highest national and international standards of quality and safety. Another chapter discussed leadership support for organizational transformation at this institution (Transformation to an Excellent Nursing Organisation: a CNO Vision and Experience). Lastly, two chapters were contributions from international authors dealing with ideas touched upon in the Concept and Evidence chapters (Productive Ward—Releasing Time to Care™: A Ward-Based Quality Improvement Intervention; Embedding Compassionate Care: A Leadership Programme in the National Health Service in Scotland).

Throughout the book, the authors and we argue that the performance of individual professionals as well as interprofessional teams needs to be supported, drawing upon empirical insights and practice-oriented theoretical frameworks rather than managerial bureaucratic theoretical approaches with weak empirical underpinning. We hope the book will inspire all healthcare workers regardless their role or function to do the best they can to work towards increasingly better (and considerably better than minimally acceptable) levels of quality and safety in care driven by patients' and families' real needs.